Recent Developments in Dental Biomaterials

Recent Developments in Dental Biomaterials

Editor: Gerard Keith

AMERICAN
MEDICAL PUBLISHERS
www.americanmedicalpublishers.com

AMERICAN MEDICAL PUBLISHERS
www.americanmedicalpublishers.com

Cataloging-in-Publication Data

Recent developments in dental biomaterials / edited by Gerard Keith.
p. cm.
Includes bibliographical references and index.
ISBN 978-1-63927-061-3
1. Dental materials. 2. Biomedical materials. 3. Dental materials--Design. 4. Dental materials--Testing.
5. Dental materials--Models. I. Keith, Gerard.
RK652.5 .D46 2022
617.695--dc23

American Medical Publishers,
41 Flatbush Avenue,
1st Floor, New York,
NY 11217, USA

ISBN 978-1-63927-061-3 (Hardback)

Contents

Preface

This book has been an outcome of determined endeavour from a group of educationists in the field. The primary objective was to involve a broad spectrum of professionals from diverse cultural background involved in the field for developing new researches. The book not only targets students but also scholars pursuing higher research for further enhancement of the theoretical and practical applications of the subject.

Biomaterials are the substances that are produced to interact with biological systems for a medical purpose. It is used in therapeutic and diagnostic medical purposes. Biomaterials are derived from nature as well as synthesized in the laboratory using various chemical methods such as utilizing metallic components, polymers, ceramics or composite materials. Biomaterials are majorly used for medical compositions such as dental applications, surgery, and drug delivery. In dentistry, they are mainly utilized for dental implantation. The fabricated biomaterials that are used in dentistry are known as dental biomaterials. Temporary dressing, cement, impression material, lining material, and restorative material are a few examples of dental biomaterials. This book covers in detail some existent theories and innovative concepts revolving around dental biomaterials. This book unravels the recent studies in the field of dental biomaterials. It strives to provide a fair idea about this discipline and to help develop a better understanding of the latest advances in this domain. Researchers and students in this field will be greatly assisted by this book.

It was an honour to edit such a profound book and also a challenging task to compile and examine all the relevant data for accuracy and originality. I wish to acknowledge the efforts of the contributors for submitting such brilliant and diverse chapters in the field and for endlessly working for the completion of the book. Last, but not the least; I thank my family for being a constant source of support in all my research endeavours.

Editor

1

The Effect of Pre-heating Silorane-based Composite Resin on Marginal Gap Formation of Class V Restorations

Alizadeh Oskoee P[a]; Ebrahimi Chaharom ME[b]; Abed Kahnemui M[c]; Mohammadi N[d]; Pournaghi Azar F[e]; Vahedpour H[f]; Saadat M[g]

[a]Professor, Department of operative dentistry, Dental School, Tabriz University of Medical Science, Tabriz, Iran
[b]Associate professor, Department of operative dentistry, Dental School, Tabriz University of Medical Science, Tabriz, Iran
[c]Associate professor, Department of operative dentistry, Dental School, Tabriz University of Medical Science, Tabriz, Iran
[d]Professor, Department of operative dentistry, Dental School, Tabriz University of Medical Science, Tabriz, Iran
[e]Assistant professor, Department of operative dentistry, research center for evidence-based medicine, Dental School, Tabriz University of medical science, Tabriz, Iran
[f]Assistant professor, Department of operative dentistry, Dental School, Urmia University of Medical Science, Urmia, Iran
[g]Postgraduate student, Department of Periodontology, Dental School, Tabriz University of Medical Science, Tabriz, Iran

ARTICLE INFO

Key words:
Gap formation
Preheating
Silorane-based composite resin

Corresponding Author:
Fatemeh Pournaghi Azar,
Assistant professor, Department of operative dentistry, research center for evidence-based medicine, Dental School, Tabriz University of medical science, Tabriz, Iran
Email: pournaghiazar@hotmail.com

Abstract

Statement of problem: Many efforts have been made to solve the problem of composite resin adaptation and reduce microleakage.

Objective: The aim of the present study was to evaluate the effect of preheating of silorane-based composite resins before photo-polymerization on gap formation at the margins of Class V restorations.

Materials and Methods: Standard Class V cavities were prepared on the labial surfaces of 46 sound bovine incisor teeth. The teeth were divided into two groups. In group 1, after application of the bonding agent of the silorane system, the cavities were restored with Filtek silorane-based composite resin stored at room temperature. In group 2, before restoring the cavities, the silorane-based composite resin was heated in a warm water bath at 54°C for 10 minutes. After 48 hours of storage in distilled water, teeth were thermocycled and sectioned bucco-lingually. Then the gaps of tooth–restoration interfaces in both incisal and gingival margins at three external, middle and internal areas were measured using a stereomicroscope. After calculation of means and standard deviations, data were analyzed with two-factor ANOVA at $\alpha=0.05$.

Results: The mean marginal gaps in non-preheated and preheated groups were 10.66±2.39 and 7.62±2.05 μm, respectively, with a statistically significant difference ($P<0.001$). However, the differences between the occlusal and gingival margins in each group were not significant ($P=0.58$). The interactive effect of preheating and margin type was not significant ($P=0.10$).

Conclusions: Heating silorane-based composite resin before light curing resulted in decreasing the gap sizes at tooth–restoration interfaces in Class V cavities.

Introduction

Despite the ever-increasing interest in using composite resins to restore tooth cavities [1], these materials still has some shortcomings including polymerization shrinkage, poor proximal contacts and adaptation with the cavity walls in some clinical conditions [2]. In Class V cavities, especially in cervical margins located in dentin, polymerization shrinkage might result in marginal gaps formation. This would cause recurrent caries, pulpal irritation, sensitivity and marginal discoloration [3].However, in order to improve the mechanical properties of composite resins modifications have been made in the size, shape and distribution of inorganic fillers and increased filler content to improve the mechanical properties of composite resins, which results in enhanced viscosity and difficulty in manipulating and proper adapting of these composite resins[4].

Many efforts have been made to solve the adaptation problem and reduce microleakage, including utilizing flowable composite resins, composite liners [2, 4], and composite inlays and onlays [3]. Flowable composite resins are not as durable as high viscous composite resins due to lower filler content. The second and third mentioned methods complicate the procedural steps [5].

In recent years, low-shrinkage resin materials that are synthesized based on siloxane and oxirane molecules' chemistry have been introduced to overcome the problems resulting from polymerization shrinkage [6]. Mitthra *et al.*[7] showed that silorane exhibited less polymerization shrinkage and shrinkage stress compared to methacrylates. Also in their study, silorane and nanohybrid composite resin showed greater wear resistance compared to microhybrid [7]. Sivakumar *et al.* [8] evaluated the microleakage of restorations using silorane-based dental composite resin and showed that in general, silorane-based microhybrid composite had less microleakage among the other materials used in this in vitro study.

Recently, many studies has reported that preheating composite resins decreases viscosity and film thickness, which enhances flowability and adaptation with the cavity walls [9-14].

Choudhary *et al* [2], reported that preheating the composite resin up to 54°C improves adaptation and decreases the total amount of gaps. Dionysopoulos *et al.* [15] showed that preheating of conventional composite resins at 54°C and 60°C reduces their film thickness, independent of the type of composite resin. Moreover, nano-hybrid and bulk fill composite resins exhibit the greatest reduction and microhybrid and packable exhibit the lowest reduction in film thickness [15]. Temperature affects the kinetics of composite resin polymerization and increases the conversion rate, as well as reduces viscosity [16] through enhancing the motility of molecules and free radicals [17-18].When the conversion rate of resin monomers increases, the polymerization shrinkage and consequently stresses may increase [19-20]. The relationship between the conversion rate and an increased temperature has been studied in a wide range of composite resin systems [21-26]. In the majority of these studies, the effect of heating methacrylate-based composite resins has been evaluated.

The importance of the interfacial bond between composite resin and the cavity walls, and the differences in the chemical structure and polymerization process in silorane-based composite resins that can possibly affect the behavior of these composite resins when preheated is concerned. Therefore, the present study was conducted to evaluate the effect of preheating silorane-based composite resins on gap formation at the gingival and occlusal margins of Class V restorations.

Materials and Methods

A list of materials used in the present study along with the properties of each material is summarized in table 1.

In the present in vitro study, 46 sound bovine incisors without any carious lesions, cracks, fractures or anomalies in the bucco-gingival region were used. The teeth were cleaned using pumice powder and rubber cups before the study and stored in 0.5% chloramine solution. Standard Class V cavities (2 mm in depth, 2 mm mesio-distally and 3 mm occluso-gingivally) were prepared on the buccal surfaces, with the occlusal and gingival margins 1.5 mm coronal and apical to the CEJ respectively(Figure1), using a sharp diamond fissure instrument in high-speed handpiece under

Table 1: The materials and devices used in the present study

Material	Description & Composition	Manufactured by
FiltekTM Silorane, low-shrink posterior restorative	A light-curing radiopaque silorane-based composite; the monomer matrix is composed of siloxane and oxirane (23% of the composition). The inorganic filler contains fine quartz particles and radiopaque yttrium fluoride (76%). Additional contents: initiator (0.9%), stabilizer (0.13%) & pigments (0.005%).	3M ESPE Dental Product USA
FiltekP90 system adhesive	A filled, light-cured component bonding agent for enamel and dentin bonding. It contains a 3M ESPE hydrophobic bifunctional monomer, camphoroquinine/ a silane-treated silico fillers, stabilizer.	3M ESPE Dental Product USA
Astralis 7	8-mm light probe	IvoclarVivadent, Liechtenstein, Austria
Stereomicroscope, SMZ1000	Parallel Optical Zoom System Zoom Range:×0.8 to ×8.0	Nikon, Tokyo,Japan
Diamond bar	TR-25F (ISO 199/016)	Japan

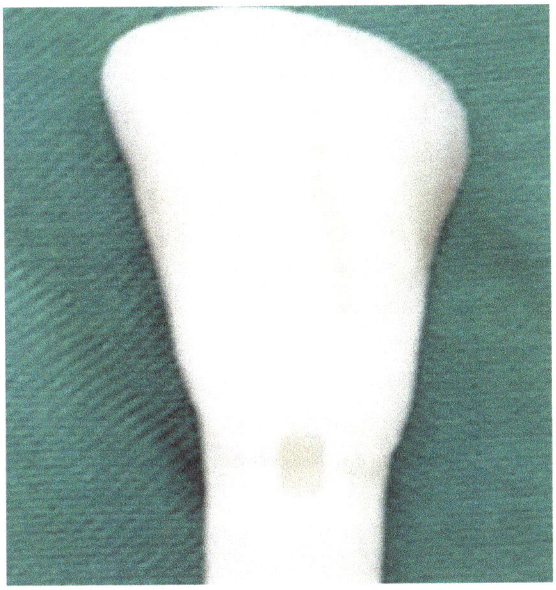

Figure 1: Class V Cavity preparation on Bovine incisor 2 mm in depth, 2 mm mesio-distally and 3 mm occluso-gingivally

air and water coolant[24].

After preparation of standard cavities, the samples were randomly assigned to two groups of 23. In the group 1, after irrigating and drying the cavities, the primer and bonding of the silorane adhesive system were applied according to manufacturer's instructions and the cavities were restored with Filtek silorane-based composite resin. They were then light-cured for 40 seconds with a tungsten halogen light-curing unit (Astralis 7; Ivoclar Vivadent, Liechtenstein, Austria) at a light intensity of 500 mW/cm2 and light-conducting tip with 8 mm light probe and perpendicular to the composite resin surface. In group 2, before restoring the cavities, Filtek silorane-based composite resin was placed in a warm thermostatically-controlled water bath(TELEDYNE HANAU, Buffalo, NY, USA) at a temperature of 54°C for 10 minutes and used to restore the cavities immediately after being retrieved from the warm environment[2]. The restorations were polished by using a diamond instrument (DiamantGmbh, D&Z, Berlin, Germany) and polishing disks (Sof-Lex TM, 3M ESPE Dental Products, St. Paul, USA) and stored in distilled water at room temperature for 48 hours. In order to simulate the oral cavity conditions, the samples underwent a thermocycling procedure in a water bath consisting of 500 cycles at 5/55°C, with a dwell time of 30 seconds and a transfer time of 10 seconds[25].

Subsequently, the samples were sectioned bucco-lingually by using diamond disks (Diamant Gmbh, D&Z, Berlin, Germany). Marginal gaps were measured using a stereomicroscope (SMZ 1500; Nikon, Tokyo, Japan) at 40× magnification. A digital camera was employed to photograph the selected areas with the use of a DS-L2 control unit

(Nikon, Tokyo, Japan). Therefore, the gaps could be measured at occlusal and gingival margins of the cavities in 3 points (Figure 2).

The gap widths were measured by using the built-in software (DS-L2 Ver 441, Nikon, Japan) in µm by determining two points on each side of the gap (one on the restoration side and one on the root side) and measuring the distance between these two points. Data were analyzed using two-way ANOVA and paired sample t- test at α=0.05.

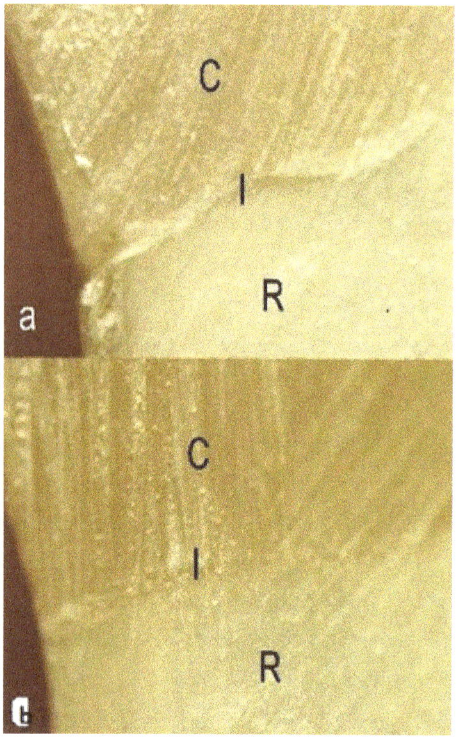

Figure 2: Marginal gap measurement (µm) with the use of the specific software program of the stereomicroscope at 40× magnification a: non-preheated,b: preheated
C: composite, I:interface,R:root

Results

Table 2 presents the means and standard deviations of marginal gap width of the study groups. The means of marginal gap width in the group 1 (non-preheated) and the group 2 (preheated) were 10.66±2.39 and 7.62±2.05µm, respectively. The results of Two-way ANOVA showed significant differences in marginal gap width of both occlusal and gingival margins between the preheated and non-preheated groups (P<0.001).

Paired sample t- test showed that there were no significant differences in marginal gaps between occlusal and gingival margins within each group (P=0.58). Two way Anova test showed that the interactive effect of preheating and margin type was not statistically significant (P=0.10).

Discussion

In the present study, the effect of preheating of silorane-based composite resin before photo-polymerization on the gap formation (at tooth–restoration interfaces) in Class V cavities was evaluated. Based on the results, the mean size of the marginal gaps at both the occlusal and gingival margins in the preheated group was significantly less than that in the control (non-preheated) group. Similarly, Fores-Salgado *et al.* [26] reported that marginal adaptation improved when composite resin was preheated. Furthermore, Choudhary *et al.* [2] showed that less marginal gaps were formed when composite resin was heated up to 54°C compared to composite resin at room

Table 2: The descriptive table (Mean±SD) of the gap width values (µm) in study groups

Group \ Margin	Occlusal	Gingival	N	P value(inter group)
Preheated	7.06±1.03	8.14±2.04	23	0.58
Non-preheated	12.91±2.56	12.57±1.45	23	0.58
P value (intra group)	0.0001*	0.0001*		

*Statistically significant

temperature or at 37°C.Demmirbuga *et al*.[27] investigated the effect of preheating on microshear bond strength of silorane and methacrylate-based composite resins to human dentin. They concluded that preheating of composite resins might be an alternative way to increase the micro-shear bond strength of composites on dentin. This finding is most likely due to increased flow and consequently better marginal adaptation to the dentin surface, which results in reduced marginal gap width [27]. However, Arslan *et al*.[6] showed that Pre-heating reduced microleakage values of Aelite LS Posterior composite, but did not significantly alter the microleakage values of Filtek Silorane composite. Alizadeh *et al*. [28] showed that repeated preheating of dimethacrylate and silorane-based composite resins decreased the marginal gap formation in class V restorations. Preheating occurs when heating composite resin up to a specific temperature before placing it in the cavity [5, 6]. Based on literature, heating composite resin decreases its viscosity by increasing molecular motility [14], therefore; as a result, the flow increases and the adaptation of the material with the cavity walls and wetting of the angled areas improves [6]. Wagner *et al*. [5] showed that preheating composite resin could improve its adaptation with tooth structures. Despite the advantages mentioned above, Lohbourer *et al*.[29] reported that preheating composite resin might have a deleterious effect on the margins of composite resin due to enhanced polymerization shrinkage . Considering the mechanical properties of preheated composite resins, some previous studies have reported an increased conversion rate and subsequently increased polymerization shrinkage [1,17-18]. Also, the thermal expansion coefficient of composite resin is 6–8 times greater than surrounding tooth structure [30] that along with polymerization shrinkage results in interfacial stresses in preheated composite resin that might affect adaptation, seal and the marginal integrity [31]. Elhejazi *et al*. [32] suggested a delay of 15 s before light curing to solve such a problem. Zhao *et al*. [33] showed that a delay in light-curing preheated composite resin results in decreasing the temperature at which the conversion rate is not affected, whereas the temperature is high enough to allow better wetting of the cavity walls. In clinical conditions and also in the present study, there was an interval between transferring the composite resin to the cavity, shaping and curing. It has been estimated that when composite resin is heated up to 60°C, its temperature drops 35-40% within 40 seconds after removal from the warm environment, with a decrease of 50% after 2 minutes [6]. Based on the results of the present study, it can be concluded that when the preheated composite resin is light-cured, its temperature reaches a level that is adequate for enhancing flow and adaptation; however, it is not adequate for increasing conversion rate, polymerization shrinkage and other mechanical properties. Deb *et al*. [31] showed that in non-isothermal conditions, the possible increased polymerization shrinkage due to temperature rise could be compensated by enhanced flow. Sharafeddin *et al*. [34] showed that flexural strength and flexural modulus of silorane based composites improved when preheating at 45°C. These two mechanical properties are fundamental for brittle materials and along with better adaptation can affect the clinical performance.The results of the present study showed that there was no significant difference in the mean gap width between the occlusal and cervical gaps in each study group, contrary to some previous studies which have shown less microleakage at occlusal margins compared to gingival margins [5, 27]. However, Deb *et al*. [31] showed no significant differences between incisal and cervical margins. Formation of marginal gap is influenced by the amount of composite resin polymerization shrinkage and presence of enamel margin and the cavity geometry [5]. In the present study, a low shrinkage composite resin was selected. The results of the study showed that using silorane-based composite resin and enhanced flow might have mitigated the negative effects of composite resin polymerization shrinkage on the occlusal and gingival margin integrity since there were no statistically significant differences between the two margins. In addition, previous studies have shown that silorane-based composite resins have better marginal integrity and performance compared to methacrylate-based composite resins [6].

Conclusions

Silorane based composite showed better marginal

adaptation when preheated due to low viscosity and wetting ability. However, there was no significant difference between occlusal and gingival margins.

Acknowledgements

This study was supported by a grant from Tabriz University of medical sciences.

Conflict of Interest: None declared.

References

1. Uctasli MB, Arisu HD, Lasilla LVJ, *et al.* Effect of preheating on the mechanical properties of resin composites. Eur J Dent. 2008; 2: 263-268.
2. Choudhary N, Kamat S, Mangala TM, *et al.* Effect of pre-heating composite resin on gap formation at three different temperatures. J Conserv Dent. 2011; 14: 191-195.
3. Acquaviva PA, Cerutti F, Adami G, *et al.* Degree of conversion of three composite materials employed in the adhesive cementation of indirect restorations: a micro-Raman analysis. J Dent. 2009; 37: 610-615.
4. Nada K, El-Mowafy O. Effect of precuring warming on mechanical properties of restorative composites. Int J Dent. 2011; 2011: 1-5.
5. Wagner WC, Aksu MN, Neme AM, *et al.* Effect of pre-heating resin composite on restoration microleakage. Oper Dent. 2008; 33: 72-78.
6. Arslan S DS, Zorba YO, Ucar FI, *et al.* The effect of pre-heating silorane and methacrylate-based composites on microleakage of class V restorations. Eur J Gen Dent. 2012; 1: 178-182.
7. Mitthra S, Rajkumar K, Mahalaxmi S . Evaluation of polymerization shrinkage, polymerization shrinkage stress, wear resistance, and compressive strength of a silorane-based composite: A finite element analysis study. Indian J Res Dent. 2017; 28:375-379.
8. Sivakumar JS, Prasad AS, Soundappan S, *et al.* A comparative evaluation of microleakage of restorations using silorane-based dental composite and methacrylate-based dental composites in Class II cavities: An in vitro study. J Pharm Bioallied Sci. 2016; 8:S81-S85.
9. Daronch M RF, Moss L, De Goes F. Clinically relevant issues related to preheating composites. Esthet Restor Dent. 2006; 18: 340-351.
10. Blalock JS,Holmes RG, Rueggeberg FA. Effect of temperature on unpolymerized composite film thickness. J Prosthet Dent. 2006; 96: 424-432.
11. Knight JS,Fraughn R, Norrington D. Effect of temperature on the flow properties of resin composite. Gen Dent.2006; 54: 14-16.
12. Freedman G, Krecji I. Warming up to composites. Compend Contin Educ Dent 2004; 25: 371-374.
13. Freedman PD. Clinical benefits of pre-warmed composites. Private Dent. 2003; 8: 111-114.
14. Daronch M,Rueggeberg FA, De Goes MF, *et al.* Polymerization kinetics of pre-heated composites. J Dent Res. 2006; 85: 38-43.
15. Dionysopoulos D, Tolidis K, Gerasimou P, *et al.* Effect of preheating on the film thickness of contemporary composite restorative materials. J Dent Sci. 2014; 9:313–319.
16. Daronch M, Rueggeberg FA, De Goes MF. Monomer conversion of preheated composite. J Dent Res.2005; 84: 663-667.
17. Trujillo M NS, Stansbury JW. Use of near-IR to monitor the influence of external heating on dental composite photopolymerization.Dent Mater. 2004;20:760-777.
18. Labella R. Lambrechts P, Van Meerbeek B, *et al.* Polymerization shrinkage and elasticity of flowable composites and filled adhesives. Dent Mater. 1997; 15:128-137.
19. Duarte S Jr, Botta AC, Meire M, *et al.* Microtensile bond strength & scanning electron microscopic evaluation of self-adhesive and self-etch resin cements to intact & etched enamel.J Prosthet Dent. 2008; 100: 203-210.
20. Lovell LG, Lu H, Elliott JE, *et al.* The effect of cure rate on the mechanical properties of dental resins. Dent Mater. 2001; 17: 504-511.
21. Lovell LG, Newman SM, Bowman CN. The effect of light intensity, temperature and comonomer composition on the polymerization behavior of dimethacrylate dental resins.J Dent Res. 1999; 78: 1469-1476.
22. Asmussen E. Factors affecting the color

stability of restorative resins. Acta Odontol Scand. 1983; 41: 11-18.

23. Schneider LF, Pfeifer CS, Consani S, *et al.*Influence of photoinitiator type on the rate of polymerization, degree of conversion, hardness and yellowing of dental resin composites. Dent Mater. 2008; 24: 1169-1177.
24. Sensi LG, Marson FC, Baratieri LN, *et al.* Effect of placement techniques on the marginal adaptation of class V composite restorations. Contemp Dent Pract. 2005; 6:17-25.
25. Buonocore MG. A simple method of increasing the adhesion of acrylic filling materials to enamel surfaces. J Dent Res. 1995; 34: 849-853.
26. Froes- Salgado NR, Maria SL, Kawano Y, *et al.*Composite pre-heating: Effects on marginal adaptation, degree of conversion and mechanical properties.Dent Mater.2010; 26: 908-914.
27. Demirbuga S, Ucar FI, Cayabatmaz M, *et al.* Microshear bond strength of preheated silorane- and methacrylate-based composite resins to dentin. Scanning. 2016; 38:63-9.
28. Alizadeh Oskoee P, Pournaghi Azar F, Jafari Navimipour E,*et al.* The effect of repeated preheating of dimethacrylate and silorane-based composite resins on marginal gap of class V restorations. J Dent Res Dent Clin Dent Prospects. 2017; 11:36-42.
29. Lohbauer U, Zenelis S, Rahiotis C, *et al.*The effect of resin composites pre-heating on monomer conversion and polymerization shrinkage. Dent Mater. 2009; 25:514-519.
30. Sidu SK, Carrick TE, McCabe JF. Temperature mediated coefficient of dimensional change of dental tooth-colored restorative materials. Dent Mater. 2004; 20: 435-440.
31. Deb S, Di Silvio L, Mackler HE, *et al.* Pre-warming of dental composite. Dent Mater. 2011; 27: e51-e59.
32. Elhejazi AA. The effects of temperature and light intensity on the polymerization shrinkage of light-cured composite filling materials. J Contemp Dent Pract. 2006; 7:12–21.
33. Zhao S, Qian Y, Liu H, *et al.* The effect of preheating on light cured resin composites. J Hard Tissue Biol 2012; 21:273-2788.
34. Sharafeddin F, Motamedi M, Fattah Z. Effect of Preheating and Precooling on the Flexural Strength and Modulus of Elasticity of Nanohybrid and Silorane-based Composite. J Dent (Shiraz). 2015;16:224-9.

2

Vital Pulp Therapy of an Immature Traumatized Permanent Tooth with External Inflammatory Root Resorption

Sahebi S[a]; Pourhatami N[b*]; Ahzan SH[b]

[a] Associate Professor, Department of Endodontics, School of Dentistry, Shiraz University of Medical Sciences, Shiraz, Iran

[b] Postgraduate Student, Department of Endodontics, School of Dentistry, Shiraz University of Medical Sciences, Shiraz, Iran

ARTICLE INFO

Key words:
External inflammatory root resorption
Dental trauma
Vital pulp therapy
Mineral trioxide aggregate

Corresponding Author:
Negar Pourhatami
Postgraduate Student,
Department of Endodontics,
School of Dentistry, Shiraz
University of Medical Sciences,
Shiraz, Iran
Email: pourhatamn@sums.ac.ir

Abstract

External inflammatory root resorption is a serious complication of a dental trauma, which leads to progressive loss of the tooth structure and destruction of periodontal tissues. Therefore, it represents a challenge in endodontic practice especially in cases of young children with incomplete root development. Vital pulp therapy (VPT) is an appropriate technique in the management of immature permanent teeth with partial pulp necrosis. This case report describes the outcome of a successful VPT in an immature traumatized permanent tooth with concurrent associated partial necrosis and external root resorption limited to the coronal part of the root in a 7-year-old boy. The tooth was treated according to the protocol suggested by American Association of Endodontics (AAE), consisted of disinfecting the root canal system beyond the resorptive lesion. Afterwards, mineral trioxide aggregate (MTA) was packed into the coronal portion of the canal and the tooth was restored with composite resin. The radiographic follow-up at 3 months showed arrest of root resorption followed by re-establishment of the periodontal space at 6 and 12 months in the absence of clinical symptoms. The satisfactory outcome of this case suggests that this conservative approach can heal a partially necrotic pulp and create a favorable environment for continued root development, and arrest of the resorptive process.

Introduction

The completion of root development and closure of the apex occur up to 3 years after eruption of the tooth in the oral cavity. Dental caries, trauma, and anomalous tooth morphology such as dens evaginatus are potential causes of pulpal and periapical diseases [1]. Most dental traumas occur in the 7 - 10 year-old age group with incomplete root development [2]. Immature traumatized teeth may become infected through crown fractures or cracks [3]. Bacterial invasion gradually promotes inflammation of the pulp tissue, and if not treated, pulp necrosis will happen, leading to destruction of odontoblasts and cessation of the root development. The outcomes of the interrupted root development include a poor crown-root ratio, a root with very thin walls, an increased risk of fracture, and an open apex [4]. External inflammatory root resorption is one of the potential consequences of trauma to the teeth and occurs when there has been loss of cementum due to damage to the external surface of the root and concurrent bacterial infection of the root canal system. The loss of cementum causes reaching intracanal bacteria and their byproducts to the adjacent periodontal ligament (PDL) and bone and this can ultimately lead to the development of the inflammatory resorptive process[5].

Conventional treatment of external inflammatory root resorption is based on eliminating bacteria and their irritants from dentinal tubules and the entire root canal system by means of thorough chemomechanical preparation of the canal space and a short-term dressing of creamy paste of calcium hydroxide for disinfection, followed by a long-term dressing with densely packed calcium hydroxide until cessation of the resorptive process [6,7]. Although documented data show that long-term calcium hydroxide therapy for this situation has a high success rate and stimulates hard tissue formation at the root apex of immature teeth with external inflammatory root resorption induced by trauma, the time-consuming nature of this method, weakening of the root structure and necrotizing effect of calcium hydroxide on PDL cells are some complicating disadvantages [8]. Regenerative endodontic therapy has been suggested to be an appropriate therapeutic technique in the management of immature permanent teeth with total pulpal necrosis. In 2004, Banchs & Trope published a case report describing this new approach for the treatment of an immature necrotic tooth and called it revascularization [9]. Vital pulp therapy (VPT) of permanent teeth includes partial/coronal extirpation of dental pulp tissue and covering the remaining wound with dental biomaterials. The ultimate goal of this approach is preservation of the healthy portion of the pulp tissue, and therefore maintaining its healing ability [10]. VPT is an ideal therapeutic technique in the management of immature permanent teeth with partial pulpal necrosis and has the potential to allow for continuation of root development and thickening of dentinal walls [11]. Thus, the objective of the current case was to determine if the presented protocol would result in the formation of a longer and thicker root in a tooth believed to exhibit a partial loss of vital pulp tissue with associated external root resorption.

Case Report

A 7-year-old boy was referred to the Department of Endodontics due to the history of impact trauma to the anterior region of maxilla three days earlier. The medical history was unremarkable. Clinical examination showed uncomplicated crown fractures with no pulpal exposures of both maxillary central incisors. Sensitivity to percussion and no response to cold and electric pulp tests were observed in both teeth. Radiographic examination revealed that the fractured teeth had immature apices (Figure 1A). Based on clinical and radiographic examinations, the treatment plan was dentin coverage with glass ionomer cement (GC, Tokyo, Japan) and permanently restoring the teeth with composite resin (Filtek Z350, 3M ESPE, St. Paul, MN, USA). Oral hygiene instruction was provided, and the patient and his parents were told that they should come to the clinic immediately if there was pain or swelling on each of the traumatized teeth. At the recall appointments (2 weeks, 1, 2, 3, and 4 months), both maxillary central incisors were asymptomatic, although none of them respond to cold and electric pulp tests. In addition, no abnormalities were found in radiographs of both teeth. When the patient was recalled 5 months after the first visit, the teeth were asymptomatic but in clinical examination, the maxillary left central incisor was sensitive to percussion and palpation and showed the probing depth of 5 mm at the distal surface of its root. No response to vitality tests was detected. Radiographic examination revealed that the tooth had still an immature apex. Moreover, external inflammatory root resorption at the coronal part of distal root wall of the mentioned tooth was obvious (Figure 1B). The initial diagnosis of pulpal necrosis was established based on clinical and radiographic examinations. The parents were informed that the prognosis of the tooth would be highly unfavorable and the treatment would be an attempt to extend the tooth life. It was decided to accomplish the treatment according to the clinical protocol recommended by AAE for the management of external inflammatory root resorption at the first appointment by chemomechanical preparation of the entire root canal system. Local anesthesia using 2 % lidocaine with 1:100000 epinephrine (DarouPakhsh, Tehran, Iran) was administered and tooth #9 was isolated with rubber dam. Access cavity preparation was made utilizing a high speed handpiece with water-coolant. While a size #15 k file (K-file, Mani Corp, Tochigi, Japan) was inserted into the coronal two thirds of the canal, hemorrhage into the pulp chamber was observed and the patient reported discomfort, potentially indicating the survival of the residual pulp tissue. The clinical diagnosis was revised from total pulpal necrosis to partial necrosis. After evaluating the treatment options, it was established that the patient would benefit greatest from maintaining the viability of the remaining portion of pulp tissue through VPT. Then parents were comprehensively informed about the benefits, complications, and alternative treatment approaches (apexification and regenerative endodontic therapy) and the relevant consent was obtained. The coronal portion of the canal was irrigated with 10 ml of 5.25% NaOCl and then rinsed with sterile saline solution. No instrumentation was performed. White mineral trioxide aggregate (MTA) (ProRoot MTA, Dentsply, Tulsa, OK, USA) was gently packed into the coronal portion of the canal beyond the resorptive lesion. The access cavity was sealed with 4 mm of cavisol (Golchai, Karaj, Iran).One day later, the temporary restoration was removed from the tooth #9, and access cavity was refined and restored with composite resin (Figure 1C). The patient returned two weeks later, asymptomatic with no sensitivity to percussion and palpation. No significant radiographic changes were noted. At the 3-month post-op visit, the patient was asymptomatic. Tests for percussion, palpation, mobility and probing depth were all within normal limits for tooth # 9. Decreasing the diameter of the apex and thickening of the radicular walls were evident radiographically in this tooth. The resorptive process was arrested, and interestingly a dentinal bridge was seen at the site of vital pulp therapy (Figure 1D). At the 4-month post-op recall, a sinus tract was observed on the buccal mucosa of tooth #8. No caries were clinically detected in this tooth. Neither teeth #8 nor #9 were sensitive to palpation, percussion and vitality tests. Radiographically, in tooth #9, the lamina dura could be traced around the entire root surface and

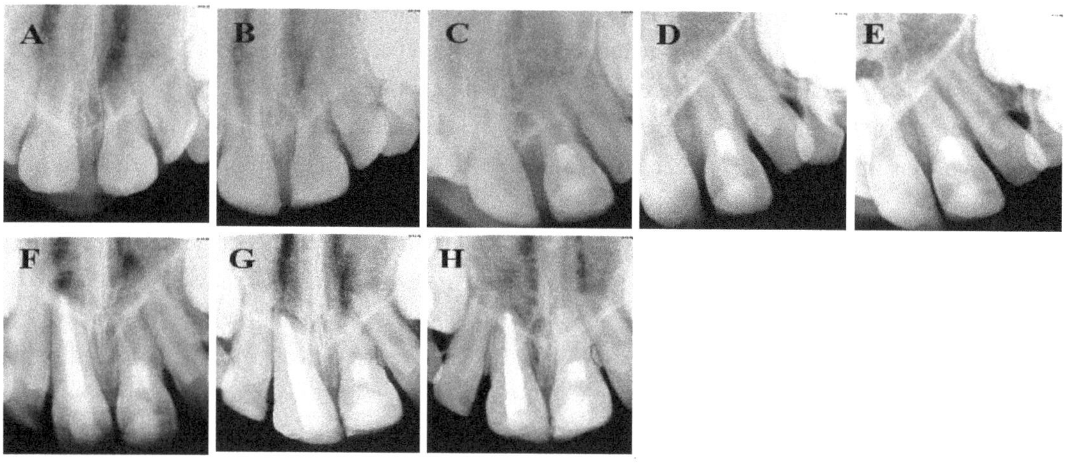

Figure 1: (A) The first-visit radiograph of teeth # 8 and # 9 with uncomplicated crown fractures. (B) Preoperative radiograph of tooth # 9 with external root resorption (C) Postoperative radiograph after VPT of tooth # 9 (D) 3-month post-op follow-up with a dentinal bridge formation at the site of VPT in tooth # 9 (E) 4-month post-op follow-up; in tooth # 9 the inflammatory root resorption was stopped and the lamina dura could be traced around the entire root surface Tooth # 8 had a radiolucent periapical lesion (F) Immediately after obturation of tooth # 8 with MTA plug and thermoplastic gutta percha (G) 6-month post-op follow-up (H) 12-month post-op follow-up; in tooth # 9, a longer and thicker root could be seen and the resorptive lacuna was filled with newly formed bone Re-establishment of a normal periodontal condition could be seen around the whole root surfaces of teeth # 8 and # 9

the periodontal ligament space was re-established. However, tooth #8 had a periapical radiolucent lesion (Figure 1E). The definitive diagnosis for tooth #8 based on clinical and radiographic examinations was total pulpal necrosis with asymptomatic apical abscess. Because of an absence of apical stop, it was decided to place an MTA plug and the rest of the canal was obturated with thermoplastic gutta percha using Obtura III gun (Courtesy Kerr, Orange, CA) (Figure 1F). At the 6- and 12-month follow up visits, no tenderness to percussion and palpation was noted in treated teeth. Periodontal pocket depths and mobility were within normal limits for both teeth. The cold and electric pulp tests were negative for tooth #9. Radiographic findings were also normal for the traumatized teeth (Figure 1G, H).

Discussion

External inflammatory root resorption is an important complication of a traumatic injury [12]. Normally an intact tooth is resistant to resorption even in the presence of inflammation. However, when an impact trauma damages the protective layer of precementum, inflammation of the pulp or periodontium will motivate root resorption. The aim of the interceptive treatment of external inflammatory root resorption is to reduce PDL inflammation, inhibit clastic cells, eliminate bacteria and their byproducts in the root canal system and encourage healing of periradicular hard tissues [5]. Historically, the conventional treatment of such cases was performed using long-term calcium hydroxide therapy to stop the resorptive process by making alkaline pH in dentinal tubules for killing bacteria and neutralizing their endotoxins, which are potent stimulators of inflammatory process [6]. Despite a high success rate, multiple patient visits, low patient compliance, probability of canal contamination between visits, and increased risk of root fracture due to dentin brittleness are some disadvantages of this protocol. Additionally, the necrotizing effect of calcium hydroxide on PDL cells might result in replacement resorption and ankylosis [8]. One-visit apexification by using MTA as an apical barrier is another alternative approach and may shorten the treatment time. Although MTA is effective in promoting new hard tissue formation in the apical area of the affected immature teeth, the risk of future fracture may still exist, because the dentin thickness will not increase. Therefore, the long-term prognosis of such teeth will be compromised [13]. In the present case, after access cavity preparation and inserting a size # 15 k file into the coronal two thirds of the canal, hemorrhage into the pulp chamber was observed, meaning that although the part of pulp tissue adjacent to the resorptive lesion was necrotic, the residual pulp tissue was vital. VPT was regarded the optional treatment choice for this case considering the stage of root development, the thin dentinal walls and the wide open apex. The interesting successful outcome in this case indicates that the management of external inflammatory root resorption in an immature tooth with partial necrosis does not necessitate the clinician to eliminate the entire pulp tissue from the root canal space, similar to what happens in regenerative endodontic therapy or the apexification process. Indeed, the conventional treatment of a tooth with external inflammatory root resorption is complete root canal therapy. However, the findings of this case report revealed that maintaining the vital apical portion of the pulp even in the presence of inflammation, in a tooth with immature apex, can improve the chance of root development and its long-term prognosis.The satisfactory outcome of the current case can be explained as the diseased residual pulp tissue, which probably had the granulation tissue nature, was healed after inflammation control and pulp protection with MTA through VPT, and subsequently promoted root end closure. In fact, VPT was selected to treat our patient because it is considered as an adequate conservative approach in a trauma victim. VPT allows further root maturation by sustaining a viable Hertwig's epithelial root sheath, which is responsible for signaling the physiological development of the root [10]. The presence of bacteria and their byproducts in the root canal system is one of the most substantial reasons for VPT failure. Therefore, a tight seal against bacterial ingress to the pulp tissue space may warrant the success of VPT [11]. Previous reports demonstrated that the pulp tissue has an inherent ability for soft tissue healing and hard tissue formation under different dental biomaterials [14, 15]. MTA was used in this study to provide an effective pulpal seal. Releasing of calcium hydroxide, exponential marginal adaptation, and inducing the release of bioactive proteins from dentin matrix, make MTA a potentially favorable biomaterial in the treatment of external inflammatory root resorption [16]. The deposition of hard tissue bridge beneath MTA in the present case, appears to be due to the stimulation of dental pulp stem cells proliferation and cell migration from stem cells of apical papilla with subsequent differentiation.

Conclusions

In conclusion, the current case report demonstrates a successful VPT of an immature traumatized permanent tooth with external inflammatory root resorption and partial necrosis based on clinical and radiographic evidence. In spite of a poor prognosis at the beginning of treatment, this approach caused healing of a progressive external root resorption within 12 months regarding the re-establishment of a normal periodontal condition, and a stronger and longer mature root. Further large-scale clinical trials with long-term follow-up periods are required to confirm this protocol.

Conflict of Interest: None declared.

References

1. Cehreli ZC, Isbitiren B, Sara S, *et al.* Regenerative endodontic treatment (revascularization) of immature necrotic molars medicated with calcium hydroxide: a case series. J Endod. 2011;37:1327-30.
2. Bastone EB, Freer TJ, McNamara JR. Epidemiology of dental trauma: a review of the literature. Aust Dent J. 2000;45:2-9.
3. Sundqvist G, Figdor D. Life as an endodontic pathogen. Endod Topics. 2003;6:3-28.
4. Cotti E, Mereu M, Lusso D. Regenerative treatment of an immature, traumatized tooth with apical periodontitis: report of a case. J Endod. 2008;34:611-6.
5. Abbott PV. Prevention and management of external inflammatory resorption following trauma to teeth. . Aust Dent J. 2016;61:82-94.
6. Fuss Z, Tsesis I, Lin S. Root resorption–diagnosis, classification and treatment choices based on stimulation factors. Dent Traumatol. 2003;19:175-82.
7. Rafter M. Apexification: a review. Dent Traumatol. 2005;21:1-8.
8. Hammarström L, Blomlöf L, Feiglin B, *et al.* Effect of calcium hydroxide treatment on periodontal repair and root resorption. Dent Traumatol. 1986;2:184-9.
9. Banchs F, Trope M. Revascularization of immature permanent teeth with apical periodontitis: new treatment protocol? J Endod. 2004;30:196-200.
10. Ingle JI, Bakland L, Baumgartner J, *et al.* Ingles endodontics 6th ed. Hamilton, ON: BC DeckerInc. 2008:1348-51.
11. JOE Editorial Board. Vital pulp therapy: an online study guide. J Endod. 2008;34:e103-6.
12. Trope M. Root resorption due to dental trauma. Endod Topics. 2002;1:79-100.
13. Steinig TH, Regan JD, Gutmann JL. The Use And Predictable Placement Of Mineral Trioxide Aggregate In One-Visit Apexification Cases. Aust Endod J. 2003;29:34-42.
14. Ford TR, Torabinejad M, Abedi HR, *et al.* Using mineral trioxide aggregate as a pulp-capping material. J Am Dent Assoc. 1996;127:1491-4.
15. Schuurs AH, Gruythuysen RJ, Wesselink PR. Pulp capping with adhesive resin-based composite vs. calcium hydroxide: a review. Endod Dent Traumatol. 2000;16:240-50.
16. Torabinejad M, Parirokh M. Mineral trioxide aggregate: a comprehensive literature review--part II: leakage and biocompatibility investigations. J Endod. 2010;36:190-202.

3

Comparison of Shear Bond Strength of Silorane and Nanohybrid Composite Resins to Calcium Enriched Mixture Cement in Different Time Periods

Koohpeima F[a*]; Sobhnamayan F[b]; Esfandiari M[c]; Siabani S[d]

[a]Assistant Professor, Department of Operative Dentistry, School of Dentistry, Shiraz University of Medical Sciences, Shiraz, Iran
[b]Assistant Professor, Department of Endodontics, School of Dentistry, Shiraz University of Medical Sciences, Shiraz, Iran
[c]Undergraduate Student, School of Dentistry, Shiraz University of Medical Sciences, Shiraz, Iran
[d]Postgraduate Student, Department of Operative Dentistry, School of Dentistry, Shiraz University of Medical Sciences, Shiraz, Iran

ARTICLE INFO

Key words:
Calcium enriched mixture
Nanohybrid
Shear bond strength
Silorane

Corresponding Author:
Fatemeh Koohpeima
Assistant Professor,
Department of Operative Dentistry, School of Dentistry,
Shiraz University of Medical Sciences, Postal Code: 1836-71345, Shiraz, Iran
Email: fkoohpeima@sums.ac.ir

Abstract

Statement of problem: It is crucial to select the best dental material for restoration of teeth that undergo vital pulp therapy after endodontic treatment.

Objectives: Adhesion of composite resin and endodontic pulp capping material affect the outcome of treatment. The aim of the present study is to evaluate the adhesion of two different composite resins to calcium enriched mixture (CEM).

Materials and Methods: We prepared a total of 60 cylindrical acrylic blocks that contained a central hole (4 mm diameter and 2 mm height). CEM cement was mixed according to the manufacturer's instructions and introduced into the holes. We stored 30 specimens for 3 days and the remaining 30 specimens were stored for 7 days at 37°C. The specimens were further divided into 2 subgroups based on the composite resins that we used. One subgroup of specimens was restored by Z350 (3M, ESP, St. Paul, MN, USA) nanohybrid and the other restored by P90 (3M, ESP, St. Paul, MN, USA) silorane based composite. Shear bond strengths were measured by a universal testing machine. Failure modes of the samples were evaluated under a stereomicroscope.

Results: At day 3, P90 had significantly higher shear bond strength than Z350 (P=0.001). On day 7, Z350 had significantly higher shear bond strength compared to P90 (P=0.004).

Conclusions: Within the limits of the present study, the best results of P90 silorane based composite filling after vital pulp therapy with CEM cement biomaterial were obtained after 3 days, whereas the Z350 nanohybrid composite showed better results on day 7.

Introduction

Composite resins are extensively used in dentistry for esthetic areas. Because of favorable esthetic results of composite restorations, they are popular among both clinicians and patients. Dental composite resins have improved since their introduction. However, despite the improvements, some of the shortcomings of composite materials have not been overcome. Numerous studies have emphasized decreasing polymerization shrinkage, which is one of the main shortcomings of the resin composites. Silorane based composite, a low-shrinkage tooth-colored restorative material, has been introduced to the market. Silorane is a hybrid biomaterial of oxirane and siloxane [1]. The functional groups of oxirane are responsible for lower shrinkage while siloxane specify the highly hydrophobic nature of the siloranes, compared to methacrylate-based composites. While methacrylate-based composites polymerize via a free-radical mechanism, Oxiranes, polymerize by a cationic ring-opening mechanism. They also show better performance in maintaining the bond interface because of their highly hydrophobic properties [2]. Developments in the manufacture of resin composites led to production of nanocomposites with better mechanical and handling characteristics, higher aesthetic aspects, and decreased polymerization shrinkage. The use of nanotechnology in production of nanocomposites has resulted in higher polishability and polish retention, high translucency, proper maintenance of physical properties, and high wear resistance [3, 4]. In the last few years, one of the most important improvements of resin composites to enhance the mechanical properties of them is the application of nanotechnology to resin composites. Nanotechnology is defined as the development of new structures and materials in the range of approximately 0.1-100 nanometers that lead to different chemical or physical characteristics. In nanohybrid composites, an increased filler load may be obtained due to the reduced dimensions of the particles and a greater size distribution of fillers and lead to decreased polymerization shrinkage and promotion of mechanical properties of composites such as tensile and compressive strength, and fracture resistance. These characteristics appear to be equivalent or sometimes higher than those of universal hybrid or microfilled composites [5-7]. Calcium enriched mixture (CEM) was introduced [8] as an endodontic material that has the same clinical applications but different chemical composition from mineral trioxide aggregate (MTA). This cement like MTA releases calcium hydroxide during and after setting [9, 10]. CEM has similar antibacterial features as calcium hydroxide, but better than MTA [11]. Its sealing ability, pH, and cytotoxic effects are similar to MTA; however, it has increased flow, decreased setting time, and film thickness. This cement has excellent biocompatibility and tremendous capacity to induce hard tissue formation in vital pulp therapies [12, 13]. CEM has shown acceptable results in pulpotomy of permanent teeth, apexogenesis , management of furcal perforation, and internal and external root resorption [14-16].

CEM cement appears to be a preferable alternative to MTA because of easier manipulation and increased thickness of the dentin bridge with CEM cement compared to MTA [13, 17]. The shear bond strength of vital pulp capping materials to restorative materials has been a critical issue in recent years. The bond strength of vital pulp capping materials and composite resins, affect the quality of filling and success of restoration. On the other hand, the proper bonding of composite resins to vital pulp capping biomaterials result in the adhesive joint to spread the stress relatively evenly over the entire surface of the bond [18].

The present study is designed to compare the shear bond strength of silorane and nanohybrid composite resin to CEM cement in two different time periods. We intend to determine whether the time of applying the composite resin on the CEM cement can affect shear bond strength of these materials.

Materials and Methods

Table 1 lists the compositions of the materials used in this study. We prepared 60 CEM cement (Yektazist Dandan, Iran, Tehran) specimens by using cylindrical acrylic blocks. Each block had a central hole that measured 4 mm in diameter and 2 mm in depth. The CEM cement was mixed according to the manufacturer's instructions, poured into the holes in the acrylic blocks, and

Table 1: Test materials, manufacturers, and composition

Name	Manufacture	Type	Composition
Silorane adhesive system primer	3M, ESP, ST. PAUL, MN, USA	Two-step self-etch acid primer	Phosphorylate methacrylates, vitrebond copolymer, bis-GMA, HEMA, water/ethanol solvent, silane treated silica fillers
Silorane adhesive system bond	3M, ESP, St. Paul, MN, USA	Two-step self-etch acid primer	Phosphorylate methacrylates, hydrophobic dimethacrylate, TEGDMA, silane treated silica fillers
Filtek^{R} P90	3M, ESP, St. Paul, MN, USA	Silorane-based composite resin	Monomers:3,4-epoxycyclohexyl-ethyl-cyclo-poly-methylsiloxane (5%-15% w/w), bis-3,4-epoxycyclohexyl-ethyl-phenyl-methylsilane (5%-15% w/w); Fillers: SiO2, YtF3(55% v, 76% w)
Etchant 37%	Ivoclar Vivadent, Germany	-	H3PO4 37%
Adper single bond II	3M, ESP, St. Paul, MN, USA	Two-step self-etch acid primer	Bis-GMA, HEMA, dimethacrylated, polyalkenoic acid copolymer, water/ethanol solvent
Filtek^{R} Z350	3M, ESP, St. Paul, MN, USA	Methacrylate-based composite resin	Monomers: Bis-GMA, UDMA, TEGDMA, PEGDMA, bis-EMA
CEM cement	Yektazist Dandan, Iran	Pulp capping material	51.75% w calcium oxide (CaO), 9.53% w sulfur trioxide (SO3), 8.49% w phosphorous pentoxide (P2O5), 6.32% w silicon dioxide (SiO2), aluminum trioxide (Al2O3), sodium oxide (Na2O), magnesium oxide (MgO), chloride (Cl)

Abbreviations; Bis-GMA: Bisphenol-a-glycidyl dimethacrylate, HEMA: Hydroxyethyl methacrylate, TEGDEMA: Tetraethyleneglycol dimethacrylate, UDMA: Urethane dimethacrylate, PEGDMA: Polyethylene glycol dimethacrylate, bis-EMA: Ethoxylated bisphenol-a-glycol dimethacrylate

covered with a moist cotton pellet and temporary filling material (Cavit; ESPE America, Norristown, PA, USA).

We stored 30 specimens for 3 days and the remaining 30 specimens were stored for 7 days at 37°C and 100% humidity. After removal of the temporary material and moist cotton, we did not rinse or polish the CEM cement surface. The specimens in each group were further divided into 2 subgroups of 15 specimens each. Preparation of the specimens was based on the type of the employed adhesive system and the time interval as follows:

Group 1 (3 day): CEM cement + acid etching + Adper Single Bond + Composite Z350

Group 2 (7 day): CEM cement + acid etching + Adper Single Bond + Composite Z350

Group 3 (3 day): CEM cement + Silorane adhesive system + Composite P90

Group 4 (7 day): CEM cement + Silorane adhesive system + Composite P90

After removing the temporary material and moist cotton, nanohybrid (Z350) and silorane (P90) composite resins were applied on the CEM cement surface by packing the materials into a split cylindrical metal mold with an internal diameter of 3 mm and a height of 2 mm. The specimens were cured with an LED curing system (Demi Plus, Kerr, Switzerland) for 20 seconds within the split mold with an 800 mW/cm2 light intensity and 20 seconds after split mold removal to ensure complete setting of the whole composite. After this process, specimens were stored at 37°C and 100% humidity for 24 hours in an incubator (Binder 7200 Tuttlingen, Germany) to encourage setting. All samples were prepared by the same operator. The specimens were mounted in a universal testing machine (Zwick/Roell Z020, Stuttgart, Germany) and we evaluated the shear force. A crosshead speed of 0.5 mm/min was applied to each specimen by a knife-edge blade until the bond between the CEM cement and composite resins failed. The values were calculated in newtons and converted into megapascals (MPa). Next, the samples were evaluated under a stereomicroscope (Motic K-500L, Motic Inc. Ltd., Hong Kong) under 40x magnification. An expert observed confirmed and categorized the failure modes as either adhesive (between two materials), cohesive (inside one of the materials), or mixed (both adhesive and cohesive).

Statistical analysis

The means and standard deviations were calculated. The mean bond strengths of the groups were compared by two-way analysis of variance (ANOVA). Two-way ANOVA was employed to assess the effect of composite resin type at different time intervals. Due to the significant interaction effect, we performed subgroup analysis by the student's t-test. $P<0.05$ was considered statistically significant.

Results

Table 2 and Figure 1 demonstrate the mean shear bond strength values and standard deviation of the two composite systems at the two time intervals. Two-way ANOVA and the student's t-test showed a significant interaction effect between composite type and time interval ($P<0.001$). Thus, the effect of time on shear bond strength depended on the type of composite resins. At day 3, shear bond strength of P90 (3.12±0.75) was significantly higher than Z350 (2.12±0.66; P=0.001). However, at day 7, Z350 (1.92±0.39) had significantly higher shear bond strength compared to P90 (1.46±0.42; P=0.004). Different time intervals affected the shear bond strength of P90 composite resins, as the mean shear bond strength of composite P90 at day 3 (3.12±0.75) was significantly higher than the mean

Table 2: Descriptive statistics of the groups and comparison of shear bond strength values (MPa; n=15)

Groups	Code	Mean±SD	Significance
1	A	2.12±0.66	A,C (P=0.004)
2	B	1.92±0.39	B,D (P=0.011)
3	C	3.12±0.75	C,D (P=0.0002), C,A (P=0.004)
4	D	1.46±0.42	D,C (P=0.0002) , D,B (P=0.011)

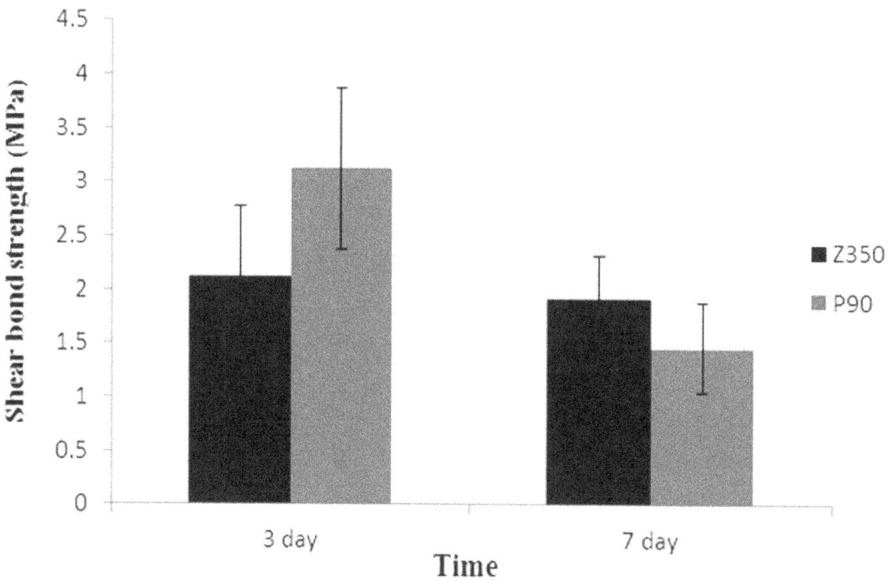

Figure 1: Mean shear bond strength (MPa) of the P90 and Z350 groups at different time periods

shear bond strength at day 7 (1.46±0.42; P<0.001). On the other hand, different time intervals did not show a significant change on the shear bond strength of Z350 (P=0.341). Evaluation with stereomicroscope showed cohesive failure in 82% and adhesive failure in 8% of the samples. Mixed failures were seen in 10% of the specimens (Table 3). Differences between cohesive and adhesive failure modes were significant. Differences between cohesive failures and mixed failures were also significant. Data were analyzed by the student's t-test (P<0.05).

Table 3: Frequency of specimen failure modality

Groups	Cohesive	Adhesive	Mixed
1	9	0	2
2	12	2	1
3	15	1	2
4	13	2	1

Discussion

One of the most important factors necessary for success of vital pulp therapy is insertion of a perfect restoration as soon as possible after endodontic treatment in order to make and maintain an acceptable seal. Composite restoration is recommended as the result of lower forces applied onto the pulp capping biomaterial during placement of restoration. Therefore the bond strength between pulp capping biomaterials and composite resins has a crucial role in quality of fillings and treatment outcome [19]. One of the most commonly used methods for evaluation the bond strength of dental materials to composite resins is the shear bond strength test [19]. Therefore, we have used the shear bond test to evaluate the adhesive joint between CEM cement biomaterial and two types of adhesive systems. The bond strength of pulp capping biomaterials such as CEM cement to composite resin depends on the physical and chemical characteristics [20, 21]. CEM cement is a hydrophilic biomaterial which sets in the presence of moisture. The main ingredients of CEM include calcium oxide, sulfur trioxide, silica, and phosphorous [10]. CEM cement is able to precipitate hydroxyapatite even when stored in normal saline. Because CEM cement does not have resin components, the bonding mechanism of it to composites is probably micromechanical and the result of penetration and interlocking of the composite adhesive system into the surface irregularities and pores [22, 23]. The polymerization reaction mechanism of composite resins is associated with polymerization shrinkage. The available composite resins have polymerization shrinkage in the range of 2.9% to 7.1%, depending on the test. Polymerization shrinkage can result in shrinkage stresses up to 7 MPa. Composite resins that do not undergo polymerization shrinkage are not available in the market. Research is underway for producing composite resins with low or no polymerization shrinkage. Presently, silorane system composites have been introduced as a new dental composite that have polymerization shrinkage of less than 1%, which may influence its bond strength [24]. Adhesion in self-etch silorane adhesive is created by acidic monomers that etch dental substrates and thus create a retention pattern for micromechanical interlocking of the cured adhesive with the tooth. They provide chemical bonding to the calcium-containing dental materials. The majority of current self-etch adhesives contain phosphorylated methacrylates as acidic monomers. Some contain carboxylic acid functionalized monomers or the combination of both. Silorane System Adhesive primer contains phosphorylated methacrylates, as well as the vitrebond copolymer with its carboxylic acid functionality used in some types of resin-modified glass ionomers and adhesives for adhesion to dentin and enamel. Comonomers, like bisphenol-a-glycidyl dimethacrylate (bis-GMA)and hydroxyethyl methacrylate (HEMA), a solvent system that consists of water and ethanol for wetting and penetrating the dental substrates, and a photoinitiator system based on camphorquinone for thorough and fast curing. A silane treated silica filler with a primary particle size of approximately 7 nm has been added to improve the mechanical strength and film-forming properties of the Silorane System Adhesive Self-Etch Primer. This filler is very finely dispersed in order to prevent settling [25]. This study showed that the shear bond strength of the P90 low shrinkage adhesive system was significantly higher than the Z350 nanohybrid composite at day 3. This finding might be due to the higher amount of the acidic primers that contain acetone or alcohol, which might affect the characteristics of the CEM cement. These acidic primers could react with the phosphorus component of CEM cement; however, after a number of days, these acidic monomers might undergo hydrolyzed degradation. The self-etch and hydrophilic nature of the silorane adhesive system is compatible with the hydrophilic nature of CEM cement. After a number of days, hydrolyzed degradation of the self-etch adhesive layer can occur and may lead to a decrease in shear bond strength. On the other hand, because of less polymerization shrinkage (about 1%) of the P90 composite, we have lesser gap formation between the composite and CEM cement that lead to increase shear bond strength. With a pH of approximately 2.7, the silorane system adhesive primer provides rather mild etching and produces a nanoetching pattern, as well as chemical bonding to the calcium and phosphate of CEM cement [26]. It can create mechanical interlocking between the bonding agent and porosity caused by mild etching of the CEM cement surface. The acid etching process in total etch adhesive systems may have some effects on setting time of the pulp capping biomaterials. This delay in setting of CEM cement may lead to lower bond strength of total etch adhesive systems at day 3. It seems that in phosphate-buffered solution, hydroxyapatite crystals are precipitated over CEM biomaterials. Although the particle sizes of CEM biomaterials differ, the pH and setting/working times are similar [27]. Previous studies with scanning electron microscope (SEM) results show that the surface gel-like amorphous structure and needle-like crystals are removed during acid etching. The selective removal of matrix from the periphery of crystals results in a spongy appearance, which can produce a good surface for bonding [28]. A few studies investigated the bonding strength of CEM cement biomaterial to silorane-based composite resins. Oskoee *et al* evaluated the bond strength of CEM cement and MTA cement with Z250 methacrylate base composite with and without acid etching. The results showed no significant differences in bond strength values of CEM cement and MTA to composite resin. They concluded that surface etching of MTA and CEM biomaterials were not mandatory prior to composite restoration using total-etch adhesive resin during vital pulp therapy [20].

It has been reported by Boushell that the silorane composite resin had significantly lower bond strength to resin modified glass ionomer (RMGI) compared to methacrylate composite resin. However, in the current study, silorane composite resin showed higher bond strength. The differences observed in this study might be related to using a silorane adhesive system with CEM cement, not with RMGI or dentin surface [29]. In accordance with our study Kasraie *et al.* showed that application of the self-etch system lead to a more significant increase in micro shear bond strength between the RMGI and composite resin compared to the total etch system [30]. Krifka *et al.* also showed that in some adhesive systems the bond strength was influenced by time [31]. The technique of a CEM cement sample preparation can affect the bond strength results. In this study, the surface of CEM cement was not rinsed or polished, which might lead to lower bond strength compared with the previous studies that investigated other cements. We did not polish the CEM cement surface, because obtaining a smooth, glazed cement surface under composite resin could not be reproduced in clinical conditions. In contrast with the current study, two studies reported no significant differences in shear bond strength between total etch and self-etch adhesive systems [31]. These findings might be due to the differences in the type of adhesives and perhaps the method for their application. One of those studies used the adhesive systems, Protect bond and SE Bond, both of which have different pH and different compositions from the silorane self-etch adhesive system. On the other hand, because of less polymerization shrinkage (approximately 1%) of the P90 composite, the gap formation decreased at first and lead to increased shear bond strength. However, in the nanohybrid Z350 composite that has a total etch hydrophobic adhesive nature, we observed more polymerization shrinkage and gaps on day 3. This perhaps led to lower shear bond strength; however, after 7 days, the moisture absorption by the total etch adhesive system might lead to decreased gaps and increased shear bond strength [4, 32, 33]. The findings of this study have shown lower bond strength between

CEM cement and composite resins compared to other studies that evaluated other dental cements. In order to fulfill a favorable restorative procedure when two different materials are used, an appropriate bond between these materials should be considered. Generally, when fracture occurs inside each material (cohesive failure) the bond is considered acceptable, rather than in the interface (adhesive failure) [34]. Nearly all failures in the present study were the cohesive type that occurred inside the materials, which might show the low cohesive strength of the materials compared to their bond strength. In a study by Oskoee *et al*, there was no significant difference between shear bond strength of MTA and CEM cement to adhesive resin cylinders using Single Bond. The researchers evaluated the shear bond strength of MTA and CEM cement to composite resin with and without the use of acid etch [20]. Another study also showed that the failure modes between CEM cement and dentin were mostly the cohesive type, which agreed with the results of the present study [35]. More studies should be conducted to investigate other aspects of bond quality and the influence of time on bond strength of pulp capping biomaterials to restorative dental materials.

Conclusions

Within the limits of the present study, we observed the best results of P90 silorane based composite filling after vital pulp therapy with CEM cement biomaterial at day 3, whereas the Z350 nanohybrid composite showed better results at day 7.

Acknowledgments

The authors would like to thank the Vice Chancellor of Shiraz University of Medical Sciences for supporting this research (Grant# 8218), which is based on the thesis by Dr. Masoud Esfandiari.

Conflict of Interest: None declared.

Refrences

1. Navarra CO, Cadenaro M , Armstrong SR , *et al*. Degree of conversion of Filtek Silorane Adhesive System and Clearfil SE Bond within the hybrid and adhesive layer: an in situ Raman analysis. Dent Mater. 2009;25:1178-1185.
2. Weinmann W, Thalacker C, Guggenberger R. Siloranes in dental composites. Dent Mater. 2005; 21: 68-74.
3. Ozel E, Korkmaz Y, Attar N. Influence of location of the gingival margin on the microleakage and internal voids of nanocomposites. J Contemp Dent Pract. 2008;9: 65-72.
4. Sharafeddin F, Nouri H, Koohpeima F. The effect of temperature on shear bond strength of Clearfil SE Bond and Adper Single Bond adhesive systems to dentin. J Dent(Shiraz). 2015;16: 10-6.
5. Moszner N, Salz U. New developments of polymeric dental composites. Prog Polym Sci. 2001; 26: 535-576.
6. Moszner N, Klapdohr S. Nanotechnology for dental composites. Int J Nanotechnol. 2004; 1: 130-156.
7. Mitra SB, Wu D, Holmes BN. An application of nanotechnology in advanced dental materials. J Am Dent Assoc. 2003; 134: 1382-1390.
8. Duarte MA, Demarchi AC, Yamashita JC , *et al*. pH and calcium ion release of 2 root-end filling materials. Oral Surg Oral Med Oral Pathol Oral Radiol Endod. 2003; 95: 345-347.
9. Asgary S, Shahabi S, Jafarzadeh T, *et al*. The properties of a new endodontic material. J Endod. 2008; 34: 990-993.
10. Asgary S, Eghbal MJ, Parirokh M, *et al*. Comparison of mineral trioxide aggregate's composition with Portland cements and a new endodontic cement. J Endod. 2009; 35: 243-250.
11. Asgary S, Kamrani FA. Antibacterial effects of five different root canal sealing materials. J Oral Sci. 2008; 50: 469-474.
12. Tabarsi B, Parirokh M, Eghbal MJ ,*et al*. A comparative study of dental pulp response to several pulpotomy agents. Int Endod J.2010; 43: 565-571.
13. Asgary S, Eghbal MJ, Parirokh M,*et al*. A comparative study of histologic response to different pulp capping materials and a novel endodontic cement. Oral Surg Oral Med Oral Pathol Oral Radiol Endod. 2008; 106: 609-614.

14. Asgary S. Furcal perforation repair using calcium enriched mixture cement. J Conserv Dent. 2010; 13: 156-158.
15. Asgary S, Ehsani S. Permanent molar pulpotomy with a new endodontic cement: A case series. J Conserv Dent. 2009; 12: 31-36.
16. Asgary S, A Nosrat, A Seifi. Management of inflammatory external root resorption by using calcium-enriched mixture cement: a case report. Journal of endodontics. 2011; 37: 411-413.
17. Asgary S, Eghbal MJ, Parirokh M. Sealing ability of a novel endodontic cement as a root-end filling material. J Biomed Mater Res A. 2008; 87: 706-709.
18. Perdigão J, Swift EJ, W R, *et al*. Fundamental concepts of enamel and dentin adhesion. Sturdevant's Art & Science of Operative Dentistry. 2013: 114-140.
19. Tunç ES, Sönmez IS, Bayrak S, *et al*. The evaluation of bond strength of a composite and a compomer to white mineral trioxide aggregate with two different bonding systems. J Endod. 2008; 34: 603-605.
20. Oskoee SS, Kimyai S, Bahari M, *et al*. Comparison of shear bond strength of calcium-enriched mixture cement and mineral trioxide aggregate to composite resin. J Contemp Dent Pract. 2011; 12: 457-462.
21. Doozaneh M, Koohpeima F, Firouzmandi M, *et al*. Shear Bond Strength of Self-Adhering Flowable Composite and Resin-modified Glass Ionomer to Two Pulp Capping Materials. Iran Endod J. 2017;12: 103-107.
22. Feilzer AJ, De Gee AJ, Davidson CL. Curing contraction of composites and glass-ionomer cements. J Prosthet Dent. 1988; 59: 297-300.
23. Jaberi-Ansari Z, Mahdilou M, Ahmadyar M, *et al*. Bond strength of composite resin to pulp capping biomaterials after application of three different bonding systems. J Dent Res Dent Clin Dent Prospects. 2013; 7: 152-156.
24. Ferracane JL. Current trends in dental composites. Crit Rev Oral Biol Med. 1995; 6: 302-318.
25. D'ALPINO PHP, FARIAS NCd, SILVA MS, *et al*. Compatibility between silorane adhesive and simplified methacrylate-based adhesive systems. Dent Mater J. 2013; 32: 263-273.
26. Rohr N, Fischer J. Tooth surface treatment strategies for adhesive cementation. J Adv Prosthodont. 2017;9: 85-92.
27. Madani ZS, Haddadi A, Mesgarani A, *et al*. Histopathologic Responses of the Dental Pulp to Calcium-Enriched Mixture (CEM) and Mineral Trioxide Aggregate (MTA) in Diabetic and Non-Diabetic Rats. Int J Mol Cell Med. 2014; 3: 263-271.
28. Kayahan MB, Nekoofar MH, Kazandağ M, *et al*. Effect of acid-etching procedure on selected physical properties of mineral trioxide aggregate. Int Endod J. 2009; 42: 1004-1014.
29. Boushell LW, Getz G, Swift EJ Jr, *et al*. Bond strengths of a silorane composite to various substrates. Am J Dent. 2011; 24: 93-96.
30. Kasraie S, Shokripour M, Safari M. Evaluation of micro-shear bond strength of resin modified glass-ionomer to composite resins using various bonding systems. J Conserv Dent. 2013;16: 550-554.
31. Krifka S, Preis V, Rosentritt M. Effect of Decontamination and Cleaning on the Shear Bond Strength of High Translucency Zirconia. Dent J. 2017; 5: 32.
32. Sharafeddin F, Salehi R, Feizi N. Effect of Dimethyl Sulfoxide on Bond Strength of a Self-Etch Primer and an Etch and Rinse Adhesive to Surface and Deep Dentin. J Dent(Shiraz). 2016; 17: 242-249.
33. Sharafeddin F, Koohpeima F, Palizian B, Evaluation of Microleakage in Class V Cavities Filled with Methacrylate-based versus Silorane-based Composites. J Dent Biomater. 2015; 2: 67-72.
34. Tate WH, Friedl KH, Powers JM. Bond strength of composites to hybrid ionomers. Oper Dent. 1996; 21: 147-152.
35. Sobhnamayan F, Adl A, Sadat Shojaee N, *et al*. The Effect of Chlorhexidine on the Push-Out Bond Strength of Calcium-Enriched Mixture Cement. Iran Endod J. 2015; 10: 59-63.

4

Influence of Er,Cr:YSGG Laser Surface Treatments on Micro Push-Out Bond Strength of Fiber Posts to Composite Resin Core Materials

Ghavami-Lahiji M[a]; Benedicenti S[b]; Karimian R[c] ; Shahabi S[d*]

[a]Ph.D. candidate for Dental Biomaterials, Research Center for Science and Technology in Medicine, Department of Dental Biomaterials, School of Dentistry,Tehran University of Medical Sciences, Tehran, Iran
[b] Professor , Department of Surgical Sciences and Integrated Diagnostics, University of Genoa, Genoa, Italy
[c]Undergraduate Student, Department of Dental Biomaterials, School of Dentistry, Tehran University of Medical Sciences, Tehran, Iran
[d]professor, Laser Research Center of Dentistry, Dentistry Research Institute, Department of Dental Biomaterials, School of Dentistry,Tehran University of Medical Sciences, Tehran, Iran

ARTICLE INFO

Key words:

Fiber post
Resin core build-up
Er,Cr:YSGG laser
Bond strength

Corresponding Author:
Sima Shahabi
professor, Laser Research Center of Dentistry, Dentistry Research Institute, Department of Dental Biomaterials, School of Dentistry,Tehran University of Medical Sciences, Tehran, Iran
Email: shahabis@tums.ac.ir

Abstract

Statement of problem: The bonding of fiber post to resin core or root dentin is challenged by limited penetration of resin material to the polymeric matrix of fiber posts.

Objectives: The purpose of this study was to investigate the effect of Er,Cr:YSGG on micro push-out bond strength of glass fiber posts to resin core material.

Materials and Methods: We used 2 commercially available fiber posts, Exacto (Angelus) and White Post DC (FGM), which had similar coronal diameters. Specimens of each fiber post (n=36) were randomly divided into three subgroups (n=12 posts per group) according to different surface treatment methods: control (no surface treatment), irradiation by 1W Er,Cr:YSGG, and irradiation by 1.5W Er,Cr:YSGG. A cylindrical plastic tube was placed around the post. Resin core material was filled into the tube and cured. Coronal portions of the posts were sectioned into 1-mm-thick slices. Then, the specimens were subjected to a thermocyling device for 3000 cycles. The micro push-out test was carried out using a Universal Testing Machine. Data were analyzed using one-way ANOVA followed by Tukey's HSD post hoc test to investigate the effect of different surface treatments on each type of fiber post.

Results: The 1.5W Er,Cr:YSGG laser statistically reduced micro push-out bond strength values in the Exacto groups ($P<0.05$). However, there was no significant difference between the control and 1W Er,Cr:YSGG groups. We observed no significant difference among different surface treatment methods in the White post DC groups ($P>0.05$). Mode of failure analysis showed that mixed failure was the predominant failure type for all surface treatment groups.

Conclusions: The beneficial effect of Er,Cr:YSGG laser application could not be confirmed based on the results of this in vitro study. Er,Cr:YSGG laser could not significantly enhance the bond strength values. However, the 1.5W laser statistically decreased micro push-out bond strength in the Exacto fiber posts.

Introduction

Endodontically treated teeth may have inadequate crown structures due to severe caries, removal of filings, or excessive wear. Therefore, we should place posts to maintain the core and reconstruct any missing tooth structure. Prefabricated posts are better than cast posts in terms of time and decreased cost [1, 2]. The excellent optical and mechanical properties of fiber posts introduce them as alternatives to casting and ceramic posts [3]. Prefabricated fiber posts are bonded to root canals to reduce microleakage and provide retention for composite resin cores [4]. Strengthening of this bond seems necessary to avoid treatment failure. Fiber posts are usually made of carbon, glass, quartz, silica or polyethylene fibers embedded in a polymer resin matrix based on methacrylate or epoxy resins. The fibers are bonded to matrix by a silane coupling agent [5]. The numbers of fibers depends on the type of post changes (between 25-35) that are parallel to the post axis; each of these fibers ranges in diameter from 6-10 μm/mm2 of cross-section area [6]. Although the fiber posts are easier to use than conventional posts, clinical and laboratory studies suggest that the bond of the fiber post to the dentine of the root canal and resin core can be problematic. The main advantage is that the elastic modulus of the fiber post is similar to dentin. This property provides appropriate stress distribution to minimize the risk of vertical root fracture [4, 7]. However, the polymeric matrix of the fiber post has substantial cross-linking and cannot react with resin composite monomers [1, 4]. Several surface treatment methods (e.g., micro-mechanical and chemical) have been introduced for the fiber posts to improve this bond [8]. Porosity of the surfaces will increase following surface treatment. Thus, resin can penetrate the porosities and micromechanical locking enhances core retention. Numerous chemical and mechanical efforts have been made to improve this bond because it is not satisfactory. For example, a silane coupling agent can modify the chemical surface and enhance wettability by forming a chemical bridge between the composite resin and glass fiber posts [9]. Micromechanical surface treatment of fiber posts with airborne-particle abrasion and hydrofluoric acid also significantly increases bond strength between the fiber posts and resin based materials [10-12]. Micromechanical surface treatments make surfaces rougher, which increases surface area and surface energy. Removal of the superficial layer of the resin matrix will expose the fibers to create a chemical bond [13, 14]. Micromechanical methods for the fiber post surface treatment are harmful. They may reduce the strength of the posts and change its shape, which subsequently affects its ability to fit the canal [2, 13].The use of lasers in dentistry has increased in recent decades. Various lasers have been used as alternatives to previous methods to increase the bond strength of dental materials. This study aimed to evaluate the effect of the Er,Cr:YSGG laser as a surface treatment for fiber posts. The null hypotheses tested in this study were: (1) Er,Cr:YSGG laser does not cause surface changes in fiber posts and (2) prior application of Er,Cr:YSGG laser on the post surface does not affect micro push-out bond strength.

Materials and Methods

In this study, we investigated the effects of the Er,Cr:YSGG laser on micro push-out bond strength of glass fiber posts to resin core material. Table 1 lists the materials used in this study. Two commercially available glass fiber posts with similar coronal diameters and smooth surfaces were used. The first group included 36 glass fiber conical intraradicular posts (Exacto size #3, Angelus, Londrina, PR, Brazil) and the second group included 36 glass fiber double tapered posts (White Post DC n. 2, FGM, Joinville, SC, Brazil). We randomly divided the specimens from each group into three subgroups of 12 posts each for a total of 6 groups, as follows: Group 1: Exacto fiber post that received no surface treatment (control group).Group 2: Exacto fiber post irradiated with an Er,Cr:YSGG laser device (Waterlase MD, Biolase, Irvine) with a MZ8 μm tip, energy level of 1W, repetition rate of 20 Hz, 140 μs pulse duration with 80% water and 60% air for 10 sec, using the non-contact mode. Group 3: Exacto fiber post irradiated with an Er,Cr:YSGG laser device (Waterlase MD, Biolase, Irvine) that had an energy level of 1.5W repetition rate of 20 Hz, 140 μs pulse duration with 80% water and 60% air for 10 sec, using the non-contact mode.

Table 1: Materials used in this study

Trade name	Type	Manufacturer	Lot number
Exacto	Glass fiber conical intraradicular post	Angelus, Londrina, PR, Brazil	S4167256
White Post DC	Glass fiber double tapered posts	FGM, Joinville, SC, Brazil	100615
Dentocore Body	Nanofil composite core build-up material, automix, dual-cure	Itena, France	5194-25QCA3
Silano	Silane	Angelus, Londrina, PR, Brazil	37069
Clearfil SE Bond	Adhesive	Kuraray Noritake Dental, Inc. Okayama, Japan	C30289
Panasil	Vinyl polysiloxane impression material	Kettenbach Gmbh & Co. KG, Germany	22699/2112

Group 4: White Post DC post that received no surface treatment (control group). Group 5: White Post DC post irradiated with an Er,Cr:YSGG laser at energy level of 1W, the same as method 2 (Figure 1A).Group 6: White Post DC post that irradiated with Er,Cr:YSGG laser, at energy level of 1.5W, the same as method 3. After the surface treatments, a single layer of the silane coupling agent was applied with a micro brush to the post surfaces for 1 min, and gently air-dried. Then, a thin layer of unfilled resin (bonding agent) was applied on the surfaces and cured with an LED light curing unit (Bluephase G2, Ivoclar Vivadent). A cylindrical plastic tube (15.0 mm length and 7.0 mm inner diameter) was placed around the post. The apical part of the post was fixed into the putty additional silicon impression material (Panasil, Germany) with the post located at the center of the tube and allowed to set (Figure 1B). Resin core material was filled into the tube and light cured for 20 s each direction of the tube. To ensure optimal polymerization of the core material, an additional light-curing was performed at the end of the specimens for 40 s. Then, the specimens were removed from the tube by sectioning with a scalpel blade and stored in distilled water at 37°C for 24 h. After the storage period, the untapered, coronal portions of the posts were sectioned perpendicular to their long axis by the diamond saw of a cutting machine (Nemopars, Iran) under cooled water with 3 slices (1±0.1 mm thickness) from each specimen. Then, the specimens were subjected to thermocycling (Dorsa, Iran) for 3000 cycles between 5-55°C water baths using a dwell time of 20 s. A compressive push-out load was applied with a Universal Testing Machine at a cross-head speed of 1 mm/min, with a load cell of 20 kgf (BONGSHIN, Model DBBP-20, Korea; Fig 1D). The load was applied in the apical-coronal direction using a 1.5 mm diameter cylindrical plunger, which was placed at the center of the post to avoid contact with the surrounding core material. The maximum load at failure was recorded in Newtons (N) and converted to MPa by dividing the applied load into the bonding area. The bonded area was calculated via the following formula: $A=2\pi rh$ Where r is the post radius, h is the thickness of each disk in mm, and $\pi=3.14$.We analyzed the morphology of the fiber post surfaces from the six groups using a field emission scanning electron microscopy (FE-SEM; TESCAN, Czech Republic). Failure modes were analyzed by a stereomicroscope (Olympus SZ51,

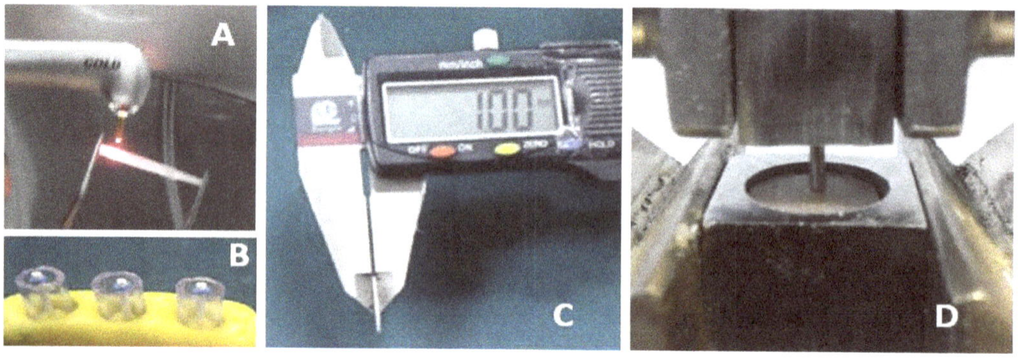

Figure 1: A) Irradiation of glass fiber posts with the Er,Cr:YSGG laser. B) Fixation of posts into the silicon impression material. C) Measuring the thickness of the specimens with a caliper. D) Applying the push-out load by using a Universal Testing Machine

Philippines) at 40x magnification and categorized according to four criteria: 1. cohesive failure within the resin core build-up material; 2. cohesive failure within the fiber post; 3. adhesive failure between the resin core build-up material and fiber post; and 4. mixed failure (a combination of the above failures). Two specimens from each group were analyzed under FE-SEM after fracture to determine the types of failure.

Statistical analysis

Two-way analysis of variance (ANOVA) was performed in order to simultaneously determine the effect of the type of post material and surface treatment on bond strength. We examined these two variables separately considering the significant interaction between surface treatment and type of post material (0.041; $P<0.05$), Therefore, the effect of different surface treatments on each type of fiber posts was analyzed by one-way ANOVA followed by Tukey's HSD post hoc test. We used the independent t-test to assess the effects of different fiber posts on each surface treatment method.

Results

Table 2 shows the mean±SD of the push-out test. The lowest mean bond strength value was observed in the White post DC irradiated with the 1W Er,Cr:YSGG laser. We observed the highest mean bond strength in the Exacto group irradiated with the 1W Er,Cr:YSGG laser 1W. We compared the effect of different surface treatments on each type of fiber post by one-way ANOVA. Post hoc Tukey's HSD test showed that the 1.5W Er,Cr:YSGG laser statistically reduced the micro push-out bond

Table 2: Mean±standard deviation (SD) of the micro push-out bond strength of the studied groups

	Control mean±SD (MPa)	1W Er,Cr:YSGG laser mean±SD (MPa)	1.5W Er,Cr:YSGG laser mean±SD (MPa)
Exacto	14.42±2.0 ^{A,a}	14.52±3.05 ^{C,a}	12.67±1.75 ^{E,b}
White post DC	11.98±1.98 ^{B,c}	11.91±2.04 ^{D,c}	12.02±1.54 ^{E,c}

Groups with different lowercase superscript letters are statistically different in the same row. Groups with different capital superscript letters are statistically different in the same column.

strength values in the Exacto groups ($P<0.05$). However, the difference between the control and 1W Er,Cr:YSGG groups did not statistically differ ($P=0.987$). Multiple comparison in the White post DC groups showed no significant difference between the different surface treatment methods ($P>0.05$). Therefore, surface pretreatment with the laser did not affect bond strength values of White post DC and could not improve bond strength. We performed the independent t-test assessment of the effect of different fiber posts on each surface treatment method. Exacto fiber posts revealed significantly higher bond strength compared to White post DC when using the 1W laser and/or no treatment ($P\leq0.001$). The two commercial fiber posts did not show a significant difference when using the 1.5W laser for surface pretreatment ($P=0.172$). Figure 2 shows photomicrographs of the six groups after surface pretreatment. FE-SEM micrographs showed that prior application of the surface with the Er,Cr:YSGG laser caused partial dissolution of the epoxy resin matrix. Removal of the epoxy resin matrix might enhance the micromechanical retention of core-build up materials. There were no damaged or cracked fibers observed in White post DC groups. However, several micro-cracks were found in Exacto posts irradiated with 1.5W Er,Cr:YSGG (Figure 2). Mode of failure after the push-out test revealed that the mixed failure mode had the most failure mode of all groups (Table 3).

Discussion

Based on the results of the present study, we rejected the first null hypothesis. The results of FE-SEM micrographs revealed that the Er,Cr:YSGG laser caused surface changes in the fiber posts because the laser partially removed the cross-linked epoxy resin matrix. Therefore, the surface roughness and porosities of the post surface increased. This might provide better penetration of resin to the porosities and micromechanical locking would improve the retention of core materials. The second null hypothesis was partially rejected. In the White post DC groups as laser irradiation had no significant effect on the micro push-out bond strength. However, the 1.5W Er,Cr:YSGG laser irradiation of the Exacto posts significantly reduced bond strength.The micro push-out bond strength is classified as shear bond strength test.

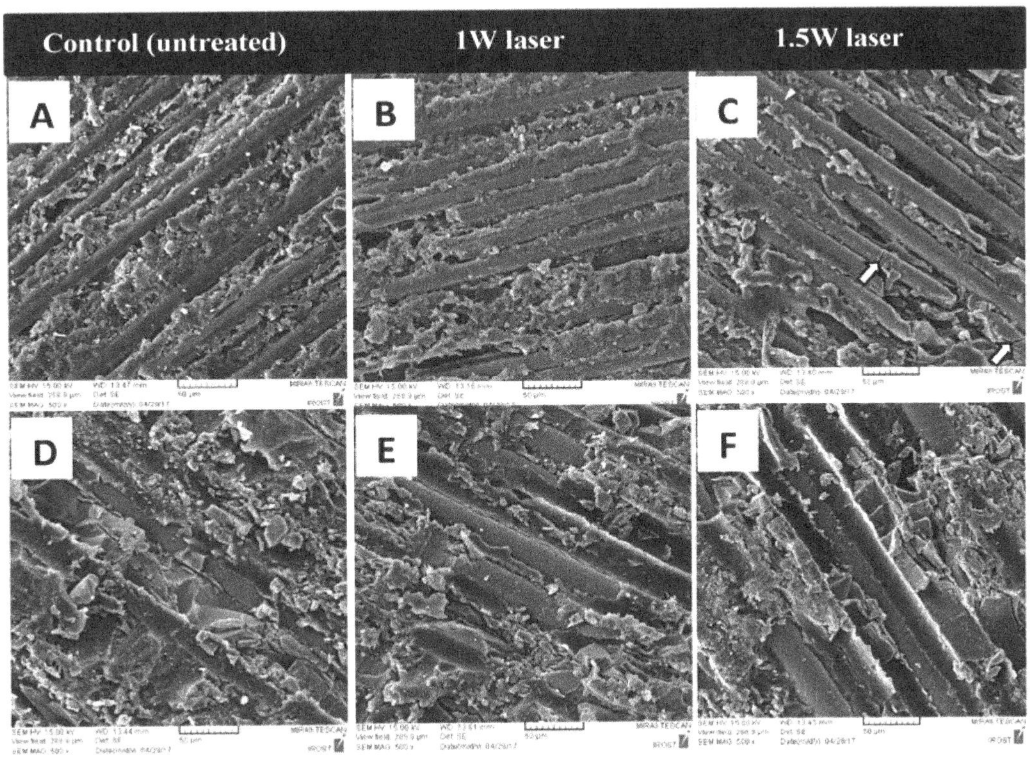

Figure 2: Field emission scanning electron microscopy (FE-SEM) micrographs of glass fiber post surface after different treatments at 500x magnification. (A-C) Exacto post, (D-F) White post DC. The differences in diameter of the fiber posts are clearly shown in the pictures. White post DC fibers are thicker than the Exacto fibers. White arrows show the cracked areas on .the surface of the fiber post

Table 3: Mode of failure distribution in the different groups

Failure mode	Group 1	Group 2	Group 3	Group 4	Group 5	Group 6	Total
1. Cohesive failure within fiber post	2	-	-	2	-	1	5
2. Cohesive failure within core build-up material	-	-	-	-	-	-	-
3. Adhesive failure between fiber post and core build-up material	2	11	6	4	3	4	30
4. Mixed failure	20	14	19	19	22	20	114
a) 1 and 2	5	2	9	2	8	8	34
b) 1 and 3	-	1	-	4	-	3	8
c) 2 and 3	5	10	8	8	8	3	42
d)1, 2, and 3	10	1	2	5	6	6	30
Specimen could not be investigated	1	-	-	-	-	-	1

Group 1: Exacto (control); Group 2: Exacto irradiated with 1W Er,Cr:YSGG laser; Group 3: Exacto irradiated with 1.5W Er,Cr:YSGG laser; Group 4: White Post DC (control); Group 5: White Post DC irradiated with 1W Er,Cr:YSGG laser; Group 6: White Post DC irradiated with 1.5W Er,Cr:YSGG laser

Using this method, the fracture occurs parallel to the bonding interface [15]. This method provides comparable results with the microtensile test with lower premature failures [16]. This method resembles the clinical condition and provides more reliable results compared to the conventional shear test [15, 17]. Furthermore, the size of specimens was decreased to provide more uniform stress distribution using micro push-out test [15]. We obtained 3-4 samples, each with a thickness of 1 mm from each post.In this study, the surfaces of fiber posts in all six groups were treated by silane. It has been reported that salinization appears to favor its use on the post surface to enhance bond strength [18, 19]. Here, we have used a flowable resin core build-up material. The low viscous materials can easily fill porosities and irregularities formed by various pretreatment methods [20-22]. It has been reported that fibers and matrix properties and the bonding between these components could affect mechanical properties. Orientation, length, and concentration of fibers can also play an important role [23]. Luiz *et al.* evaluated the mechanical properties of the two commercial fiber posts used in the present study. They found no statistically significant differences between the two kinds of posts in terms of fracture resistance and two point bending flexural strength. FE-SEM micrographs showed the larger diameter and lower quantity of White post DC fibers compared to Exacto posts [24]. This could possibly explain the more frequent occurrence of cohesive fractures within the post, at least in some areas in the White post DC (Figure 3). Lower bond strength values of the White post DC in the current study could be explained by the fact that the distance between fibers in the White post DC was more than the Exacto; in addition, the direction of the applied force in mico-push-out was parallel to the fibers [24] than the tests used in the Luiz study. Therefore rupture in the area between fibers was observed in most specimens from the White post DC group.The treatment of fibers of these two posts differs during the manufacturing process. Exacto fibers are pre-stressed under tension during the manufacturing process followed by soaking in resin, after which the resin is polymerized. When the resin is finally cured, the tension in the fibers is released. Thus, the glass fibers

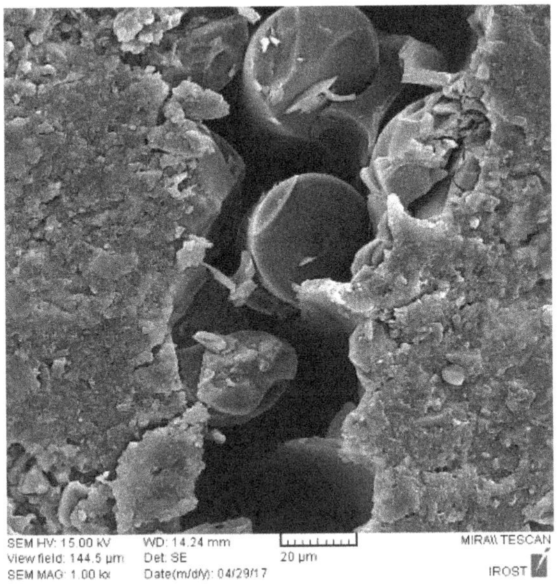

Figure 3: Field emission scanning electron microscopy (FE-SEM) micrographs of White post DC shows a cohesive fracture within the fiber post. The fractures within the fiber posts were observed in more specimens from the White post DC groups, which was probably due to the higher fiber diameters

are placed under compression which enables them to absorb tensile stresses while the post is placed under forces [25]. However, White post DCs are not pre-stressed during the manufacturing process [24]. This factor can be a possible reason for the higher strength of the Exacto fiber posts.Several manufacturers silanize fibers prior to embedding in the resin matrix to ensure adequate fiber/matrix adhesion. If there is adequate interfacial bonding between the fiber and resin matrix, the load can transfer from the resin matrix to the fibers. This would improve both the mechanical properties and integrity of the fiber posts [26]. The commercial fiber posts that have been used in this study were composed of pre-silanized glass fibers. Therefore, this factor did not affect the results. Laser technology has been utilized for different dental procedures in recent years. Surface treatment of dental tissues and dental materials, decreasing of tooth hypersensitivity, and caries removal are some laser applications in the field of dentistry [27-29]. According to the literature, various types of lasers (Nd:YAG, Er:YAG, and Er,Cr:YSGG) have been investigated to increase the bond strength of fiber posts to root dentin, resin cements or resin core materials. Among these, Er:YAG (2.94 nm) and Er,Cr:YSGG (2.78 nm) have similar wavelengths and may cause similar effects. Arslan *et al.* stated that Er:YAG irradiation (450 mJ at 10Hz) on the fiber post surface increased the bond strength of posts to core materials [29]. However, Kurt *et al.* found that prior application of Er:YAG (500 mJ, 2Hz) on the fiber post surface resulted in decreased bond strength [30]. This might be attributed to different parameters (pulse mode, repetition rate, irradiation time, energy density) and type of devices used in those studies.. Another study by Křižnar revealed that methacrylate-based fiber posts significantly decreased bond strength compared to epoxy resin-based fiber posts after Er:YAG pretreatment [22]. The Er,Cr:YSGG laser has been used to improve the bond strength of fiber posts to root dentin. Studies of dentin pretreated with an Er,Cr:YSGG laser showed contradictory results. In a study conducted by Kirmali *et al.*, an Er,Cr:YSGG laser with different power outputs was used as a surface treatment method for root dentin. They reported that push-out bond strength of fiber posts to the treated dentin surface were not enhanced by laser irradiation [31]. However, Mohammadi *et al.* reported a significant increase in bond strength value [32]. Nagase *et al.* found that root dentin irradiation with an Er,Cr:YSGG laser did not cause any statistically significant difference compared to the control group whereas Nd:YAG laser significantly decreased bond strenght value [33]. There is little information about the effects of Er,Cr:YSGG laser irradiation on fiber post surface. Therefore, the current study has evaluated the effects of an Er,Cr:YSGG laser on micro push-out bond strength of two commercial glass fiber posts to resin core build-up material. Only one study conducted by Kurtulmus-Yilmaz *et al.* investigated the Er,Cr:YSGG laser on micro push-out bond strengths between quartz and glass fiber posts and resin core material. They reported that the 1W and 1.5W lasers significantly increased bond strength between the post and resinous core material in both types of posts compared to the control and 2W laser [17]. These results contradicted the current study.

We observed no significant difference in the White post DC groups. The Exacto groups showed no significant difference between the 1W laser and control groups. However, we observed significant reduction in bond strength value in the 1.5W laser group. One explanation could be the different materials (structural characteristics and chemical composition of post and core) used in our study. The second reason was the lack of thermocycling in the study by Kurtulmus-Yilmaz *et al*. However, restorations are exposed to temperature variations in the oral cavity. Hence, the thermocycling procedure was performed as an artificial aging method in the current study. We ignored the 2W laser according to the results reported by Kurtulmus-Yilmaz *et al*. In addition, the authors suggested microscopic evaluations in further research. The influence of the 1 and 1.5W lasers on post surfaces was evaluated under SEM in our study. The reduction in bond strength of the composite resin to the 1.5W Er,Cr:YSGG-treated Exacto posts could be explained by the fact that 1.5W laser irradiation of the post surface partially removed the epoxy resin and resulted in fiber micro-cracking (Figure 2). For the Exacto post, high power output (1.5W) might influence the integrity of the fiber post and have a weakening effect. It could reduce the bonding ability with silane and bonding agent and core material. According to Siqueira *et al*., Er,Cr:YSGG (1.5W) increased the roughness of the fiber post surface and reduced the mechanical properties of fiber posts such as flexural strength and elastic modulus. However, they determined this reduction to be in the acceptable range [34]. The 1.5W laser irradiation of Exacto post in our study compromised the results because of micro-cracking. Hashemikamangar *et al*. reported that 1W Er,Cr:YSGG laser irradiation significantly enhanced the bond strength of fiber posts to core buildup materials compared to that of the control group [35]. The number of fiber posts in each group (n=3) was not sufficient for adequate assessment. However, the difference in the current study was not statistically significant. Mode of failure analysis showed that mixed failure was the predominant failure type for all surface treatment groups. The highest percentages of adhesive failure between post and core material was observed in the 1W Exacto post group (44%; Table 3). Evaluation of fracture revealed that most specimens in the White post DC groups had areas of fracture within the fiber post (Figures 3,4). This might be due to higher diameters of the fibers. This finding correlated with the lower bond strength values of the White post DC groups. Fractures in the composite core are easily treatable in the clinic. Fractures that occur within the post necessitate the removal of the post for re-treatment of the tooth, which is challenging [35]. Strong adhesion between the post and resin core material is needed. Debonding of posts from the core is the most desirable mode of failure in clinical situations [17, 35]. For future research, it is recommended to study different fiber posts with methacrylate-based resin matrix and other parameters of the Er,Cr:YSGG laser in order to find an optimized power output since SEM micrographs in this in vitro study showed that the laser could partially remove the resin matrix.

Conclusions

Based on the results of this in vitro study, we

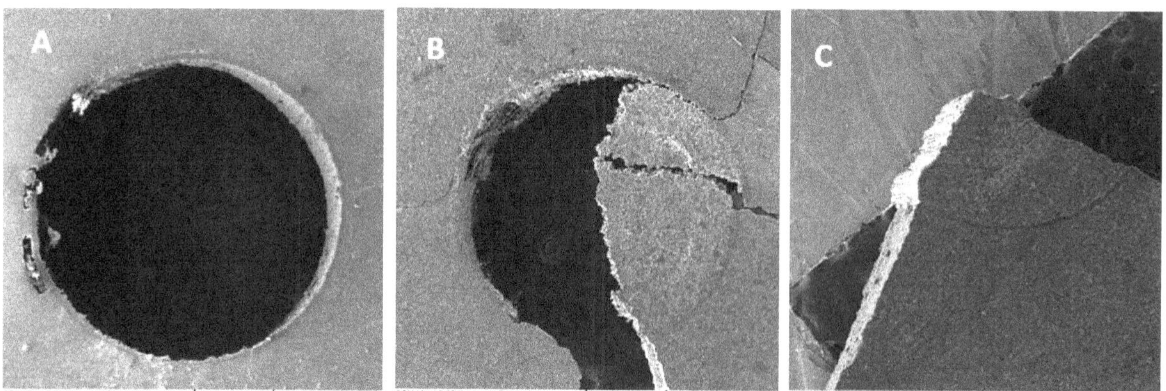

Figure 4: Adhesive (A), mixed (B), and cohesive failure (C) within post and core under field emission scanning electron microscopy (FE-SEM)

conclude that there is a difference in micro push-out bond strength of the core build-up material in the White post DC compared to the Exacto post. This might be attributed to structural characteristics, and the diameters and densities of the fibers. The beneficial effect of an Er,Cr:YSGG laser application could not be confirmed according to the results of this in vitro study. The Er,Cr:YSGG laser did not have a significant effect on bond strength values. However, the 1.5W laser statistically decreased micro push-out bond strength in the Exacto fiber posts ($P<0.05$).

Acknowledgments

This article has been financially supported by grant no: 31821 from Tehran University of Medical Sciences.

Conflict of Interest: None declared.

References

1. Choi Y, Pae A, Park EJ, *et al.* The effect of surface treatment of fiber-reinforced posts on adhesion of a resin-based luting agent. J Prosthet Dent. 2010;103:362-8.
2. Soares CJ, Santana FR, Pereira JC, *et al.* Influence of airborne-particle abrasion on mechanical properties and bond strength of carbon/epoxy and glass/bis-GMA fiber-reinforced resin posts. J Prosthet Dent. 2008;99:444-54.
3. Liu C, Liu H, Qian YT, *et al.* The influence of four dual-cure resin cements and surface treatment selection to bond strength of fiber post. Int J Oral Sci. 2014;6:56-60.
4. Schwartz RS, Robbins JW. Post placement and restoration of endodontically treated teeth: a literature review. J Endod. 2004;30:289-301.
5. Baba NZ, Golden G, Goodacre CJ. Nonmetallic prefabricated dowels: a review of compositions, properties, laboratory, and clinical test results. J Prosthodont. 2009;18:527-36.
6. Goracci C, Ferrari M. Current perspectives on post systems: a literature review. Aust Dent J. 2011;56:77-83.
7. Lassila LV, Tanner J, Le Bell AM, *et al.* Flexural properties of fiber reinforced root canal posts. Dent Mater. 2004;20:29-36.
8. Mazzitelli C, Ferrari M, Toledano M, *et al.* Surface roughness analysis of fiber post conditioning processes. J Dent Res. 2008;87:186-90.
9. Zicari F, De Munck J, Scotti R, *et al.* Factors affecting the cement–post interface. Dent Mater. 2012;28:287-97.
10. Güler AU, Kurt M, Duran I, *et al.* Effects of different acids and etching times on the bond strength of glass fiber-reinforced composite root canal posts to composite core material. Quintessence International. 2012;43:e1-8.
11. Schmage P, Cakir FY, Nergiz I, *et al.* Effect of surface conditioning on the retentive bond strengths of fiberreinforced composite posts. J Prosthet Dent. 2009;102:368-77.
12. Sipahi C, Piskin B, Akin GE, *et al.* Adhesion between glass fiber posts and resin cement: evaluation of bond strength after various pre-treatments. Acta Odontol Scand. 2014;72:509-15.
13. Monticelli F, Osorio R, Sadek FT, *et al.* Surface treatments for improving bond strength to prefabricated fiber posts: a literature review. Oper Dent. 2008;33:346-55.
14. Bitter K, Priehn K, Martus P, *et al.* In vitro evaluation of push-out bond strengths of various luting agents to tooth-colored posts. J Prosthet Dent. 2006;95:302-10.
15. Cekic-Nagas I, Sukuroglu E, Canay S. Does the surface treatment affect the bond strength of various fibre-post systems to resin-core materials? J Dent. 2011;39:171-9.
16. Goracci C, Tavares AU, Fabianelli A, *et al.* The adhesion between fiber posts and root canal walls: comparison between microtensile and push-out bond strength measurements. Eur J Oral Sci. 2004;112:353-61.
17. Kurtulmus-Yilmaz S, Cengiz E, Ozan O, *et al.* The effect of Er,Cr:YSGG laser application on the micropush-out bond strength of fiber posts to resin core material. Photomed Laser Surg. 2014;32:574-81.
18. Goracci C, Raffaelli O, Monticelli F, *et al.* The adhesion between prefabricated FRC posts and composite resin cores: microtensile bond strength with and without post-silanization. Dent Mater. 2005;21:437-44.

19. Albaladejo A, Osorio R, Papacchini F, *et al.* Post silanization improves bond strength of translucent posts to flowable composite resins. J Biomed Mater Res B Appl Biomater. 2007;82:320-4.
20. Salameh Z, Papacchini F, Ounsi HF, *et al.* Adhesion between prefabricated fiber-reinforced posts and different composite resin cores: a microtensile bond strength evaluation. J Adhes Dent. 2006;8:113-7.
21. Ounsi HF, Salameh Z, Carvalho CA, *et al.* Bond strength of composite core build-up materials to fiber-reinforced posts: a microtensile comparison between conventional and wet-ethanol bonding systems. J Adhes Dent. 2009;11:375-80.
22. Kriznar I, Jevnikar P, Fidler A. Effect of Er:YAG laser pretreatment on bond strength of a composite core build-up material to fiber posts. Lasers Med Sci. 2015;30:733-40.
23. Ulbrich NL, Franco APGdO, Zielak JC, *et al.* The stress evaluation of root posts using the finite element analysis. RSBO (Online). 2011;8:189-93.
24. Luiz BKM, Mattei FP, Francisco KRM, *et al.* Fracture resistance, two point bending strength and morphological characteristics of pulpless teeth restored with fiber-reinforced composite posts. RSBO (Online). 2012;9:272-9.
25. Seefeld F, Wenz HJ, Ludwig K, *et al.* Resistance to fracture and structural characteristics of different fiber reinforced post systems. Dent Mater. 2007;23:265-71.
26. Grandini S, Goracci C, Monticelli F, *et al.* Fatigue resistance and structural characteristics of fiber posts: three-point bending test and SEM evaluation. Dent Mater. 2005;21:75-82.
27. Shiu P, De Souza-Zaroni WC, Eduardo Cde P, *et al.* Effect of feldspathic ceramic surface treatments on bond strength to resin cement. Photomed Laser Surg. 2007;25:291-6.
28. Arslan H, Barutcigil C, Yilmaz CB, *et al.* Push-out bond strength between composite core buildup and fiber-reinforced posts after different surface treatments. Photomed Laser Surg. 2013;31:328-33.
29. Kurt M, Güler AU, Duran İ, *et al.* Effects of different surface treatments on the bond strength of glass fiber-reinforced composite root canal posts to composite core material. J Dent Sci. 2012;7(1):20-5.
30. Kirmali O, Kustarci A, Kapdan A, *et al.* Effects of dentin surface treatments including Er, Cr: YSGG laser irradiation with different intensities on the push-out bond strength of the glass fiber posts to root dentin. Acta Odontologica Scandinavica. 2015;73:380-6.
31. Mohammadi N, Savadi Oskoee S, Abed Kahnamoui M, *et al.* Effect of Er,Cr:YSGG pretreatment on bond strength of fiber posts to root canal dentin using a self-adhesive resin cement. Lasers Med Sci. 2013;28:65-9.
32. Nagase DY, de Freitas PM, Morimoto S, *et al.* Influence of laser irradiation on fiber post retention. Lasers Med Sci. 2011;26:377-80.
33. Barbosa Siqueira C, Spadini de Faria N, Raucci-Neto W, *et al.* Evaluation of Mechanical Properties of Glass Fiber Posts Subjected to Laser Surface Treatments. Photomed Laser Surg. 2016;34:460-6.
34. HashemiKamangar SS, Tabatabaii MH, Kalantari S, *et al.* Bond Strength of Fiber Posts to Composite Core: Effect of Surface Treatment With Er, Cr: YSGG Laser and Thermocycling. J Lasers Med Sci. 2017;9:36-42.
35. Mannocci F, Machmouridou E, Watson TF, *et al.* Microtensile bond strength of resin-post interfaces created with interpenetrating polymer network posts or cross-linked posts. Med Oral Patol Oral Cir Bucal. 2008;13:E745-52.

5

Novel User-friendly Device for Human Bite Force Measurement

Khaghaninejad MS[a]; Peyravi A[b*]; Khosravifard A[c]; Peyravi E[d]; Eftekharian HR[e]; Peyravi MR[f]

[a]Assistant Professor, Department of Oral and Maxillofacial Surgery, School of Dentistry, Shiraz University of Medical Sciences, Shiraz, Iran

[b]Undergraduate Student, Student Research Committee, School of Dentistry, Shiraz University of Medical Sciences, Shiraz, Iran

[c]Assistant Professor, Department of Solid Mechanics, School of Mechanical Engineering, Shiraz University, Shiraz, Iran

[d]Undergraduate Student, Student Research Committee, School of Medicine, Shiraz University of Medical Sciences, Shiraz, Iran

[e]Associate professor, Department of Oral and maxillofacial surgery, School of Dentistry, Shiraz University of Medical Sciences, Shiraz, Iran

[f]Assistant Professor, Department of Health in Emergencies and Disasters, School of Management and Medical Informatics, Shiraz University of Medical Sciences, Shiraz, Iran

ARTICLE INFO

Key words:
Bite Force
Strain Gauge
Force Sensitive Resistor
Sensor

Corresponding Author:
Ali Peyravi
Undergraduate Student,
Student Research Committee,
School of Dentistry, Shiraz
University of Medical
Sciences, Shiraz, Iran
Email: ali.peyravi110@gmail.com

Abstract

Statement of Problem: Bite force is generated due to the consonance between different parts of the masticatory system. In dentistry, measurement of the bite force is quite common through several methods and devices.

Objective: The aim was to present a novel bite force-measuring device that could help reducing the costs.

Materials and Methods:This study presented the design, fabrication, and calibration method of a novel low-cost bite force-measuring device based on a force-sensitive resistor and application of strain gages. The FSR 402 was the selected sensor, which was suitable in size for placement in mouth, sterilizable for reuse, and contained biocompatible material.It could measure a large bite force of up to 90 kg with high repeatability.The device had a liquid crystal display (LCD) for immediate visualization of the results and a system for quick calibration of the device in office. To assess the accuracy of the device, some forces were applied to the sensor in nine values from11 to 80kg. The mean of measured force, absolute error, and error percentage were measured and recorded.

Results: The mean relative error was almost 2% within the range of 11-80kg. The lowest error percentage was 0.46% at the load of 52kg and the highest error percentage was 3.97% at the load of 28 kg.Error percentage was 2.51% in the lowest range (11kg) and 2.65% in the highest range (80kg).The relative error in different ranges did not follow a particular trend.

Conclusions:The bite force-measuring device is an economical and user-friendly appliance that can be simply used for routine practice in the office. The device shows good linearity and repeatability. It also has a calibration apparatus that can help maintaining the device accuracy.

Introduction

Among the several performance indicators of the masticatory system is the bite force [1-6], that is generated due to the consonance between different parts of the masticatory system [7]. Determination of the bite force is widely used in dentistry, especially for deliberation of prosthetic appliances [8], or before and after bilateral sagittal split ramus osteotomy and orthognathic surgery in patients with mandibular prognathism [9-10]. Castelo *et al.* [11] studied the relation of masticatory muscle thickness, bite force, and occlusal contacts in young children with unilateral posterior cross bite. Bite force is also known as a significant factor in diagnosis of the temporomandibular disorders (TMD) [7].

Bite force is generally affected by the subject's anatomical and physiological characteristics. Meanwhile, there are several other influential factors including the subject's age and sex, position of the measurement device on the teeth, use of acrylic splints [12], and the side involved in recording [2]. Many studies reported that the effect of bilateral clenching was higher than the unilateral clenching [2, 13].

Methods of bite force measurement are mainly divided into direct and indirect [10]. In the literature, several methods and devices have been presented for bite force measurement [12,14-16]. One of the most accessible and reliable methods is T-scan III, which is made of a horseshoe-shaped bite foil of pressure-sensitive film that can perform a full arch analysis [17-20]. Nevertheless, it is considered a costly system when full arch analysis is not needed [4].

The currently used sensitive electronic devices work based on the electrical resistance strain gages and are accurate enough for measuring the usual forces [8]. Gnathodynamometer were long used for measuring bite forces [14]. Kogawa *et al.* [21] used digital dynamometer for measuring the maximum bite force in patients with TMD. Floystrand *et al.* [12] introduced a new miniature device for recording the bite force. The calibration test of this device showed that the bite force to be reliable within 10-1000 N [12]. Waltim and Kononen [22] introduced a quartz force transducer as a sensitive unit that displayed the result of biting on a liquid crystal display (LCD). They reported that bite forces ranging from 113 to 1692 N could be reliably recorded with this device [22].

Another option of choice for bite force measurement is Flexi Force, which is a thin flexible printed circuit [23]. Flexi Force and Force Sensitive Resistors (FSR) are quite precise in bite force measurement [24-25]. FSR is one of the force sensors that balances force and an electric variable, and then, measures the applied force through using the available measurement circuits. The low cost and ease of use of FSR are the main reasons for its wide application in biomechanics, measurements, and body scan systems.

Considering the limited available space in the oral cavity for inserting the force measurement system, it is important to choose an appropriate device that can transform the bite force to measurable signals, measure forces up to 90 Kg, is accurate, of suitable size for placement in mouth, easily inserted, and sterilizable for reuse. However, such a device is costly and unavailable in Iran. Thus, it seemed necessary to propose a simple cost-effective system that could instantly provide the clinicians with the required data. Accordingly, this research aimed to present the design, fabrication, and calibration method of a novel low-cost bite force-measuring device based on FSR and application of strain gauges.

Materials and Methods

The device designed for bite force measurement was made of a sensor for receiving the bite force, a liquid crystal display (LCD) for immediate display of the results, and a system for quick calibration of the device in office. FSR-402 sensor (Interlink Electronics; USA) was selected due to their availability in the market and the range of required force. The sensor was suitable in size for placement in the mouth, sterilizable for reuse, and contained biocompatible material. It was also capable of measuring large bite force range up to 90 kg with high repeatability. Table 1 shows the characteristics of the applied sensor and Figure 1 displays the force-resistance curve.

According to previous reports, the bite force would possibly reach 90 kg, which was beyond the manufacturer's recommended range for FSR

Table 1: The characteristics of the applied sensor

Parameter	Value
Force sensitivity range	<100 g to >10 kg, depending on mechanics
Pressure sensitivity range	<0.1 kg/cm^2 to >10 kg/cm^2, depending on mechanics
Part-to-part repeatability	±15% to ±25% of established nominal resistance [a]
Single part repeatability	±2% to ±5% of established nominal resistance [a]
Cutoff frequency	500 Hz
Device rise time	1-2 msec
Resolution	0.5% full scale
Current consumption	FSR-400: 0.2 mA, FSR-402: 1.3 mA
Power draw	FSR-400: 0.66 mw, FSR-402: 4.3 mW
Lifetime	>10 million actuations
Package size	FSR-400: 7.5 mm × 38.1 mm, 0.30 mm thickness FSR-402: 18.3 mm × 54.1 mm, 0.46 mm thickness

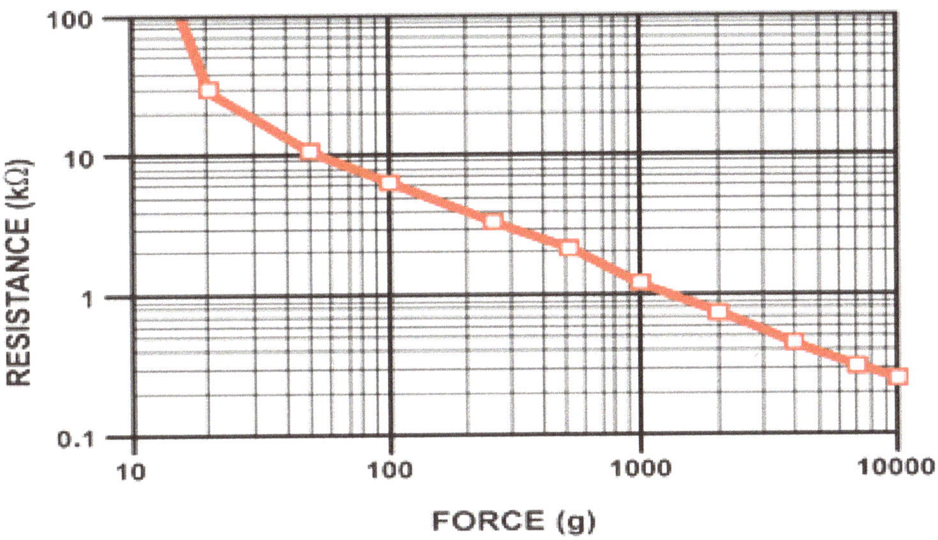

Figure 1: Force-Resistance curve of FSR-402

sensor and would result in nonlinear behavior in resistance variation. Thus, the sensor needed to be calibrated before each use through methods such as lookup table or embedded calibration relationships by using a processor for converting the resistance to force.

In addition, the circuits proposed for establishing the sensor needed to be investigated so that actuating the sensor in a range higher than its usual range would not damage the sensor. Resistance variations of the sensor were measured in initial experiments and the results are shown in Figure 2. According to the manufacturer's proposed circuit, the actuation resistance was approximately set to 250 ohms. Low startup resistances were used in this circuit to yield proper variations of the output voltage within the variation range of input force, so that the measurement would be done at high accuracy. (Figure 3)

To provide a secure current range for the sensor operation, the sensor was replaced and the resistance was actuated through changing the structure of the circuits proposed by the manufacturer. The values measured by the sensor were instantly displayed on the 2-inch color LCD (Figure 4).

A platform was also required to be designed so that

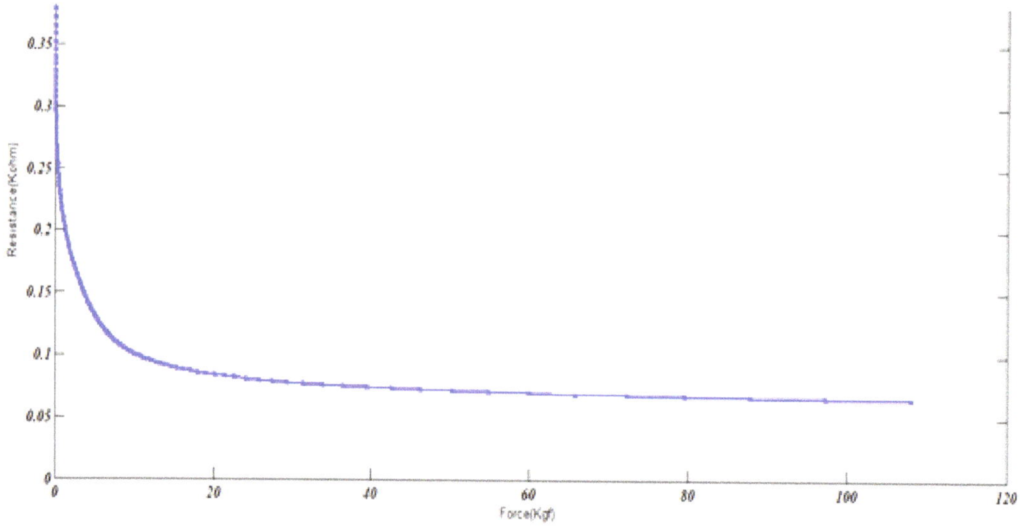

Figure 2: Resistance variations vs. force applied to the sensor

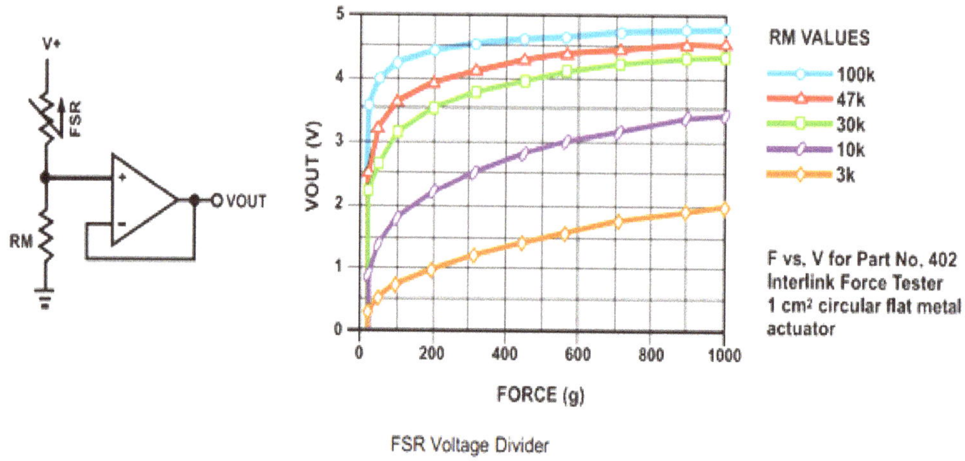

Figure 3: Circuit proposed by the manufacturer for driving FSR-402

it could embed the force measurement sensor. The accurate 3D printer used for making the sheath, not only met the tolerances required for the dimensional optimality, but also could stand higher forces. In order to apply the initial force, distribute it on the sensitive surface of the sensor, and increase the sensor stability, Neodymium magnets were used to connect both sides of the sensor sheath to the surface of sensor; then, the force was applied to both sides of the sensor.

For better distribution of force and creating a proper effective contact area, a thin stereolithographic apparatus (SLA) polymer layer was inserted between the magnets and FSR sensor. Polymer layers were necessary for transmitting the force with respect to the sensor structure and the manufacturer suggested instruction. O-ring sealing was used to prevent fluids penetration into the sensor and to allow sensor sterilization. Figure 5 illustrates the general scheme of the sensor sheath and cross section of the sheath.

In order to calibrate the sensor, a manual calibration system was connected to a PC and the force required to apply pressure onto the sensor was created by using actuation jack. Having pumped the oil in the oil jack and displacing the moving heads of the device, the load cell measured the force applied to the sensor by the jack and transferred it to the computer calibration program through the computer interface circuit.

The force values of force measurement, which were transmitted to the computer through the sensor data logger, were used as the inputs of curve fitting program. Figure 6 shows the voltage

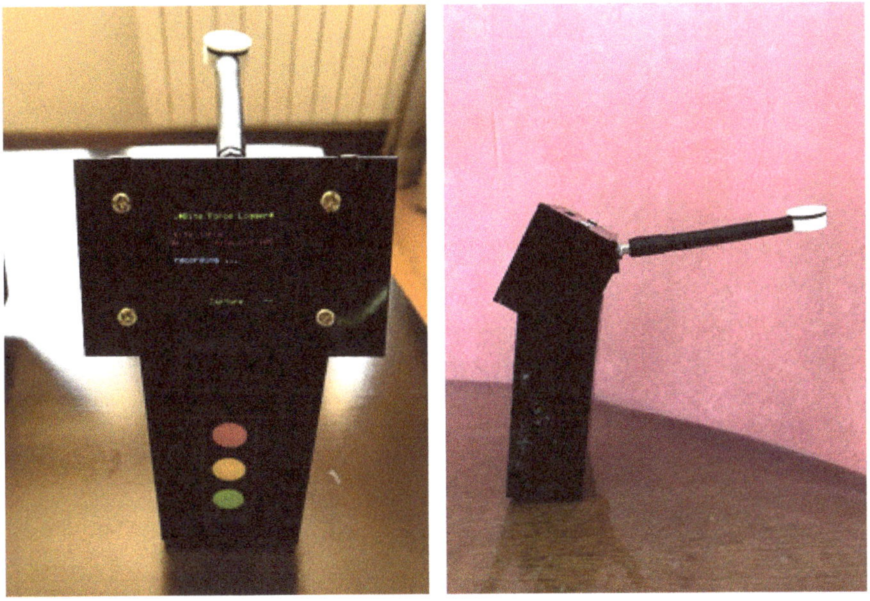

Figure 4: bite force measuring device

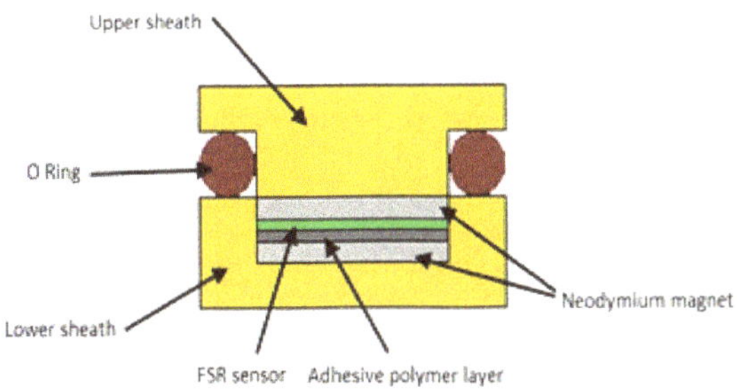

(a)

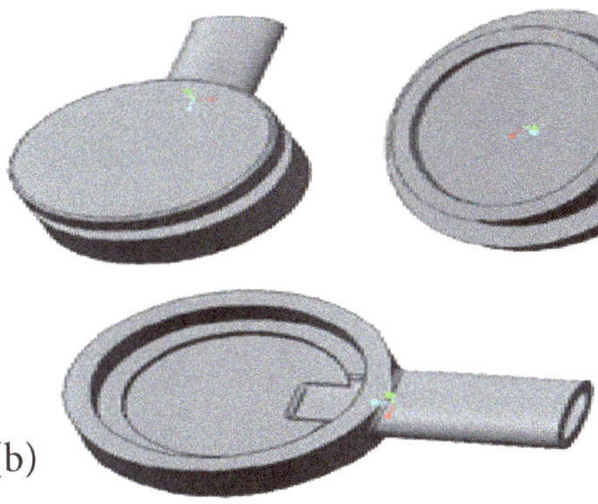

(b)

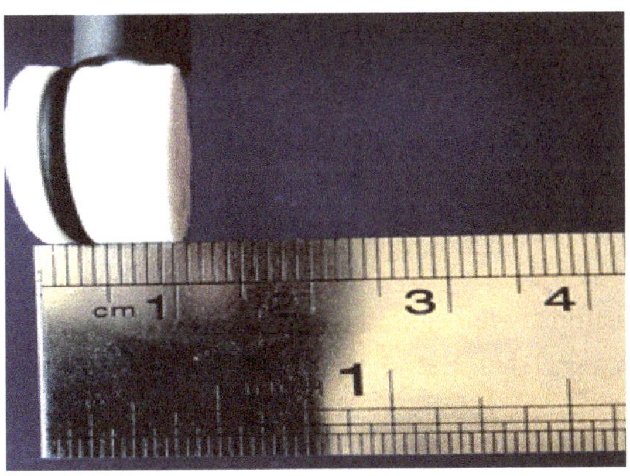

(c)

Figure 5: (a) General scheme, (b) schematic of the sensor sheath's cross section, (c) sensor diameter

variations of the input versus the applied force and fitting parameters of the mathematical model. The calibrator used in this study was built based on the range of applied forces (Figure 6). In order to reduce the costs, the manual oil jack that actuated the moving heads of the device was used to apply force to the sensor. The design of the sensor allowed simultaneous receiving and recording of the input force and the data from the logger (Figure 7).

By using the input data and computer software and according to the calibration-fitting program, calibration factors were calculated and transferred to the logger. Accordingly, the logger measured the force applied to the sensor, which was transmitted to the computer for calibration. A user interface program was designed for calibration to calculate the calibration factors automatically upon receiving the measured data from the data logger and calibrator. The measured data were then transmitted to the data logger of the sensor upon verification of the user. Consequently, this would update the calibration factors of the internal microprocessor.

According to the calibration data obtained from the calibration device, the associated force was calculated. In order to confirm the validity and reliability of the device, a digital dynamometer and a load cell (3-500 kg) were used to apply force on the sensor in nine values from 110 to 800 N twice. Finally, the ideal force, mean measured force, absolute error, and error percentage were determined.

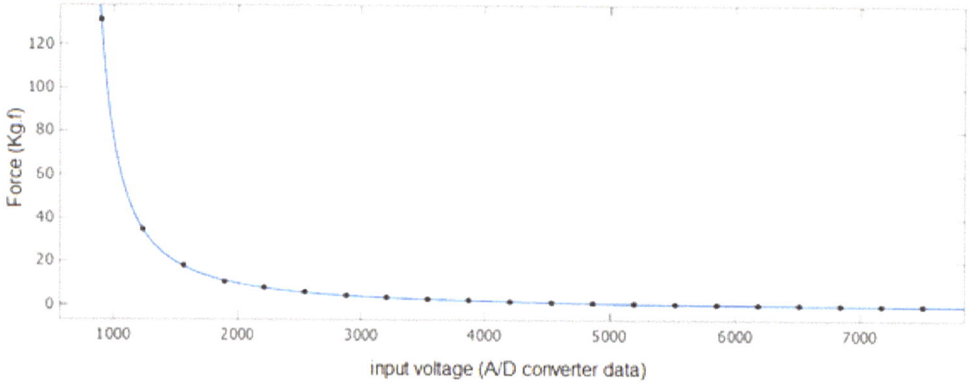

General model	Coeff. "a"	Coeff. "b"	Goodness of fit: SSE:	Goodness of fit: R-square:
f(x) = a*exp(b/x)	0.005064	1.71e+04	0.1456	0.9908

Figure 6: nonlinear variations of the applied voltage vs. force and table of mathematical model agreement with experimental data

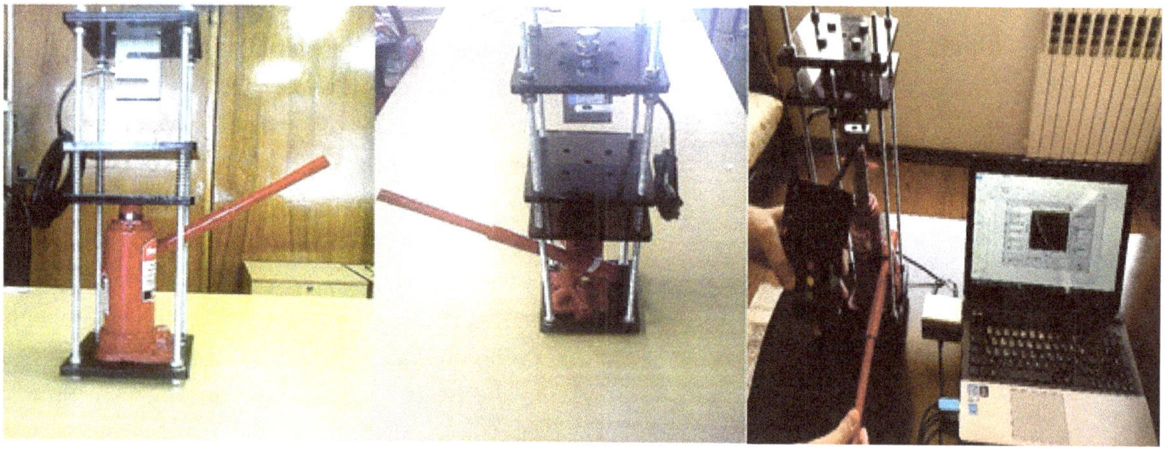

Figure 7: Calibration device built for this study

Results

Table 2 demonstrates the bite force intensity. Accordingly, the mean relative error within the 11-80-kg range was about 2%. The lowest error percentage was 0.46% at 52-kg load and the highest was 3.97% at 28-kg load. The error percentage was 2.51% in the lowest range (11 kg) and 2.65% in the highest range (80 kg). Figure 8 shows the relation between the applied load and percentage error. Accordingly, the error percentage in different ranges did not follow a particular trend. Figure 9 demonstrates the relation between the measured load and the applied load; the line slope is approximately 1.

Discussion

This study presented the construction of a novel bite force-measuring device. The experiment approved the potential of the mentioned device for bite force measurement. The paramount superiority of this device is its low price, which makes it quite cost-effective. The device can be simply calibrated with a user-friendly appliance in the office; which facilitates the calibration process and help saving times and cost. Another advantage is the LCD that shows the results of measurement immediately. It can also measure the forces up to 90 kg with high precision. Moreover, the sensor size is suitable for placement in mouth and it can be sterilized.

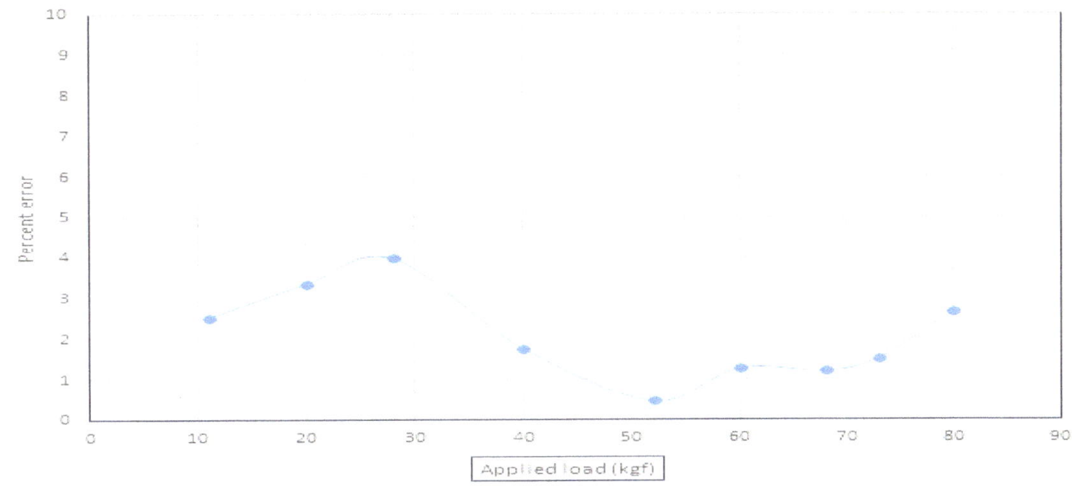

Figure 8: Measurement error

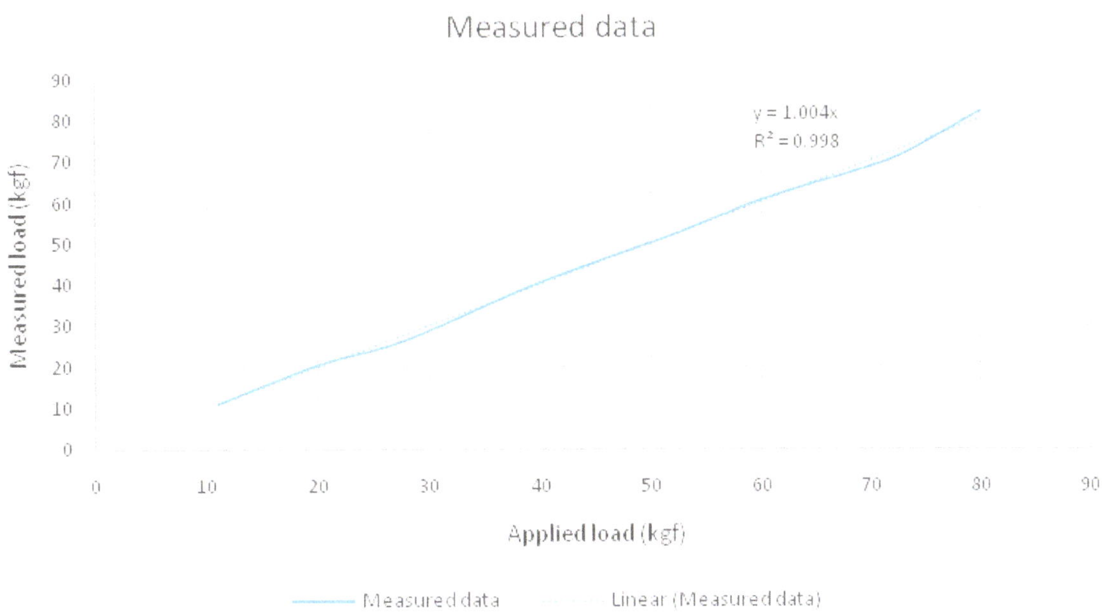

Figure 9: Measured load versus the applied load

Table 2: Ideal force versus errors

Ideal force	Mean of measured force	Absolute error	Error percentage
11	11.27	0.27	2.51
20	20.67	0.67	3.35
28	26.89	1.11	3.97
40	40.7	0.7	1.75
52	52.24	0.24	0.46
60	60.76	0.76	1.26
68	67.19	0.81	1.20
73	71.89	1.11	1.52
80	82.12	2.12	2.65

Although T-Scan III is among the most common and well-known systems for bite force measurement, is not valid enough for measuring absolute values of occlusal force. The bite force applied on this system depends on the patient's position and the location of the occlusal contacts. Therefore, it may record different values each time and show misleading bite force values [26]. T-Scan III is not reliable for measuring relative force [27], and is costly when full arch analysis is not required [16]. Furthermore, T-Scan III needs a USB wire to connect to the PC for setting up system [28]. Whereas, our device is wireless and does not need a PC during measurement, since the clinician can observe the bite force value on the LCD of the device.

The Dental Prescale System (Fuji Film; Tokyo, Japan) consists of a horseshoe-shaped pressure sensitive sheet (50H, R type) and a computerized scanning system (FPD705) [29]. Unlike the device presented in this study, Dental Prescale System is a costly system and does not provide information instantly. This novel measuring bite force device can measure absolute bite force with 2% error. Yet, further studies are suggested to reduce the error percentage and decrease the sensor sheath size.

Conclusions

With respect to the ease of calibration, cost-effectiveness, and accuracy of measurement, the proposed device is considered a user-friendly appliance, which can be simply used, in routine practice.

Acknowledgments

The authors thank the vice-chancellery for research and technology of Shiraz University of Medical Sciences, for supporting the research (Grant#13632). This paper is extracted from a thesis by Dr. Ali Peyravi.

Conflict of Interest: None declared.

References

1. Umesh S, Padma S, Asokan S, *et al.* Fiber Bragg grating based bite force measurement. JBiomech. 2016;49:2877-2881.
2. Van Der Bilt A, Tekamp A, Van Der Glas H, *et al.* Bite force and electromyograpy during maximum unilateral and bilateral clenching. EurJOral Sci. 2008;116:217-222.
3. Yen CI, Mao SH, Chen CH, *et al.* The correlation between surface electromyography and bite force of mastication muscles in Asian young adults. Ann Plast Surg. 2015;74:168-172.
4. Cerna M, Ferreira R, Zaror C, *et al.* Validity and reliability of the T-Scan® III for measuring force under laboratory conditions. J Oral Rehab. 2015;42:544-551.
5. Owais AI, Shaweesh M, Abu Alhaija ES. Maximum occlusal bite force for children in different dentition stages.EurJOrthod. 2013;35:427-433.
6. Sun KT, Chen SC, Li YF, *et al.* Bite-force difference among obese adolescents in central Taiwan. J Formos Med Assoc. 2016;115:404-410.
7. Calderon PS, Kogawa EM, Lauris JR, *et al.* The influence of gender and bruxism on the human maximum bite force. J Appl Oral Sci. 2006;14:448-453.
8. Fernandes CP, Glantz PO, Svensson SA, *et al.* A novel sensor for bite force determinations. Dent Mater. 2003;19:118-126.
9. Harada K, Watanabe M, Ohkura K, *et al.* Measure of bite force and occlusal contact area before and after bilateral sagittal split ramus osteotomy of the mandible using a new pressure-sensitive device: a preliminary report. J Oral MaxillofacSurg. 2000;58:370-373.
10. Ueki K, Marukawa K, Shimada M, *et al.* Changes in occlusal force after mandibular ramus osteotomy with and without Le Fort I osteotomy. Int JOral MaxillofacSurg. 2007;36:301-304.
11. Castelo PM, Gavião MB, Pereira LJ, *et al.* Masticatory muscle thickness, bite force, and occlusal contacts in young children with unilateral posterior crossbite. Eur J Orthod. 2007;29:149-156.
12. Koc D, Dogan A, Bek B. Bite force and influential factors on bite force measurements: a literature review.Eur J Dent. 2010;4:223-

232.
13. Shinogaya T, Bakke M, Thomsen CE, *et al*. Bite force and occlusal load in healthy young subjects--a methodological study. Eur JProsthodontRestor Dent. 2000;8:11-15.
14. Rane V, Hamde S, Agrawal A. Development of computerized masticatory force measurement system. J Med Eng Technol. 2017;41:65-71.
15. Testa M, Di Marco A, Pertusio R, *et al*. A validation study of a new instrument for low cost bite force measurement. J Electromyog Kinesiology. 2016;30:243-248.
16. Fastier-Wooller J, Phan HP, Dinh T, *et al*. Novel low-cost sensor for human bite force measurement. Sensors. 2016;16:1244.
17. Kerstein RB. Articulating paper mark misconceptions and computerized occlusal analysis technology. DentImplantolUpdate. 2008;19:41-46.
18. Baltrusaityte A, Surna A, Pileicikiene G, *et al*. The relationship between unilateral mandibular angle fracture and temporomandibular joint function.Stomatologija. 2014;16:87-93.
19. Liu CW, Chang YM, ShenYF, *et al*. Using the T-scan III system to analyze occlusal function in mandibular reconstruction patients: A pilot study. Biomed J. 2015;38:52-57.
20. Lila-KrasniqiZD, Shala KS, Pustina-Krasniqi T, *et al*. Differences between centric relation and maximum intercuspation as possible cause for development of temporomandibulardisorder analyzed with T-scan III. Eur JDent. 2015;9:573.
21. Kogawa E, Calderon P, Lauris J, *et al*. Evaluation of maximal bite force in temporomandibular disorders patients.J Oral Rehab. 2006;33:559-565.
22. Waltimo A, Könönen M. A novel bite force recorder and maximal isometric bite force values for healthy young adults. EurJournal Oral Sci. 1993;101:171-175.
23. Tekscan Force Sensors for Design. (accessed on 10 March 2016) Available at: [https://www.tekscan.com/sites/default/files/FLX-Force-Sensors-For-Design.pdf].
24. Diaz Lantada A, Gonzalez Bris C, Lafont Morgado P, *et al*. Novel system for bite-force sensing and monitoring based on magnetic near field communication. Sensors. 2012;12:11544-11558.
25. Bousdras VA, Cunningham JL, Ferguson-Pell M, *et al*. A novel approach to bite force measurements in a porcine model in vivo.Int JOral Maxillofac Surg. 2006;35:663-667.
26. Lee SM, Lee JW. Computerized occlusal analysis: correlation with occlusal indexes to assess the outcome of orthodontic treatment or the severity of malocculusion. Korean J Orthod. 2016;46:27-35.
27. Cerna M, Ferreira R, Zaror C, *et al*. In vitro evaluation of T-Scan® III through study of the sensels.CRANIO®. 2015;33:300-306.
28. Kerstein RB. History of the T-Scan system development from 1984 to the present day. Handbook of Research on Computerized Occlusal Analysis Technology Applications in Dental Medicine 2015; 1-35.
29. Kwon HK, Yoo JH, Kwon YS, *et al*.Comparison of bite force with dental prescale and unilateral bite force recorder in healthy subjects.J Korean AcadProsthodont. 2006;44:103-111.

6

Effect of Different Bleaching Techniques on Microleakage under Orthodontic Brackets: In Vitro Study

Salehi P[a]; Malekpour B[b]; Roshan A[c*]; Hamedani Sh[d]

[a]Professor, Orthodontics Research Center, Department of Orthodontics, School of Dentistry, Shiraz University of Medical Sciences, Shiraz, Iran
[b]Postgraduate Student, Department of Orthodontics, School of Dentistry, Shiraz University of Medical Sciences, Shiraz, Iran
[c]Postgraduate Student, Department of Orthodontics, School of Dentistry, Shiraz University of Medical Sciences, Shiraz, Iran
[d]Dental Research Development Center, School of Dentistry, Shiraz University of Medical Sciences, Shiraz, Iran

ARTICLE INFO

Key words:
Bleaching
Microleakage
Orthodontic

Corresponding Author:
Ali Roshan
Postgraduate Student,
Department of Orthodontics,
School of Dentistry, Shiraz
University of Medical
Sciences, Shiraz, Iran
Email: ali.roshan1111@gmail.com

Abstract

Statement of problem: Numerous studies report significant changes in tooth color that occur during orthodontic treatment. The adverse effects of bleaching procedures during orthodontic treatments have not been studied comprehensively.
Objectives: This study investigated the effects of two methods of dental bleaching on the degree of microleakage beneath orthodontic brackets.
Materials and Methods: We selected 45 extracted premolar teeth and bonded them to orthodontic brackets. These teeth were stored in normal saline for 24 hours and thermocycled. We randomly divided the samples into 3 groups of 15 teeth per group. The first group (control) received no bleach treatment; the second group (office bleaching) was treated with 35% hydrogen peroxide (Whiteness HP Maxx); and the third group (home bleaching) was treated with 22% carbamide peroxide (Whiteness Perfect). The apices were sealed with sticky wax, rinsed in tap water, and air-dried. We applied nail varnish to the entire surface of each tooth, except for an area approximately 1 mm away from the brackets. The samples were immersed in basic fuchsine and cleaned after 24 hours. Microleakage was determined by direct measurement using a stereomicroscope. Kruskal-Wallis and Dunn post-hoc statistical tests, and SPSS software were used for statistical analysis. The significance level was set at $P \leq 0.05$.
Results: The office bleaching group had significantly more microleakage scores under the brackets at both the occlusal ($P=0.04$) and gingival ($P=0.040$) margins of the brackets compared to the home bleaching group. The home bleaching group showed statistically more significant microleakage scores than the control group in both the gingival ($P=0.006$) and occlusal ($P=0.014$) margins of the brackets. All three groups had statistically more significant microleakage at the gingival margins of the brackets than the occlusal margins.
Conclusions: Office bleaching caused the most microleakage under the brackets and home bleaching caused more microleakage than the control group. We observed more microleakage at the gingival margins of the brackets compared to the occlusal margins.

Introduction

Tooth bleaching is considered the first option to improve tooth color since it is a minimally invasive approach with acceptable esthetic results compared with other esthetic procedures such as crowns or veneers [1]. Dental bleaching can be performed directly by the dentist in a clinic (in-office bleaching), by the patient at home with professional supervision (in-home bleaching), or without professional supervision with over-the-counter products (over-the-counter). Many studies have reported that significant tooth color changes could occur during orthodontic treatment [2-4]. Fixed orthodontic treatment, particularly in young patients, provokes greater accumulation of plaque and stain deposition on teeth surfaces [5]. Currently, many orthodontic patients request tooth whitening procedures [6]. However, ideal tooth whitening should be performed after the removal of brackets at the end of orthodontic treatment [7]. Dental professionals presume that a bleaching procedure during orthodontic treatment is not possible because of the presence of the brackets, which interferes with peroxide diffusion into the labial surfaces of the teeth [8, 9]. The whitening treatment is usually performed after orthodontic treatment when bracket removal would permit bleaching agents to have better access and function on the facial surfaces of the teeth. The mechanism of the dental bleaching agent is a redox reaction that releases active oxygen, which diffuses through the tooth structure. Owing to its low molecular weight, hydrogen peroxide reduces the organic pigments that impregnate in enamel groves and dentin, and consequently leads to their elimination [10]. Studies [5, 7, 9] have evaluated the effectiveness of bleaching treatments during orthodontic treatment. However, there is limited evidence about the adverse effects of bleaching procedures during these treatments, such as the effects on the enamel-adhesive bond under the brackets. A number of reports have discussed the interaction between bleaching agent and bond efficacy of composite resins or orthodontic adhesives to bleached enamel. The authors reported a substantial reduction in the bond strength of the composite resin to bleached enamel compared to unbleached enamel [11-13]. Some studies concluded that residual peroxide or oxygen on the tooth structure might be responsible for the decrease in bond strength [14]. The enamel acts as a semipermeable membrane. It has been concluded that the bleaching agent and by-products that result from its decomposition are able to disperse proximally within the tooth structure, even at the presence of a fixed orthodontic appliance [5]. Jadad *et al.* [15] showed the effectiveness of an 8% hydrogen peroxide-based whitening agent in cases with fixed orthodontic appliances [15]. Arboleda-Lopez *et al.* [7] reported that the bleaching technique was effective and changed the shade of the teeth in the presence and absence of orthodontic brackets. Akin *et al.* [16] found that 10% carbamide peroxide bleaching did not significantly decrease shear bond strength values of orthodontic brackets. Comparably, 38% hydrogen peroxide bleaching significantly reduced these values. Mullins *et al.* [17] stated that brackets bonded within 24 hours following bleaching had a higher possibility for bond failure. Orthodontic bonding should be deferred for 2–3 weeks when patients have a history of in-office bleaching with 38% hydrogen peroxide. These studies evaluated the enamel that was bleached before the bonding procedures, which followed the bleaching procedures. In the abovementioned studies, the enamel under bleaching treatment did not have any bracket, nor was there composite restoration bonded to the enamel. To the best of the authors' knowledge, no study evaluated the effects of bleaching agents on bond strength and microleakage scores on enamel bonded to composite restorations or orthodontic brackets. Microleakage of dental restorative materials is an imperative problem in clinical dentistry [18]. Microleakage can be demarcated as the clinically undetectable dissemination of bacteria, fluids, molecules, or ions between a cavity wall and the restorative material [19]. Microleakage enables the transfer of bacteria from the oral cavity by gap formation [20]. It may cause enamel discoloration, corrosion, decreased bond strength, recurrent caries, and pulpal injury [18, 21]. This in vitro study has investigated the effects of two methods of dental bleaching on the degree of microleakage beneath orthodontic brackets. The null hypothesis advocates that there is an equal degree of microleakage under orthodontic brackets in specimens with and without bleaching procedures.

Materials and Methods

Sample preparation

This in vitro study assessed 45 premolars previously extracted for orthodontic purposes. The samples were intact and did not have any cracks, restoration, white spots, gross irregularities, decays, fractures, previous bracket bonding, or enamel hypoplasia. The teeth were scaled and washed to remove any covered blood, soft tissue, or debris. Next, they were immersed in 10% formalin solution for two weeks for sterilization [22]. The teeth were kept in saline solution at 37°C for no more than one month. The normal saline was changed weekly to prevent bacterial growth.

Bonding procedure

Before the etching procedure, the buccal surfaces of the teeth were cleaned using fluoride-free pumice paste and a rubber cup in a low-speed hand piece. Next, they were rinsed with water and air-dried. All samples were etched with a 37% phosphoric acid gel (3M Unitek, Monrovia, CA, USA) for 30 seconds. After application of the acid, the buccal surfaces were rinsed thoroughly for 15 seconds and dried with oil- and moisture-free air until a frosty white appearance was achieved. After the etching process, we applied a thin layer of Transbond™ XT primer (3M Unitek, Monrovia, CA, USA) onto the surfaces of the teeth with a brush, light cured with an LED light unit (BlueLEX GT-1200W, San Chong, Taipei County, Taiwan) for 10 seconds. Transbond XT adhesive paste (3m Unitek, Monrovia, CA, USA) was applied to the bracket base (American Orthodontics, MBT, 022, Sheboygan, WI, USA), and the bracket was placed on the FA point on the tooth. The FA point is described as the middle of the clinical crown occluso-gingivally and mesiodistally, following the long axis of the crown. The excessive composite resin was removed with a dental explorer. Each tooth was light-cured for 30 seconds- 15 seconds from the mesial, and 15 seconds from the distal.

Thermocycling

After the bonding procedure, the teeth were stored at room temperature in normal saline for 24 hours. Thermocycling was performed at 5±2°C to 55±2°C for 1000 cycles with a dwell time of 30 seconds and a transfer time of 5 seconds.

Bleaching procedure

We randomly divided the samples into three groups of 15 per group by random selection.

The first group (control) received no bleaching treatment. In the second group (office bleaching), the teeth were bleached with a 35% hydrogen peroxide gel (Whiteness HP Maxx, FGM Dental Products, Joinville, SC, Brazil). In the third group (home bleaching), the teeth were bleached with a 22% carbamide peroxide gel (Whiteness Perfect, FGM Dental Products, Joinville, SC, Brazil). In the second group, we applied the 35% hydrogen peroxide gel to the entire facial surface of the teeth according to the manufacturer's instructions. Three courses of a 15-minute application were performed for each bleaching session for three bleaching sessions, each 45 minutes with no interval. In the home bleach group, we applied a 22% carbamide peroxide gel to the facial surface of the teeth without using a dental tray. The gel remained for one hour on the tooth's surface during each bleaching session. In total, there were 12 bleaching sessions with no interval. In both groups, after each tooth whitening session, the gel was removed, and the surface was washed with tap water and dried with compressed air.

Evaluation of microleakage

The apices were sealed with sticky wax, rinsed in tap water, and air-dried. Then, two layers of nail varnish were applied to the entire surface of the tooth, except for an area approximately 1 mm away from the brackets, which was marked with a black pencil. Next, the samples were immersed for 24 hours at room temperature in a 0.5% solution of basic fuchsine (0.5 g powder in 100 ml of distilled water) that covered the entire teeth and brackets. After 24 hours, the superficial dyes were removed from the samples by a low speed handpiece and bristle brushes. A buccolingual directed cut was made on the midline of the brackets on samples with a low-speed diamond disc (Brasseler, Lemgo, Germany). Next, we used a stereomicroscope (BS 3060, China, 40X magnifications) to record the microleakage scores in millimeters. Microleakage was determined by direct measurement using the image analyzer software of the stereomicroscope (scope image: 9X, magnification: 40x). Half of the samples were randomly re-examined to evaluate for intra-observer error of measurement. Occlusal and gingival margins of the brackets were assessed for leakage scores in the tooth-adhesive interfaces.

Statistical analysis

We used the Kruskal-Wallis and Dunn post-hoc statistical tests, and SPSS software (version 22, Chicago, IL, USA). The significance level was set at P≤0.05 for all tests.

Results

A comparison of the microleakage scores (mm) for all specimens according to the Kruskal-Wallis test in both the occlusal and gingival margins showed statistically significant differences (P<0.001). The bleaching procedures caused increased microleakage scores under the orthodontic brackets. The results of the post-hoc test showed that the office bleaching group had significantly more microleakage scores under the brackets at both the occlusal (P=0.04) and gingival (P =0.040) margins of the brackets compared to the home bleaching group. The home bleaching group showed statistically more significant microleakage scores than the control group in both the gingival (P=0.006) and occlusal (P=0.014) margins of the brackets. A comparison of the gingival margins of the brackets to the occlusal margins showed significantly more microleakage in all three groups – office bleaching (P=0.009), home bleaching (P=0.007), and control (P=0.049). One-way ANOVA showed no significant intra-observer differences. Table 1 summarizes the study results. Figure 1 shows the microleakage at the gingival and occlusal sides (magnification: 40X).

Discussion

This study evaluated the effects of bleaching procedures on microleakage at the enamel-adhesive interface from the occlusal and gingival margins of brackets in patients who undergo orthodontic treatments. The enamel surfaces and enamel-adhesive interfaces were treated chemically with the aim to break the adhesion at the composite-enamel interface. The specimens have been subjected to a microleakage test. Orthodontic treatments and bleaching procedures both have the potential to increase the risk of microleakage by affecting the enamel surface and enamel-adhesive interface [23, 24]. Hence, the current study has intended to determine the safety of bleaching teeth during orthodontic treatment. Hydrogen peroxide and carbamide peroxide dissolution products are low molecular-weight molecules that easily diffuse into the lamellae, grooves, fissures, and depression areas in enamel structures [8]. If the bleaching agent spreads through the enamel pores and diffuses into the dentinal tubular structure, so the bleaching

Table 1: Median and Mean±Standard deviation (SD) of microleakage (mm) at the enamel-adhesive interface measured from the occlusal and gingival margins of the bracket base

		Office bleaching	Home bleaching	Control	P-value
Gingival	Mean ± SD	0.34±0.17	0.14±0.11	0.02±0.016	P <0.001
	Median	0.3200	0.1000	0.0200	
Occlusal	Mean ± SD	0.18±0.14	0.05±0.05	0.01±0.01	P <0.001
	Median	0.1100	0.0200	0.0100	

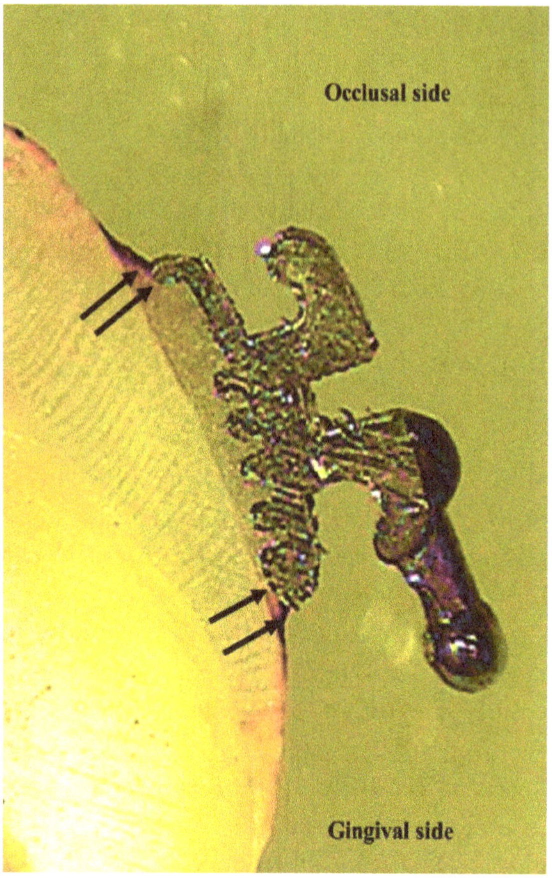

Figure 1: Arrows show microleakage at the gingival and occlusal sides (magnification: 40X)

process can be done in patients with orthodontic devices. Free radicals from hydrogen peroxide can disseminate in all directions throughout dental structures located under the bracket adhesive interface. Therefore, they have the potential to spread through the enamel-adhesive interface and, consequently, affect the resin tags and bond efficacy under the brackets. They may also break the organic stain molecules present throughout the labial surface of the teeth [5]. Several techniques have been introduced to evaluate microleakage in dentistry. The easiest and most frequently used method involves exposure of the samples to a dye solution before viewing cross-sections under a light microscope [25]. We have chosen dye penetration for this study since it provides a simple, relatively inexpensive quantitative and comparable method for evaluation of possible microleakage. To the best of the authors' knowledge, this study was the first that investigated the effect of bleaching on microleakage values of enamel adhesive interface under orthodontic brackets. The results showed that all bleaching procedures adversely affected the bond efficacy of orthodontic brackets to the enamel with increased microleakage scores. However, we observed significantly increased microleakage values among the specimens from the office bleaching group. Hence, this bleaching technique might have the most destructive effects on the enamel- adhesive interface and resin tags. This concern should be considered for patients who request to bleach their teeth during the orthodontic treatments. Patients should be informed that an increased rate of white spots, decalcifications, staining, and numerous other adverse effects would be expected consequent to increased microleakage scores under the brackets. However, if the patient insists on bleaching during orthodontic treatment, home bleaching is the technique of choice due to its apparently less adverse effects. The office bleaching group had more microleakage than the home bleaching group; hence, the impact of bleaching agents on microleakage could be considered to be concentration-dependent. In addition, the influence of the bleaching procedure on the morphology and hardness of the enamel surface depended on the concentrations of the active ingredients [26]. The gingival margin generally exhibited a higher microleakage value compared with the occlusal margin of the enamel-adhesive interfaces. However, the difference was statistically significant for any of the study groups. Several studies [27-30] reported statistically greater microleakage in the gingival rather than the occlusal margins. This finding was attributed to either the surface curvature anatomy which might result in relatively thicker adhesive at the gingival side [27, 29] or to the curing method that emitted light only from the occlusal side [28, 30]. The relatively greater microleakage obtained from gingival enamel probably resulted from its aprismatic structure, which appeared to be more resistant to dissolution in acids compared to the prismatic mid-coronal enamel [31]. It seemed that the difference in microleakage values between gingival and occlusal margins of the brackets was irrelevant for the bleaching procedures and unbleached specimens. The microleakage values in the gingival margin of the brackets were greater than the occlusal margin.m Perhaps, with a larger number of specimens the outcomes could be unequivocally different. Therefore, we suggest that further studies be conducted with larger numbers of samples.

Conclusions

The office bleaching group showed the most microleakage values under the brackets, whereas the home bleaching group had more microleakage compared to the control group. We observed microleakage at the gingival margins of the brackets compared to the occlusal margins.

Acknowledgements

We express our appreciation to Dr. Vosough, Dental Research Development Center, School of Dentistry, for the statistical analysis.

Conflict of Interest: None declared

Refrences

1. Basting RT, Amaral FLB, França FMG, *et al.* Clinical comparative study of the effectiveness of and tooth sensitivity to 10% and 20% carbamide peroxide home-use and 35% and 38% hydrogen peroxide in-office bleaching materials containing desensitizing agents. Oper Dent. 2012;37:464-73.
2. Çörekçi B, Irgın C, Malkoç S, *et al.* Effects of staining solutions on the discoloration of orthodontic adhesives: an in-vitro study. Am J Orthod Dentofacial Orthop. 2010;138:741-6.
3. Karamouzos A, Athanasiou AE, Papadopoulos MA, *et al.* Tooth-color assessment after orthodontic treatment: a prospective clinical trial. Am J Orthod Dentofacial Orthop. 2010;138:537.e1-8.
4. Trakyalı G, Özdemir FI, Arun T. Enamel colour changes at debonding and after finishing procedures using five different adhesives. Eur J Orthod. 2009;31:397-401.
5. Gomes MN, Dutra H, Morais A, *et al.* In-Office Bleaching During Orthodontic Treatment. J Esthet Restor Dent. 2017;29:83-92.
6. Slack ME, Swift EJ, Rossouw PE, *et al.* Tooth whitening in the orthodontic practice: A survey of orthodontists. Am J Orthod Dentofacial Orthop. 2013;143: S64-S71
7. Arboleda-Lopez C, Manasse RJ, Viana G, *et al.* Tooth Whitening during Orthodontic Treatment: A Six-Month In vitro Assessment of Effectiveness and Stability. Int J Dent Oral Health. 2015;1:1-4.
8. Consolaro A, Consolaro RB, Francischone L. Clarifications, guidelines and questions about the dental bleaching" associated" with orthodontic treatment. Dental press J orthod. 2013;18:4-10.
9. Lunardi N, Correr AB, Rastelli AN, *et al.* Spectrophotometric evaluation of dental bleaching under orthodontic bracket in enamel and dentin. J Clin Exp Dent. 2014;6: e321-e326.
10. Kawamoto K, Tsujimoto Y. Effects of the hydroxyl radical and hydrogen peroxide on tooth bleaching. J Endod. 2004;30:45-50.
11. Ben-Amar A, Liberman R, Gorfil C, *et al.* Effect of mouthguard bleaching on enamel surface. Am J Dent. 1995;8:29-32.
12. Josey AL, Meyers IA, Romaniuk K, *et al.* The effect of a vital bleaching technique on enamel surface morphology and the bonding of composite resin to enamel. J oral rehabil. 1996;23:244-50.
13. Sung EC, Chan SM, Mito R, *et al.* Effect of carbamide peroxide bleaching on the shear bond strength of composite to dental bonding agent enhanced enamel. J Prosthet Dent. 1999;82:595-9.
14. Torneck CD, Titley KC, Smith DC, *et al.* The influence of time of hydrogen peroxide exposure on the adhesion of composite resin to bleached bovine enamel. J Endod. 1990;16:123-8.
15. Jadad E, Montoya J, Arana G, *et al.* Spectrophotometric evaluation of color alterations with a new dental bleaching product in patients wearing orthodontic appliances. Am J Orthod Dentofacial Orthop. 2011;140: e43-e7.
16. Akin M, Aksakalli S, Basciftci FA, *et al.* The effect of tooth bleaching on the shear bond strength of orthodontic brackets using self-etching primer systems. Eur J Dent. 2013;7:55-60.
17. Mullins JM, Kao EC, Martin CA, *et al.* Tooth whitening effects on bracket bond strength in vivo. Angle Orthod. 2009;79:777-83.

18. Mali P, Deshpande S, Singh A. Microleakage of restorative materials: an in vitro study. J Indian Soc Pedod Prev Dent. 2006;24:15-8.
19. Fabianelli A, Pollington S, Davidson CL, *et al*. The relevance of microleakage studies. International Dentistry SA. 2007;9:64-74.
20. St Georges AJ, Wilder AD Jr , Perdigão J, *et al*. Microleakage of Class V composites using different placement and curing techniques: an in vitro study. Am J Dent. 2002;15:244-7.
21. Alkis H, Turkkahraman H, Adanir N. Microleakage under orthodontic brackets bonded with different adhesive systems. Eur J Dent. 2015;9:117-21.
22. Lee JJ, Nettey-Marbell AN, Cook Jr A, *et al*. Using extracted teeth for research: the effect of storage medium and sterilization on dentin bond strengths. J Am Dent Assoc. 2007;138:1599-603.
23. Türkün M, Türkün LS. Effect of nonvital bleaching with 10% carbamide peroxide on sealing ability of resin composite restorations. Int Endod J. 2004;37:52-60.
24. Shinohara MS, Rodrigues JA, Pimenta LA. In vitro microleakage of composite restorations after nonvital bleaching. Quintessence Int. 2001;32:413-7.
25. Nilgun Ozturk A, Usumez A, Ozturk B, *et al*. Influence of different light sources on microleakage of class V composite resin restorations. J Oral Rehabil. 2004;31:500-4.
26. Abouassi T, Wolkewitz M, Hahn P. Effect of carbamide peroxide and hydrogen peroxide on enamel surface: an in vitro study. Clin Oral Investig. 2011;15:673-80.
27. Arhun N, Arman A, Çehreli SB, *et al*. Microleakage beneath ceramic and metal brackets bonded with a conventional and an antibacterial adhesive system. Angle Orthod. 2006;76:1028-34.
28. Ulker M, Uysal T, Ramoglu SI, *et al*. Microleakage under orthodontic brackets using high-intensity curing lights. Angle Orthod. 2009;79:144-9.
29. Ramoglu SI, Uysal T, Ulker M, *et al*. Microleakage under ceramic and metallic brackets bonded with resin-modified glass ionomer. Angle Orthod. 2009;79:138-43.
30. Uysal T, Ulker M, Ramoglu SI, *et al*. Microleakage under metallic and ceramic brackets bonded with orthodontic self-etching primer systems. Angle orthod. 2008;78:1089-94.
31. Galil KA, Wright GZ. Acid etching pattern on buccal surfaces of permanent teeth. Pediatric Dent.1979;1:230–234.

7

Efficacy of Endodontic Files with Different Metallurgical Characterization in Removing Root Canal Filling Material

Topcuoglu HS[a]; Sener I[b]; Demirbuga S[c]; Çakir NN[d]*; Topcuoglu G[e]

[a]DDS, PhD Department of Endodontics, Faculty of Dentistry, Erciyes University, Kayseri, Turkey
[b]DDS, Department of Endodontics, Faculty of Dentistry, Erciyes University, Kayseri, Turkey
[c]DDS, PhD Department of Restorative Dentistry, Erciyes University, Kayseri, Turkey
[d]DDS, PhD Department of Restorative Dentistry, Kayseri, Turkey
[e]DDS, PhD Oral and Dental Health Hospital, Kayseri, Turkey

ARTICLE INFO

Key words:
Root canal filling
Retreatment
Endodontics

Corresponding Author:
Nazire Nurdan Çakır
Department of Restorative Dentistry, Faculty of Dentistry, Erciyes University, 38039, Melikgazi, Kayseri, Turkey.
Email: nurdanncakir@hotmail.com

Abstract

Statement of problem: Safe and efficient removal of all root filling materials from the canal system is essential for optimal nonsurgical retreatment, because it provides effective cleaning, shaping, and re-filling of the root canal system.

Objectives: This study compares the effectiveness of Reciproc Blue, HyFlex CM, Reciproc, and ProTaper Universal retreatment files (PTUR) in removing root canal filling material (RCFM).

Materials and methods: Sixty human upper central incisors were shaped with Revo-S files up to apical size 40 and were obturated using the cold lateral compaction technique. After two weeks, the RCFMs were removed with Reciproc Blue, HyFlex CM, Reciproc, or PTUR (ProTaper Universal Retreatment) files. Teeth were cleaved longitudinally, and digital images were then captured. The amounts of RCFMs in the obtained images were analyzed using ImageJ software, and the time required to remove the RCFM was recorded. Data were analyzed using a one-way of variance (ANOVA) test.

Results: There was no significant difference among the files in the coronal third ($P>0.05$). In contrast, in the middle and apical thirds, the amount of remaining RCFM was significantly higher in HyFlex CM and Reciproc Blue groups than that of PTUR and Reciproc groups ($P<0.05$); however, there is no significant difference between the HyFlex CM and Reciproc Blue groups ($P>0.05$). Furthermore, there is no difference between the Reciproc and PTUR files regarding the amount of remaining RCFM ($P>0.05$). The Reciproc file removed the RCFM in a shorter time than the other groups ($P<0.05$). However, there is no difference among the other three groups ($P>0.05$).

Conclusions: None of the tested files could completely remove the RCFM. Under the limitation of this study, the files with shape memory (Reciproc and PTUR files) exhibited better performance than the files with reduced shape memory (Reciproc Blue) and controlled memory (HyFlex CM) in removing the RCFM.

Introduction

Nonsurgical endodontic retreatment procedures are performed as the first choice to eliminate or reduce the microbial infection when the initial root canal treatment fails [1]. Safe and efficient removal of all root-filling materials from the canal system is essential for optimal nonsurgical retreatment, because it provides effective cleaning, shaping, and re-filling of the root canal system [2]. Mechanical removal of root canal filling material (RCFM) is routinely performed by using hand files, rotary files, ultrasonic tips, or heating devices [3]. In particular, nickel-titanium (NiTi) rotary files are often used in endodontic retreatments because of their safety, efficiency, and ability to remove RCFM faster than hand files [4]. In many previous studies, the efficacy of traditional rotary NiTi files have been tested for removing RCFM and determined that the rotary NiTi files are effective in removing RCFM [5, 6]. Some of them are Reciproc (VDW, Munich, Germany), HyFlex CM (Coltène Whaledent, Altstätten, Switzerland), Reciproc Blue (VDW, Munich, Germany), and PTUR (Dentsply Maillefer, Ballaigues, Switzerland). Reciproc Blue (VDW) has been one of the new generations of Reciproc-instruments introduced recently. The manufacturer of this new file claims that it is much more flexible, and has an even lower fracture risk than the Reciproc file. Because of the special temperature protocol, the Reciproc Blue file can also be present to better access curved canals. The ProTaper Universal Retreatment system (Dentsply, Maillefer) was specifically developed for removal of root canal filling material and includes three instruments as follows: D1 (size 30/.09 taper), D2 (size 25/.08 taper) and D3 (size 20/.07 taper) [7]. The PTUR instruments have a convex cross-section design [8]. Several studies have determined that ProTaper retreatment instruments are more effective in removing root-filling material when compared to hand files [6, 9]. A new reciprocating motion approach was introduced for instrumentation using nickel–titanium instruments with an M-Wire alloy, which is considered more resistant than conventional alloys. Reciproc (VDW) is based on this motion. The Reciproc system consists of three files: R25 (25/0.08 in the first millimeters), R40 (40/0.06 in the first millimeters) and R50 (50/0.05 in the first millimeters) [10]. The effectiveness of instruments that work with a reciprocating motion in the removal of root canal filling material have been evaluated and determined to be effective [4]. Several studies have evaluated the amount of apically extruded debris during removal of root canal filling material using hand files, rotary and reciprocating systems [11-13]. The findings of these studies showed that all techniques caused apical extrusion of debris during the removal of canal filling material. HyFlex CM (Coltène Whaledent) files are manufactured from a CM alloy using a special thermomechanical method, which increases their resistance to cyclic fatigue by conferring extreme flexibility on the files [14, 15]. HyFlex CM contains a smaller percentage of nickel than other systems [16]. The reduction of nickel content generates a metal that is softer, i.e., exhibits lower hardness [17]. The processing of these files also affects the metal properties, such as the thermal changes that occur during the manufacturing of the HyFlex CM file, which results in a martensitic metal phase. The martensitic phase is a more flexible form of yarn that results in greater elasticity and resistance to cyclic fatigue [18].

It has been stated that thermomechanical treatment (M-wire, CM-wire, or Blue technology) of the NiTi files compared to traditional NiTi files provides significant benefits with regard the efficacy and safety of endodontic files [19, 20]. However, there are limited studies about the efficacy of M-wire and CM-wire files in removing the RCFM [21-23]. Moreover, there has been no study evaluating the efficacy of Reciproc Blue and HyFlex CM files manufactured with Blue technology and CM-wire, respectively. Therefore, this study evaluates of the effectiveness of the Reciproc, HyFlex CM, Reciproc Blue, and PTUR files in removing RCFM.

Materials and Methods

Based on data from a previous study [24], power calculations indicated that the sample size for each group must be a minimum of 12 specimens. Thus, 60 extracted single-rooted human upper central incisors were selected for this study and were stored at 4°C in distilled water up to experimental procedures. Preoperative radiographs were taken to verify the presence of a single canal, and the criteria for tooth selection included a completely formed apex and the absence of previous root filling, resorption, or calcifications. The length of the teeth was standardized to 21 mm by trimming the crowns of teeth with silicon carbide abrasive paper. The teeth were completely not decoronated, and the crowns served as a reservoir for the irrigation solution. Endodontic access cavities were prepared using diamond burs (Dentsply Maillefer, Ballaigues, Switzerland) with a high-speed handpiece under water-cooling. A K-file (#10, Dentsply Maillefer) was inserted into each canal until its tip was just visible at the apical foramen, and the length was then measured. The working length (WL) was established by subtracting 1 mm from this measurement, and the root canals were instrumented to a master apical size 40 with using SC1, SC2, SCU, AS30 and AS40 Revo-S files (Micro-Mega, Besancon, France) respectively. SC1 was used to enlarge the coronal two-thirds of the canal. SC2, SCU, AS30, AS35, and AS40 instruments were used to the WL. The canals were then irrigated with 1 mL 2.5% sodium hypochlorite (NaOCl) between each file size by using a syringe and a 29-G needle (NaviTip; Ultradent, South Jordan, UT). After the instrumentation, the canals were irrigated with 2 mL 17% EDTA for 1 minute and subsequently rinsed with 2 mL distilled water. Then all root canals were dried with paper point.

Root Canal Obturation

Sixty root canals were obturated with a resin-based sealer (MM-Seal; Micro-Mega, Besançon, France) and gutta-percha cones by using the cold lateral compaction technique. MM-Seal was introduced into the root canal by using a lentulo spiral filler (Dentsply Maillefer), and a # 40/0.02 taper master gutta-percha cone with good tug-back was coated with the sealer and slowly inserted into the canal until the WL was reached. Then, accessory cones were inserted in the same manner and laterally compacted using a # 25 finger-spreader. Excess material was seared and condensed with a plugger 1 mm below the canal opening, and the root canal openings of all specimens were sealed with temporary filling material (Cavit; 3M ESPE, Seefeld, Germany). Radiographs were then taken from the buccolingual and mesiodistal directions to ensure quality of the obturation, and the specimens were then stored at 37°C in 100% humidity for two weeks to allow complete setting of the sealer.

Experimental Groups and Retreatment Procedures

All rotary NiTi files were used with a torque and speed controlled motor (X-Smart Plus, Dentsply Maillefer), and the files were used at the torque and speed recommended by the manufacturer for each specific system. Sixty extracted single-rooted human upper central incisors were randomly divided into four groups. Root filling materials were then removed using the following techniques.

ProTaper Universal Retreatment (Dentsply Maillefer, Ballaigues, Switzerland) (PTUR) Group (n = 15)

RCFMs were removed using the D1 (#30/0.09 taper), D2 (#25/0.08 taper), and D3 (# 20/0.07 taper) retreatment files at 2-Ncm torque and 500-rpm speed. The files were used with a brushing action against the canal walls in a crown-down direction until the WL was reached. D1 was used in the cervical third, D2 in the middle third, and D3 throughout the entire WL. Finally, apical preparation was performed with a ProTaper F5 file (#50/0.05 taper) at 300 rpm. The root canals were irrigated after each file size using 2.5% NaOCl for 30 seconds.

Reciproc Group (n = 15)

RCFMs were removed using the Reciproc R25 (#25/0.08 taper, VDW, Munich, Germany) file at RECIPROC mode of endodontic motor (X Smart Plus; Dentsply Maillefer). Reciproc R25 was used in a slow in-and-out pecking motion with a 3-mm amplitude limit, and gentle apical pressure was combined with a brushing motion against the lateral walls of the root canal. After three complete pecking movements, the file was removed from the canal, and its flutes were cleaned. R25 file was then used for removing the filling material until the WL was reached followed by apical enlargement with R40 (#40/0.06 taper) and R50 (#50/0.05 taper) files. The root canals were irrigated after the pecking motion and each file size using 2.5% NaOCl for 30 seconds.

Reciproc Blue Group (n = 15)

In this group, RCFMs were removed with the same procedure as the Reciproc group, but the Reciproc Blue R25 (#25/0.08 taper, VDW, Munich, Germany) file was used to remove the root canal filling material. Final apical enlargement was completed by then using Reciproc Blue R40 (#40/0.06 taper) and R50 (#50/0.05 taper) files. The root canals were irrigated after the pecking motion and each file size using 2.5% NaOCl for 30 seconds.

HyFlex CM Group (n= 15)

RCFMs were removed using HyFlex CM (Coltène Whaledent, Altstätten, Switzerland) at a speed of 500 rpm and at 2.5 Ncm torque. HyFlex CM files were used in a crown-down sequence using #25/0.08 taper (at 2/3 of the WL), #20/0.06 taper, #30/0.06 taper, and #40/0.06 (at full WL). Additional apical preparation was performed using HyFlex CM (#45/0.04 and #50/0.04 taper) files, and the root canals were irrigated after each file size using 2.5% NaOCl for 30 seconds.

RCFM removal was conducted by one operator, and each instrument was used in one canal in all groups. Irrigation was performed using a total of 15 mL of 2.5% NaOCl for each tooth using a syringe and a 29-G side-port needle (NaviTip; Ultradent). The removal RCFM procedure was deemed complete when no debris of gutta-percha and sealer was invisible on the file surfaces and when canal walls were smooth. Working time for removal of RCFM was recorded and irrigation times were subtracted from total working time. A final rinse was performed with 2 mL 17% EDTA for 1 minute followed by 2 mL distilled water for 1 minute, and the canals were dried with paper points (Dentsply Maillefer). A dental operating microscope (Zeiss Opmi; Carl Zeiss, Jena, Germany) was used throughout the RCFM removal procedure.

Evaluation of the Removal of Canal Filling Material

Grooves were prepared with a water-cooled diamond bur on the buccal and lingual tooth surfaces, and teeth were split along their long axis in a buccolingual direction using a hammer and chisel. Digital images of the both halves were captured at 8x magnification using a digital camera (DP-70; Olympus, Tokyo, Japan) attached to a stereomicroscope (BX60; Olympus). The images were then transferred to imaging software (ImageJ; Wayne Rasband, NIH, MD, USA). The remaining RCFM on the root canal walls were measured using ImageJ software (Figure 1), and the specimens were evaluated by one operator blinded to groups tested for the removal of RCFM. The measurements were repeated to ensure reproducibility, and mean values were determined and compared. The percentage of RCFM remaining (A) was calculated using the following equation: A = (area of the remaining x 100)/area of the root canal [25].

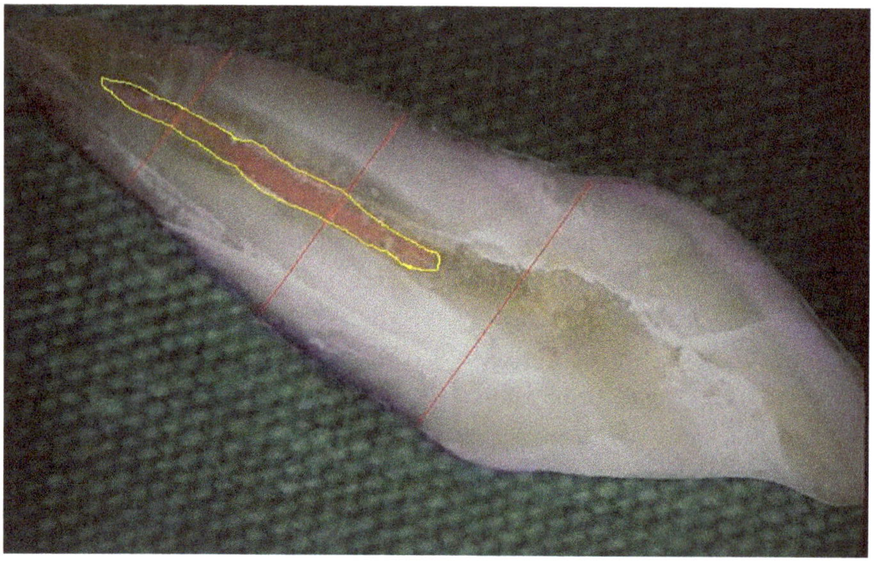

Figure 1: An image obtained to measure the amount of remaining canal filling material on root canal walls

Statistical Analysis

The data were normally distributed (Shapiro-Wilk test, $p > .05$) and homogeneity of variance (Levene test, $p > .05$). Thus, the area of the remaining RCFM and were analyzed with one-way ANOVA and Tukey post hoc tests to determine the working time. Statistical analysis was performed with SPSS Statistics Version 20 for Windows (IBM, Chicago, IL, USA), and a p value lower than 0.05 was regarded as statistically significant.

Results

The means of the percentage of remaining RCFM are shown in Table 1. None of the files could completely remove the RCFM, but statistical analysis showed the percentage of remaining RCFM was the lowest at the coronal third in all groups ($P<0.05$). However, there was no significant difference among the files in the coronal third ($P>0.05$). In the middle and apical thirds, HyFlex CM and Reciproc Blue groups exhibited higher percentages of remaining RCFM than PTUR and Reciproc groups ($P<0.05$), but there is no significance difference between HyFlex CM and Reciproc Blue groups ($P>0.05$). Reciproc and PTUR files had similar values regarding the remaining RCFM ($P>0.05$).
The Reciproc file reached the WL significantly faster than the other systems ($P<0.05$). In addition, the required total time to remove the RCFMs was shorter with the Reciproc group compared to the other groups ($P<0.05$). There is no significant difference among Reciproc Blue, HyFlex CM, and PTUR files regarding the required time to reach the WL and to remove the RCFM ($P>0.05$).

Discussion

The complete removal of RCFM is necessary to allow an effective cleaning, disinfection, and re-obturation of the root canal when initial endodontic therapy fails. However, several studies have shown that it is impossible to remove the RCFM completely, regardless of the different instruments and protocols already proposed for the non-surgical endodontic retreatment [26]. The review of the endodontic literature shows there are few studies evaluated the performance of files with different metallurgical characterizations during the removal of the RCFM [27]. Therefore, this study compared the effectiveness of the files with different metallurgical characterization in removing the RCFM.
In the current study, maxillary central incisors with similar length were used to simplify the standardization of the specimens and were initially prepared to a #40/0.06 file. During the removal of the RCFM, no solvents were used to allow for sole evaluation of the effect of the different files. The RCFM removal procedure was performed using new files in each tooth to avoid instrument separation. None of the files separated during the removal of the RCFM. Teeth were split longitudinally for evaluation, which is similar to previous studies that used single-rooted and canalled teeth [28]. Maciel *et al* [29] stated that measurements that are more accurate could be obtained with longitudinal sectioning method when compared with conventional radiographs, because

Table 1: Mean percentages and standard deviations of remaining canal filling material in each section and time to perform the procedure

Group	Apical	Middle	Coronal	T1	T2
Reciproc	15.2 ± 2.4^a	14.3 ± 4.6^a	8.2 ± 1.3^a	34.52 ± 3.2^a	62.44 ± 5.1^a
Reciproc Blue	24.1 ± 4.1^b	25.6 ± 6.3^b	7.4 ± 2.6^a	48.17 ± 3.5^b	91.73 ± 4.3^b
PTUR	12.4 ± 4.6^a	12.5 ± 2.1^a	9.2 ± 3.1^a	50.22 ± 2.4^b	87.38 ± 3.2^b
HyFlex CM	28.3 ± 3.2^b	24.6 ± 3.5^b	11.1 ± 2.4^a	51.37 ± 4.8^b	89.56 ± 4.4^b

T1: time to reach the working length, T2: time to remove the canal filling material. Values with the same superscript letters show that there is no statistical difference.

the latter may be subject to magnification or distortion. In the present study, images were traced using ImageJ software to assess the presence of the remaining RCFM on the canal walls quantitatively. In addition, no attempt was made to distinguish between remaining sealer and gutta-percha [28].

It has been stated that after retreatment procedures, the apical part generally has a greater percentage of the RCFM than the middle and coronal parts of the root canal because of the increased anatomic variability and the difficulty of instrumentation in the apical part of the root [30]. Therefore, in the present study, the additional instrumentation was performed to #50 file in all the groups.

The current study determined that none of the tested files could produce canal walls completely free of the RCFM. This finding is compatible with several studies comparing the efficacy of the rotary NiTi files in removing the RCFM [31, 32]. However, there is no consensus regarding whether the motion type of the endodontic files is an important factor in removing the RCFM. Several previous studies showed that the motion type of the files could not be an important factor when the efficacy of files is evaluated in removing the RCFM. Zuolo *et al* [32] evaluated the efficacy of files working with rotary (TRUShape) or reciprocating (Reciproc) motion in removing the RCFM and determined that there is no significant difference between the two files. Rios Mde *et al* [3] assessed the efficacy of the two reciprocating systems compared with a rotary system in the removing the RCFM in maxillary incisor teeth. They also found that the reciprocating systems (Reciproc and WaveOne) were as effective as rotary file (PTUR file).

In contrast, a few studies showed that motion type might be an important factor in removing RCFM. Capar *et al* [33] determined that the use of PTUR files with adaptive motion left significantly less RCFM than the rotational motion. In addition, Bernardes *et al* [27] evaluated the amount of remaining RCFM after the use of different techniques (Hand files, Reciproc, and PTUR files) and found that Reciproc file removed more RCFM than the other techniques. Reciproc and Reciproc Blue files employ a reciprocating motion, whereas HyFlex CM and PTUR files employ a rotational motion. The findings of the current study showed that in the middle and apical part of the root canal, Reciproc and PTUR files removed more RCFM than Reciproc Blue and HyFlex CM files. Based on these findings, the motion types of the files may not have affected the results in the current study.

In the current study, given that the two files (Reciproc and Reciproc Blue) have the same cross-sectional exhibited different retreatment efficacy, the alloy type of the file (M-wire or Blue technology) should be considered as a significant factor when the performances of the files in the retreatment process are evaluated. Reciproc Blue and HyFlex CM files are more flexible than Reciproc and PTUR files. According to the findings of this study, Reciproc Blue and HyFlex CM files showed similar abilities to removing RCFM during retreatment procedures of teeth with straight canal. Under the limitations of this study, as the flexibility of the files increases, their performance in removing the RCFM could decrease.

Considering the time needed to remove the RCFM, Reciproc was shown to take shorter retreatment times than other systems in straight root canals when removing the RCFM, because fewer files in the Reciproc group were used compared to other groups (HyFlex CM and PTUR file). However, more time is required in the Reciproc Blue group compared to the Reciproc group because of the different metallurgical properties of the Reciproc file.

Conclusions

Based on the findings of this study, none of the files could completely remove the RCFM. In addition, Reciproc and PTUR files had better performance than Reciproc Blue and HyFlex CM files regarding the removal of the RCFM in the middle and apical sections.

Conflict of Interest: None declared.

References

1. Alves FR, Marceliano-Alves MF, Sousa JC3, et al. Removal of Root Canal Fillings in Curved Canals Using Either Reciprocating Single- or Rotary Multi-instrument Systems and a Supplementary Step with the XP-Endo Finisher. J Endod. 2016;42:1114-9.

2. Rodríguez G, Patel S, Durán-Sindreu F, et al. Influence of Cone-beam Computed Tomography on Endodontic Retreatment Strategies among General Dental Practitioners and Endodontists. J Endod. 2017;43:1433-7.
3. Rios MD, Villela AM, Cunha RS, et al. Efficacy of 2 reciprocating systems compared with a rotary retreatment system for gutta-percha removal. J Endod. 2012;40:543–6.
4. Zuolo AS, Mello JE Jr, Cunha RS, et al. Efficacy of reciprocating and rotary techniques for removing filling material during root canal retreatment. Int Endod J. 2013;46:947–53.
5. Martinho FC, Freitas LF, Nascimento GG, et al. Endodontic retreatment: clinical comparison of reciprocating systems versus rotary system in disinfecting root canals. Clin Oral Investig. 2015;19:1411–7.
6. Marques da Silva B, Baratto-Filho F, Leonardi DP, et al. Effectiveness of ProTaper, D-RaCe, and Mtwo retreatment files with and without supplementary instruments in the removal of root canal filling material. Int Endod J. 2012;45:927-32.
7. VDW. Reciproc Blue. Available at: http://www.vdw-dental.com/en/ presse/ produktmeldungen/reciproc-blue.html. Accessed 12 Apr 2017.
8. Gu LS, Ling JQ, Wei X, et al. Efficacy of ProTaper Universal rotary retreatment system for gutta-percha removal from root canals. Int Endod J. 2008;41:288-95.
9. Kfir A, Tsesis I, Yakirevich E, et al. The efficacy of five techniques for removing root filling material: microscopic versus radiographic evaluation. Int Endod J. 2012;45:35–41.
10. Capar ID, Ertas H, Ok E, et al. Comparison of single cone obturation performance of different novel nickel-titanium rotary systems. Acta Odontol Scand. 2014;72:537–42.
11. Lu Y, Wang R, Zhang L, et al. Apically extruded debris and irrigant with two Ni-Ti systems and hand files when removing root fillings: a laboratory study. Int Endod J. 2013;46:1125–30.
12. Çanakçi BC, Ustun Y, Er O, et al. Evaluation of apically extruded debris from curved root canal filling removal using 5 nickel-titanium systems. J Endod. 2016;42:1101–04.
13. Somma F, Cammarota G, Plotino G, et al. The effectiveness of manual and mechanical instrumentation for the retreatment of three different root canal filling materials. J Endod. 2008;34:466–9.
14. Braga LCM, Silva ACF, Buono VTL, et al. Impact of heat treatments on the fatigue resistance of differ- ent rotary nickel-titanium instruments. J Endod. 2014;40:1494–7.
15. Plotino G, Testarelli L, Al-Sudani D, et al. Fatigue resistance of rotary instruments manufactured using different nickel-titanium alloys: a comparative study. Odontology. 2014;102:31–5.
16. Zinelis S, Eliades T, Eliades G. A metallurgical characterization of ten endodontic Ni-Ti instruments: assessing the clinical relevance of shape memory and superelastic properties of Ni-Ti endodontic instruments. Int. Endod. J. 2010;43:125–34.
17. Gao Y, Gutmann JL, Wilkinson K, et al. Evaluation of the impact of raw materials on the fatigue and mechanical properties of ProFile Vortex rotary instruments. J. Endod. 2012;38:398–401.
18. Testarelli L, Plotino G, Al-Sudani D, et al. Bending properties of a new nickel-titanium alloy with a lower percent by weight of nickel. J. Endod. 2011;37:1293–5.
19. Bürklein S, Börjes L, Schäfer E. Comparison of preparation of curved root canals with Hyflex CM and Revo-S rotary nickel-titanium instruments. Int Endod J. 2014;47:470-6.
20. De-Deus G, Silva EJ, Vieira VT, et al. Blue Thermomechanical Treatment Optimizes Fatigue Resistance and Flexibility of the Reciproc Files. J Endod. 2017;43:462-6.
21. Niemi TK, Marchesan MA, Lloyd A, et al. Effect of Instrument Design and Access Outlines on the Removal of Root Canal Obturation Materials in Oval-shaped Canals. J Endod. 2016;42:1550-4.
22. Nevares G, de Albuquerque DS, Freire LG, et al. Efficacy of ProTaper NEXT Compared with Reciproc in Removing Obturation Material from Severely Curved Root Canals: A Micro-Computed Tomography Study. J Endod. 2016;42:803-8.
23. Rodrigues CT, Duarte MA, de Almeida MM,

et al. Efficacy of CM-Wire, M-Wire, and Nickel-Titanium Instruments for Removing Filling Material from Curved Root Canals: A Micro-Computed Tomography Study. J Endod. 2016;42:1651-5.

24. Yürüker S, Görduysus M, Küçükkaya S, et al. Efficacy of Combined Use of Different Nickel-Titanium Files on Removing Root Canal Filling Materials. J Endod. 2016;42:487-92.
25. Colaco AS, Pai VA. Comparative Evaluation of the Efficiency of Manual and Rotary Gutta-percha Removal Techniques. J Endod. 2015;41:1871-4.
26. Rossi-Fedele G, Ahmed HM. Assessment of Root Canal Filling Removal Effectiveness Using Micro-computed Tomography: A Systematic Review. J Endod. 2017;43:520-6.
27. Bernardes RA, Duarte MA, Vivan RR, et al. Comparison of three retreatment techniques with ultrasonic activation in flattened canals using micro-computed tomography and scanning electron microscopy. Int Endod J. 2015 Aug 17. doi: 10.1111/iej.12522. [Epub ahead of print].
28. Özyürek T, Demiryürek EÖ. Efficacy of Different Nickel-Titanium Instruments in Removing Gutta-percha during Root Canal Retreatment. J Endod. 2016;42:646-9.
29. de Carvalho Maciel AC, Zaccaro Scelza MF. Efficacy of automated versus hand instrumentation during root canal retreatment: an ex vivo study. Int Endod J. 2006;39:779-84.
30. Gergi R, Sabbagh C. Effectiveness of two nickel-titanium rotary instruments and a hand file for removing gutta-percha in severely curved root canals during retreatment: an ex vivo study. Int Endod J. 2007;40:532-7.
31. Monguilhott Crozeta B, Damião de Sousa-Neto M, Bianchi Leoni G1, et al. A micro-computed tomography assessment of the efficacy of rotary and reciprocating techniques for filling material removal in root canal retreatment. Clin Oral Investig. 2016;20:2235-40.
32. de Siqueira Zuolo A, Zuolo ML, da Silveira Bueno CE, et al. Evaluation of the Efficacy of TRUShape and Reciproc File Systems in the Removal of Root Filling Material: An Ex Vivo Micro-Computed Tomographic Study. J Endod 2016;42:315-9.
33. Capar ID, Arslan H, Ertas H, et al. Effectiveness of ProTaper Universal retreatment instruments used with rotary or reciprocating adaptive motion in the removal of root canal filling material. Int Endod J. 2015;48:79-83.

8

Cone Beam CT Evaluation of the Prevalence and Characteristics of the Retro-Molar Canal

Movahhedian N[a]; Shahidi SH[b]; Bahadori Jahromi M[C]

[a]Assistant Professor, Department of Oral and Maxillofacial Radiology, School of Dentistry, Shiraz University of Medial Science, Shiraz, Iran
[b]Professor, Department of Oral and Maxillofacial Radiology, School of Dentistry, Shiraz University of Medial Science, Shiraz, Iran
[c]Undergraduate Student, Student Research Committee, School of Dentistry, Shiraz University of Medical Sciences, Shiraz, Iran

ARTICLE INFO

Key words:
CBCT
Mandibular anatomy
Retromolar canal
Accessory canal

Corresponding Author:
Shoaleh Shahidi
Professor,Department of Oral and Maxillofacial Radiology, School of Dentistry, Shiraz University of Medial Science, Shiraz, Iran
Email: shoalehshahidi@yahoo.com

Abstract

Statement of problem: Retro-molar canal (RMC) is of clinical significance because of its neurovascular content, which may be at risk of damage during the surgical procedures of the area.

Objectives: The aim of the present study was to evaluate the frequency and anatomic characteristics of RMC by using cone beam computed tomography (CBCT).

Materials and Methods: The sample of this study consisted of 500 CBCT images (1000 sides), evaluated for the presence, type, and width of RMC. The canals were categorized into five groups based on their course as A_1 (vertical), A_2 (vertical with a horizontal branch), B_1 (curved), B_2 (curved with a horizontal branch), and C (horizontal).

Results: The study showed that 57 (11.4%) subjects and 67 (6.7%) sides had RMC in which 47 (9.4 %) were unilateral and 10 (2%) were bilateral. There was no statistically significant difference between male and female individuals in the occurrence of RMC (10.2% and 12.7%, respectively) (P-value=0.387). The most common morphologic types were B_1 (50.7%) and A_1 (23.9%), while A_2 (3%) and B_2 (4.5%) were the least frequent types. The mean width of the mandibular canal and RMC were 3.51 ± 0.55 mm and 1.30 ± 0.47 mm, respectively. These dimensions were not significantly influenced by gender (P-value=0.440, 0.569, respectively).

Conclusions: The results of the present investigation showed that the RMC was a common anatomic structure. Therefore, because of its clinical significance, it is highly recommended that dental practitioners consider this structure in pre-surgical evaluations of the region in order to avoid related complications.

Introduction

Accessory canals are the canals branching off the main neurovascular canal and running in different courses through the bone. There are many accessory canals in the mandible, some of which are still unspecified [1]. Accessory canal injuries can be the cause for a number of post-operative complications [2, 3].

Retro-molar canal (RMC) has been found to be the second most frequent type of accessory canals in the mandible after the forward canal [4]. RMC branches off from the inferior alveolar nerve canal, behind the third molar, toward the retro- molar area [2, 5, 6].

RMC is of clinical significance because of its neurovascular contents. Several studies have demonstrated the RMC's contents to be small arteries, venules and myelinated nerve fibers [7, 8]. These elements may be at risk of damage during the surgical removal of the third molars, dental implants insertion, bone harvesting procedures, or even under the pressure of prosthetic denture in a resorbed ridge [5, 9]. Damage to the RMC might be responsible for excessive bleeding during surgical procedures, failure in the inferior alveolar nerve block, paresthesia of the gingival tissue posterior to the canine tooth, or even post-surgical hematoma or traumatic neuroma [5, 7, 9-11].

The increasing need to surgical procedures including implant insertion and removal of impacted teeth has multiplied the need for evaluating the RMC. In recent years, the use of cone beam computed tomography (CBCT) has enabled dental professionals to evaluate the desired structure through high-resolution three-dimensional images, in detail and free from superimposition [3,5,10]. A study comparing the diagnostic ability of panoramic radiography and CBCT regarding RMC showed that panoramic radiography was able to identify only 7 RMC out of 31 as diagnosed by CBCT [6]. Identification of this anatomic variation may be useful to avoid some of the post-surgical complications. Since there has not been enough information about RMC, particularly in the Iranian population, this study aimed to evaluate the frequency and anatomic characteristics of RMC by using CBCT. To the best of our knowledge, the current study used the largest sample size among CBCT studies to evaluate this structure.

Materials and Methods

The sample of this retrospective study consisted of 500 CBCT images taken for various clinical indications, during a 2-year period (from March 2014 to June 2016) in a private oral and maxillofacial radiology center in Shiraz, Iran. A NewTom VGi Cone Beam CT machine (QR SRL Company, Verona, Italy) with basic voxel size of 0.3mm obtained all the images. The examinations were performed at 4.71 mA and 110 kVp, with a scanning time of 3.6 seconds. The subjects with a history of craniofacial malformation or syndrome, trauma, orthogenetic surgery or presence of any lesion in the retromolar area were excluded from the study.

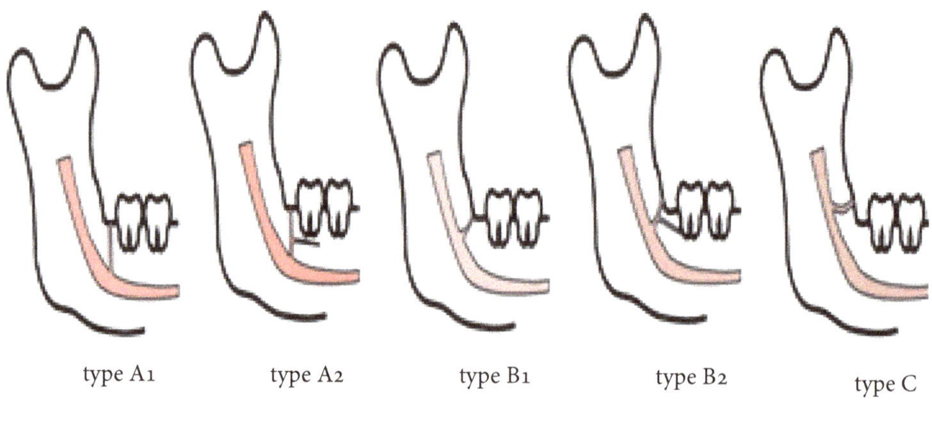

Figure 1: Schematic demonstration of retromolar canal classification

Two oral and maxillofacial radiologists evaluated the images in all three orthogonal planes (sagittal, coronal and axial) for the presence and type of RMC with consensus. The width of the mandibular canal and RMC was also measured at the point of bifurcation.

The types of the canals were categorized based on the course and morphology [6] as A_1 (vertical course), A_2 (vertical course with a horizontal branch), B_1 (curved course), B_2 (curved course with a horizontal branch), and C(horizontal course). (Figures 1 , 2)

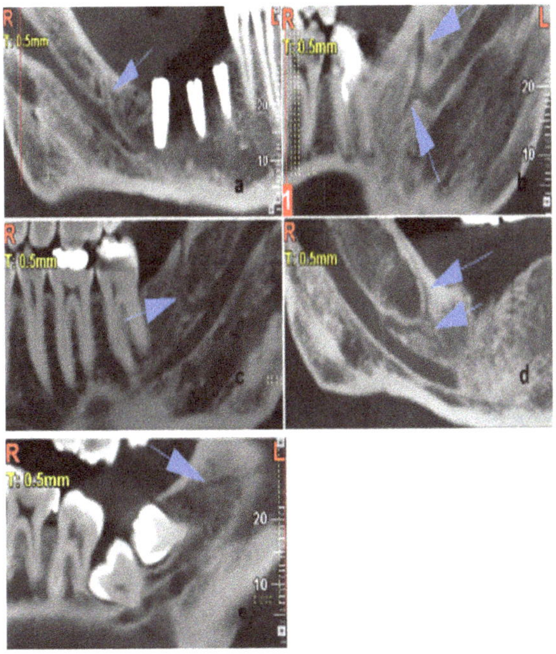

Figure 2: Sagittal CBCT plans showing different types of retromolar canal. (a) type A_1 (b) type A_2 (c) type B_1 (d) type B_2 (e) type C

Statistical analysis

Chi-square and Student's t-tests were employed to assess the relationship between the variables. SPSS version 18.0 (SPSS Inc., Chicago, IL, USA) was adopted for statistical analysis. A p-value < 0.05 was considered statistically significant.

Table Frequency (percentage) of retromolar canal

	Subjects (n=500) (%)	Sides (n=1000) (%)
Presence	57 (11.4)	67(6.7)
Unilaterally	47 (9.4)	47(4.7)
In right	27 (5.4)	27(2.7)
In left	20 (4)	20(2)
Bilaterally	10 (2)	20(2)

Results

CBCT images of 500 subjects (1000 sides) were evaluated retrospectively for this study. 57 (11.4%) subjects and 67 (6.7%) sides were found to have RMC. Among these subjects, 47 (9.4%) were found to have RMC unilaterally and 10 (2%) bilaterally (Table 1). There was no statistically significant difference between the male and female subjects in the occurrence of RMC (10.2% and 12.7%, respectively) (P-value=0.387) (Table 2). The most common morphologic types were B_1 (50.7%) and A_1 (23.9%) and the least common ones were A_2 (3%) and B_2 (4.5%). (Table 3)

The mean width of the mandibular canal and RMC were 3.51 ± .55 mm and 1.30 ± .47 mm respectively, and type B (B_1 and B_2) was found to be the widest. These dimensions were not significantly influenced by gender (P-value=0.440, 0.569, respectively) (Tables 4 and 5).

Discussion

The reported prevalence rates for RMC and retromolar foramen (RMF) has been different among different studies (Table 6). This variety may be due to the ethnicity, different evaluation techniques, different scoring criteria, and sample sizes.

Studies on RMC have been conducted on dry mandibles, panoramic radiographs, CT (computerized tomography) and CBCT examinations. The study of von Arx *et al.* [6] reported a prevalence of 25.6% of RMC in CBCT and showed that among 31 RMCs detected in

	Male (n=255)(%)	Female (n=245)(%)	P-value*
Absence	229 (89.8)	214 (87.3)	
Presence	26 (10.2)	31 (12.7)	0.387

*Chi-square

Table 3: The distribution of retromolar canals based on type for both sides and gender

Type	n	percentage	number in side		number in Gender	
			right	left	male	Female
A_1	16	23.9	8	8	8	8
A_2	2	3	1	1	0	2
B_1	34	50.7	17	17	17	17
B_2	3	0.5	3	0	1	2
C	12	17.9	8	4	6	6
Total	67	100	37	30	32	35

Table 4: Comparison of mandibular and retromolar canals width in different genders

	Total	Male	Female	P-value*
Retromolar canal width (mm)	1.30±0.47	1.26±0.46	1.34±0.49	0.569
Mandibular canal width (mm)	3.51±0.55	3.75±0.52	3.45±0.75	0.440
Ratio	0.38±0.10	0.36±0.10	0.39±0.10	0.199

*student's t test

Table 5: Comparison of the width of mandibular and retromolar canals in different genders (n=67)

Type	Mean width (mm)	number in Gender	
		Male	Female
A_1	0.9±0.43	0.96±0.52	0.84±0.37
A_2	1.05±0.07	-----	1.05±0.07
B_1	1.51±0.42	1.44±0.42	1.58±0.43
B_2	1.5±0.17	1.7	1.4
C	1.24±0.38	1.07±0.24	1.42±0.44

CBCT, panoramic radiographs were able to identify just 7 cases (5.7% of samples). Similarly, Muinelo-Lorenzo *et al.* [3] observed the RMF prevalence to be 12.4% in CBCT images (8.8% of sides), but at the same time panoramic radiographs could identify the RMFs in only 5.3% of the samples (2.8% of sides). In other words, only 32.5% of RMFs found on CBCT images were visible on panoramic examinations. Additionally, Sisman *et al.* [18] examined CBCT images of 947 sides and detected 253 RMC (26.7%), but only 29 RMC were traceable on panoramic radiographs (3.1%). These studies concluded that panoramic radiography was not sufficient for evaluation of RMC and the foramen due to the superimposition of various structures over the area including the airways, soft palate, ghost image of the contralateral side, while CBCT study provided the opportunity of evaluating the desired structures in all orthogonal planes free from superimpositions and with a higher resolution. Studies on dry mandibles obtained varying rates of prevalence ranging from 16% to 72% , probably due to dissimilar methodologies [13-17]. Besides, most of these studies have evaluated RMF instead of RMC. In a study on 2500 dry mandibles, Ossenberg [13] found different prevalence rates of RMC among different populations. His study reported higher prevalence in native American population compared to Africa, Europe, India, and north East Asia [13]. Priya *et al.* [15] showed this prevalence to be 17.8% (5.1% bilateral, 12.7% unilateral) in South India. In another study on the same ethnic population, Tiwari *et al.* [16] reported almost similar results as 16% (3% bilateral, 13% unilateral). These two studies could confirm the idea of the influence of ethnicity on the incidence of RMC. Furthermore, CBCT studies showed the prevalence of 8.5% in Korean [10], 28.1% in Turkish [4] and 52% (37% of sides) in the Japanese population [5].

Different scoring criteria can also contribute to different reported prevalence rates. For example, studies conducted on dry mandibles may consider 0.5 mm [13] or 1mm [12] as the minimum size of the RMF. Additionally, studies have used different classifications of RMC. Patil *et al.* [2], which reported a prevalence of 65.3%, included the canals which connected the third molar to the retromolar fossa as well. On the other hand, Han and Hwang [10] included a type of RMC in their studies that was not branched off the inferior alveolar nerve but originated from a separate foramen in the ramus. In the present study, RMC was defined as the canals branching off the inferior alveolar nerve and coursing into the retromolar fossa. Our result showed that 11.4% of the samples (9.4% unilaterally and 2% bilaterally) and 6.7% of sides (67/1000) had RMC.

Most of the RMCs in the present study were found to be in type B_1 with a frequency of 50.7% of all RMC, followed by A_1 (23.9%) and C (17.9%). A similar classification was used with von Arx *et al.* [6] They reported the frequency of the types in the following order: A_1 (41.9%), B_1 (29%) and A_2 (16.1%). Both studies showed that A_1 and B_1 are the most common types and the difference in the

Table 6: Summary and comparison of the present study with other studies on retromolar canal

	Study	Sample size Subjects/sides	Prevalence Total/side	Population
CBCT studies	The present study(2016)	500/1000	11.4% / 6.7%	Iran
	Thomas von Arx(2011)	100/121	----/ 25.6%	
	Giuseppe Lizio(2012)	187/233	16% / 14.6%	
	Seema Patil(2013)	171/----	75.4% / ----	
	Muinelo-Lorenzo(2014)	225 / 450	36.8% / 22.8%	Korea
	Sang-Sun Han(2014)	446 / 892	8.5% / 5.0%	Japan
	Kaan Orhan(2011)	242 / 484	66.5% / 46.5%	
Cadaver studies	Ossenberg NS.(1987)	2500/----	72% /----	Africa, Europe, India northeast Asia
	Narayana K.(2002)	242/----	21.9% /----	South India
	Priya R.(2005)	157/----	17.8% /----	South India
	Tiwari S(2015)	100/----	16% /----	India
	Rossi, Ana Claudia(2012)	100/----	16% /----	Brazil
Panoramic versus CBCT studies	Thomas von Arx(2011)	100 / 121	----/ 5.8%	
	Muinelo-Lorenzo(2014)	225 / 450	16.8% / 9.3%	
	Sisman(2015)	632 / 947	---- / 3.1%	

reported values could be explained by the influence of ethnicity. Such information is hardly comparable in studies due to the differences in classification criteria.

In the present study, the mean width of RMC was found to be 1.30 ± .47mm with type B (B_1 and B_2) as the widest type (1.51 ± .42). Although the findings showed that this width is slightly greater in females, the difference is not statistically significant. Similar findings were reported by previous studies. Han and Hwang [10] and von Arx [6] reported a mean width of 1.13mm and .99mm, respectively. However, Narayana *et al.* [14] reported a relatively greater width (1.5-4.35mm). This inconsistency can be justifies as their study was conducted on cadavers; moreover, the study did not specify the exact level of measurements.

The findings of the present investigation showed that there was not any gender predication for the occurrence of RMC. Similar findings were reported by most of the previous studies [2, 6, 7, 13-15], while Pyle *et al.* [19] witnessed a higher prevalence of RMF in male dry mandibles (9.6%) compared to those the females (6.1%).

As mentioned earlier, RMC has clinical importance because of its content. Damage to the RMC during different surgical procedures can lead to significant post-operative complications [5, 10, 20, 21].

Conclusions

The present study showed that the RMC was a common anatomic structure. Thus, because of its clinical significance, it is highly recommended that dental practitioners consider this structure in pre-surgical evaluations of the region in order to avoid the allied complications.

Acknowledgements

The authors would like to thank Shiraz University of Medical Sciences, Shiraz, Iran and Center for Development of Clinical Research of Namazi Hospital;and Dr. Nasrin Shokrpour for editorial assistance.

Conflict of Interest: None declared.

References

1. Murlimanju BV, Prakash KG, Samiullah D, *et al.* Accessory neurovascular foramina on the lingual surface of mandible: incidence, topography, and clinical implications. Indian J Dent Res. 2012; 23: 433.
2. Patil S, Matsuda Y, Nakajima K, *et al.* Retromolar canals as observed on cone-beam computed tomography: their incidence, course, and characteristics. Oral Surg oral Med oral Mathol and oral Radiol. 2013; 115: 692-9.
3. Muinelo-Lorenzo J, Suárez-Quintanilla JA, Fernández-Alonso A, *et al.* Descriptive study of the bifid mandibular canals and retromolar foramina: cone beam CT vs panoramic radiography. Dentomaxillofac Radiol. 2014; 43: 20140090.
4. Orhan K, Aksoy S, Bilecenoglu B, *et al.* Evaluation of bifid mandibular canals with cone-beam computed tomography in a Turkish adult population: a retrospective study. Surg Radiol Anat. 2011; 33: 501-7.
5. Kawai T, Asaumi R, Sato I, *et al.* Observation of the retromolar foramen and canal of the mandible: a CBCT and macroscopic study. Oral Radiol. 2012; 28: 10-4.
6. von Arx T, Hänni A, Sendi P, *et al.* Radiographic study of the mandibular retromolar canal: an anatomic structure with clinical importance. J Endod. 2011;37:1630-5.
7. Bilecenoglu B, Tuncer N. Clinical and anatomical study of retromolar foramen and canal. J Oral Maxillofac Surg. 2006; 64: 1493-7.
8. Schejtman R, Devoto FC, Arias NH. The origin and distribution of the elements of the human mandibular retromolar canal. Arch Oral Biol. 1967; 12: 1261-8.
9. Silva FM, Cortez AL, Moreira RW, *et al.* Complications of intraoral donor site for bone grafting prior to implant placement. Implant Dent. 2006; 15: 420-6.
10. Han SS, Hwang YS. Cone beam CT findings of retromolar canals in a Korean population. Surg Radiol Anat. 2014; 36: 871-6.
11. Galdámes IS, Matamala DZ, López MC, *et al.*Retromolar Canal and Forame prevalence in dried mandibles and clinical implications. Int J

Odontostomat. 2008; 2: 183-7.

12. Lizio G, Pelliccioni GA, Ghigi G, *et al.* Radiographic assessment of the mandibular retromolar canal using cone-beam computed tomography. Acta Odontol Scand. 2013; 71: 650-5.
13. Ossenberg NS. Rctromolar foramen of the human mandible. Am J phys Anthropol. 1987; 73: 119-28.
14. Narayana K, Nayak UA, Ahmed WN, *et al.* The retromolar foramen and canal in South Indian dry mandibles. Eur J Anat. 2002; 6: 141-6.
15. Priya R, Manjunath KY, Balasubramanyam. Retromolar foramen. Indian J Dent Res. 2005; 16: 15-6.
16. Tiwari S, Ramakrishna R, Sangeeta M. A study on the incidence of retromolar foramen in South Indian adult dried human mandibles and its clinical relevance. Int J Res Med Sci. 2015; 3: 1383-7.
17. Rossi AC, Freire AR, Prado GB, *et al.* Incidence of retromolar foramen in human mandibles: ethnic and clinical aspects. Int J Morphol. 2012; 30: 1074-8.
18. Sisman Y, Ercan-Sekerci A, Payveren-Arıkan M, *et al.* Diagnostic accuracy of cone-beam CT compared with panoramic images in predicting retromolar canal during extraction of impacted mandibular third molars. Med oral Patol oral y Cir Bucal. 2015;20: e74-e81.
19. Pyle M, Jasinevicius T, Lalumandier J, *et al.* Prevalence and implications of accessory retromolar foramina in clinical dentistry. Gen Dent. 1999; 47:500-3.
20. Kuribayashi A, Watanabe H, Imaizumi A, *et al.* Bifid mandibular canals: cone beam computed tomography evaluation. Dentomaxillofac Radiol. 2010; 39: 235-9.
21. Kodera H, Hashimoto I. A case of mandibular retromolar canal: elements of nerves and arteries in this canal. Kaibogaku Zasshi. 1995; 70: 23-30.

9

A One-Year Evaluation of a Free Fissure Sealant Program

Bakhtiar M[a], Azadi N[b], Golkari A[a*]

[a]Oral and Dental Disease Research Center, and Department of Dental Public Health, School of Dentistry, Shiraz University of Medical Sciences, Shiraz, Iran

[b]Student Research Committee, School of Dentistry, Shiraz University of Medical Sciences, Shiraz, Iran

ARTICLE INFO

Key words:
Pit and Fissure Sealants
Preventive Dentistry
Molar

Corresponding Author:
Ali Golkari
Oral and Dental Disease Research Center, and Department of Dental Public Health, School of Dentistry, Shiraz University of Medical Sciences, Shiraz, Iran
E-mail: golkaria@sums.ac.ir

Abstract

Statement of Problem: Pit and fissure sealant therapy has been approved as an effective measure in the prevention of occlusal dental caries. Resin based materials are the most common materials used worldwide. A variety of resin based fissure sealants are produced and used. Most of them have been presented with ideal results in research environment. However, their effectiveness in the real life, especially in a mass application program such as Iran's oral health reform plan is not clear.

Objectives: To evaluate the longevity of different fissure sealant applied in Iran's oral health reform plan in Fars Province (south of Iran) after one year.

Materials and Methods: Seven counties were selected. One hundred 6- to 8-year-old school children who had undergone fissure sealant therapy in spring 2015 were randomly selected from each county. Their first molars were examined to evaluate the status of the fissure sealants which were applied one year ago. Data on the type/brand of fissure sealant materials, type and experience of clinicians who applied them, existence of a chair-side assistant, and whether the children were caries-free at the time of fissure sealant application were collected from the existing reports.

Results: Data of 1974 teeth from 598 children were used for the final analysis. The effects of type/brand of the material was significant on the final results and remained significant ($p < 0.001$) after adjustments for the level of fluoride, urban/rural area, upper/lower jaw, type of clinician who applied the sealant, existence of a chair-side assistant, and child's gender, age, and being caries-free.

Conclusions: Many factors affect the success rate of a fissure sealant therapy program. The type/brand of the material remained significantly related to the success rate of the fissure sealant even after adjustments for other influencing factors. In this study, Clinpro™ Sealant (3M/ESPE, USA) showed better longevity after one year of application.

Introduction

It is well recognized that a higher prevalence of dental caries start from pits and fissures, compared to the smooth surfaces. In children, about 90 percent of decays of the permanent teeth start from pits and fissures. And a considerable number of them remain in these surfaces for the person's life [1,2].

Fissure sealant (FS) therapy was introduced in the 1960s and has been widely used since then [2,3]. Resin based sealants are more commonly used currently. The preventive effects of resin based pit and fissure sealants have been demonstrated in several studies [1,4]. They can reduce the occurrence of tooth decay by more than 50% in the first through five years after the application when each tooth is sealed only once with no follow up treatment. In cases that the sealed teeth are regularly (annually for instance) examined and the defected or lost fissure sealants are renewed, the chance of caries could be reduced by 75% up to four years [5].

With all proven preventive benefits of fissure sealant therapy, it is still difficult to convince people to request their dentist to perform it, or accept their dentist's suggestion for it. Unfortunately consumers, health service providers (such as health ministry), and health insurers all resist paying for preventive oral care [6,7] . However, in Iran, an oral care program was established in 2015 as part of the national health reform plan which started in 2014 [8,9]. In this program, the state health system was obliged to provide oral health prevention services to all primary school children through primary care trusts. It included regular oral examinations, oral hygiene instruction, scaling and cleaning teeth, fluoride therapy, and application of fissure sealants [9].

Although the effectiveness of pit and fissure sealants is well established, most studies confirming that have been conducted in an ideal environment. This means the method of application has been closely supervised in such an environment. However, the results of mass application of sealants, when several children are called and treated in a day, might be different [10]. In the new program in Iran, parents do not pay for sealants, and in some cases they are not even given enough information about sealing their children's teeth. Therefore, it is possible to think that the results of sealant therapy might not be as good as what is seen in both in-vitro and in-vivo experimental conditions.

It is understandable that FS material would gradually fade away by both physical (mastication forces) and chemical means. However, good evidence is available showing that, if properly applied, FS should remain on the tooth surface (covering pits and fissures in an acceptable condition) for several years [11].

One of the main reasons for early loss of FS is contamination of the tooth surface with saliva during FS application [12]. This is of special importance as FS is usually applied to children's (who might be less cooperative) teeth which might not be fully erupted [13]. Apart from that, the most important factor related to the success rate of FS in the first year of application is the type/brand of the material [11,14]. As mentioned above, the fissure sealant materials are usually tested either in factory laboratories or in the most ideal clinical environment. But how would they work under the real life conditions?

The current study was, therefore, designed and conducted to evaluate the success rate of the fissure sealants applied to the first permanent molars of six to eight year old school children of Fars province (south of Iran) under the health reform plan after one year of application. The main objective of this study was to test the efficacy of different fissure sealant materials in such conditions.

Materials and Methods

The free fissure sealant program started in the early 2015 as a national program targeting the primary school children in Iran. In Fars province, south of Iran, 28 counties (cities/towns plus their politically related villages) plus Shiraz (the capital city of Fars province) participated in the program. The approval was obtained by the Ethical Committee of Shiraz University of Medical Sciences (Grant # 95-01-03-13031). Shiraz and six randomly selected counties were included in the current study. Three counties were selected by simple randomization from those with low or optimal level of fluoride in water. Three other counties were selected from areas with high (> 1.5 ppm) level of fluoride in the tap water. Shiraz was added to the low/optimal fluoride level group. Therefore, seven counties were assessed in this study.

In each county, a list of 6- to 8-year-old children who received free fissure sealant therapy during spring 2015 was obtained from the existing documents, which were prepared for a report to the Ministry of Health. In each county, 50 children were selected from the urban and 50 from the rural areas. Stratified random sampling (educational zone, sex, school, pupil) was used for samples selection from the city of Shiraz and its rural areas. A simple randomization was used in the other six counties.

Those children with at least one of their first permanent molars undergoing fissure sealant therapy in the reports were included. Consent form was signed by the parents to allow and access to the previous information and to examine the selected children. Information on children's age and sex, type of residential area (rural/urban), dental health status, type of fissure sealant, method of application, type of the clinician who applied the fissure sealant, and existence of a chair-side assistant was obtained from the records. The types of clinicians were as follows: dental hygienist, recently graduated dentist in their vocational training (VT), dentists with less than five years of experience (not in their VT), and dentists with more experience.

A general dental practitioner was invited to the study from each of seven areas. They were trained and calibrated to act as examiners for this study. Examinations took place in spring 2016, approximately one year after the FS application. The selected children were examined in their schools using disposable gloves, mirrors and tongue blades. A head light was used in adjunct with the natural classroom lights. Occlusal surfaces of their teeth were taken into account only. The condition of the first molars, which had FS applied to them one year ago, was registered as: sound with good FS in place, sound with partial FS, sound with defected FS, sound with no FS, decayed with FS, decayed with no FS, and filled. Those with full coverage, such as a stainless steel crown, were considered as filled.

For some analysis, tooth condition was transformed into a binary variable of successful and failed. For this purpose, only those teeth that were sound and had a good FS in place were considered successful.

Those children who did not attend the examination session for any reason, had changed their school, and had undergone fixed orthodontic treatment were excluded. The examiners were allowed to mark a tooth as "questionable" if they could not reach a definite diagnosis about the condition of the tooth. The questionable teeth were also excluded from the final analysis. All information were gathered and kept highly confidential.

SPSS statistical software (version 20) was used for data entry and analysis. Each examined tooth was considered as an independent sample during analysis. Frequency and percentage of each type of tooth condition was calculated. The condition of the examined teeth was compared between urban and rural areas, areas with low/optimal and high levels of fluoride in water, boys and girls, caries-free children and those with caries in their other teeth at the time of FS application, upper and lower teeth, existence and absence of a chair-side assistant, type of clinician, and type/brand of fissure sealant, using a Chi-square test. The relationship between children's age at which an FS was placed with the success rate of FS was assessed using an ANOVA test. Logistic regression was used to assess the independent effect of the brand of the material on the outcome.

Results

Data of 1974 teeth from 598 children were used for the final analysis. As it was mentioned above, each tooth was considered as an independent sample. Demographic variables of the samples are presented in Table 1. About 60% of the examined teeth were from counties with low or optimal level of fluoride in water and the other 40% were from areas with high fluoride level (> 1.5 ppm). Only 13.6% of the examined teeth were in children who were reported as caries-free at the time of the fissure sealant application. More than half (52.6%) of the fissure sealants were conducted by general dental practitioners in their compulsory vocational training. Relatively good proportions were seen in other factors such as urban/rural area, gender, upper/lower jaw, and existence of chair-side assistance at the time of FS application.

Six types of fissure sealants were used. Each of them was used for between 13.4 and 20.2 percent of the examined teeth (Table 2). The condition of the examined teeth, at the time of examination (which was around one year after the fissure sealant application), is presented in Table 3. Only 47% (N = 927) of the examined teeth had a good fissure sealant in place. This means less than half of the teeth reported to be sealed were still in good shape and condition. None of the examined teeth was extracted.

There was a significant difference in the results based on the type of the clinicians who applied the fissure sealant ($p < 0.001$). If we consider the teeth with a good fissure sealant in place with no decay in their occlusal surface as successful, dentists with less than five years of experience who were not in their compulsory VT had the highest success rate (64%). That is while the dental hygienists had the lowest rate

Table 1: Demographic characteristics of the included teeth (N=1972)

Variable	Value	Frequency	Percentage
Level of fluoride	Low/optimal	1183	59.9
	High	791	40.1
Area	Rural	886	44.9
	Urban	1088	55.1
Gender	Boy	1051	53.2
	Girl	923	46.8
Caries free (at the time of FS application)	No	1702	86.2
	Yes	268	13.6
	Not recorded	7	0.2
Jaw	Upper	945	47.9
	Lower	1029	52.1
Existence of a chaireside assistance	Yes	937	47.5
	No	1037	52.5
Type of clinician	Dentist in VT	1039	52.6
	Dentist with < 5 years of experience	203	10.3
	Dentist with > 5 years of Experience	444	22.5
	Dental hygienist	288	14.6

Table 2: Types of fissure sealant material used and the number of teeth treated with each of them

Fissure sealant material	Manufacturer	Number of teeth treated with	% of teeth treated with
Master-Dent™ Pit and Fissure Sealant- light curing- Opaque	Dentonics (USA)	360	18.2
Seal-Rite™ Pit and Fissure Sealant	Pulpdent Corporation (USA)	286	14.5
Wet-Bond™ Pit and Fissure Sealant	Pulpdent Corporation (USA)	264	13.4
Eco-S™ Pit and Fissure Sealant	Vericom Co. Ltd. (Korea)	398	20.2
Seal-It	Spident Co. Ltd. (Korea)	368	18.6
Clinpro™ Sealant	3M ESPE Co. (USA)	298	15.1
Total	--	1974	100

Table 3: Condition of the teeth when examined one year after fissure sealant application (N=1974)

Code	Condition of teeth	Number of teeth	% of teeth
1	Sound with good FS in place	927	47.0
2	Sound with partial FS in place	116	5.9
3	Sound with defected FS	129	6.5
4	Sound with no FS detected	597	30.2
5	Decayed with partial or defected FS	33	1.7
6	Decayed with no FS detected	115	5.8
7	Filled	57	2.9
8	Extracted	None	0

(34.6%). On the other hand, dental hygienists had the highest number of teeth with no detectable fissure sealant (sound with no FS + decayed with no FS = 57.3%). Dentists with more than five years of experience had the highest percentage of the teeth which were filled (4.7%) (Table 4).

There was also a significant difference in the results between those in low/optimal level of fluoride and those in high level of fluoride in their water ($p < 0.001$). A higher percentage of sound teeth with good FS in place (55.2% vs. 41.4%) and a lower percentage of filled teeth (1.5% vs. 3.8%) were seen in areas with high level of fluoride. The difference between rural and urban areas was also statistically significant ($p < 0.001$). There was a markedly lower percentage of sound with good FS teeth (44.1% vs. 49.3%) and markedly lower percentage of filled teeth (0.9% vs. 4.5%) in those from rural areas.

In terms of being caries-free at the time of fissure sealant therapy, there was a significantly higher percentage of sound with good FS (59.3% vs. 45.1%) and significantly lower percentage of sound with no FS (20.5% vs. 31.7%) in caries-free children, compared with others ($p < 0.001$). It seemed that the upper jaw teeth were more likely to remain sound. There was a higher percentage of sound with good FS (53.4% vs. 41.0%), a lower percentage of decay with no FS (2.9% vs. 8.6%), and a lower number of filled teeth (2.0% vs. 3.7%) in the upper jaws ($p < 0.001$).

When a chair-side assistant was available, a higher number of sound with good FS, a higher number of sound with partial FS, a higher number of sound with defected FS, and much lower numbers of sound with no FS, and decay with no FS were seen ($p < 0.001$).

In terms of the effects of types of fissure sealant material, percentage of successful results (sound with good FS in place) was much higher when Clinpro™ (3M ESPE, USA) was used (67.4%). This was significantly higher than the success rate of between 38 and 51 percent in other types ($p < 0.001$). Moreover, the percentage of sound with no FS was several folds higher in any other material (22%-45%) when compared with 9.7% in Clinpro™ Sealant ($p < 0.001$). Clinpro™ was among lower percentages in other failed cases, too (Table 5).

Among other types, Pulpdent's conventional Seal-Rite™ (USA), which uses a dry bond system, had one of the highest percentages of sound with partial FS, and the highest percentage in two other failed tooth conditions: sound with the defected FS and filled teeth. Pulpdent's Wet-BondTM (USA) showed the highest proportion of decayed teeth with no FS, Masterdent and Spident had high numbers of sound with no FS.

To make sure that the differences in the results of using different materials are truly related to the type/brand of FS, the effects of other factors were eliminated by adjusting through using a logistic regression modeling. It was revealed that the difference between the six types of FS was independent from the other factors ($p < 0.001$), although they remained significant in the equation (Table 6). The effect of the type of area (urban/rural) was reversed in the regression model, showing that those living in rural areas had a better chance of success in FS after adjustments for other factors.

Discussions

Iran's Health Reform Plan started in 2014. It initially targeted the tertiary care in hospitals to make sure everybody enjoys a better quality treatment in hospitals with less out of pocket costs. All Iranians were offered a health insurance regardless of their working status. This was happening for the first time in Iran [8,9]. Considering the high costs of this plan and the fact that no previous Iranian government allocated such budget to health, it was regarded as "Rouhani Care" in global media referring to Iran president's heed towards better health insurance coverage [15,16].

Attention to primary care was added to Iran's Health Reform Plan one year after its start date. Regarding the oral health care, the plan focused mainly on preventive measures which were officially introduced in April 2015. Children in primary schools were placed as the target group. They were offered oral examination, oral hygiene instruction, fluoride therapy, extraction of infected teeth, and fissure sealant therapy free of charge. The latter was done by either dentists or dental hygienists in a mass application in which several (or even a whole class of) children were taken to a dental setting in a single day and fissure sealants were applied to all their eligible teeth. As one may predict, quality of services might fall in such mass service provision. The objective of the current study was, therefore, to evaluate the effectiveness of fissure sealant application in such non-ideal conditions. It was designed to see what types of fissure sealant materials were used in this program and to compare their effectiveness in such conditions. As different materials were used in different places, it was necessary to observe and

Table 4: Condition of the examined teeth by the type of clinician applying the fissure sealant around one year ago

	Type of clinician who applied the FS	Present tooth condition							Total
		sound with good FS	Sound with partial FS	Sound with defected FS	Sound with no FS	Decayed with FS	Decayed with no FS	Filled	
Clinician who applied the FS	Dentist in V	476 (45.8%)	67 (6.4%)	77 (7.4%)	305 (29.4%)	12 (1.2%)	71 (6.8%)	31 (3.0%)	1039 (100.0%)
	Dentist with less experience	130 (64.0%)	19 (9.4%)	9 (4.4%)	37 (18.2%)	2 (1.0%)	2 (1.0%)	4 (2.0%)	203 (100.0%)
	Dentist with more experience	227 (51.1%)	21 (4.7%)	27 (6.1%)	104 (23.4%)	16 (3.6%)	28 (6.3%)	21 (4.7%)	444 (100.0%)
	Dental hygienist	94 (32.6%)	9 (3.1%)	16 (5.6%)	151 (52.4%)	3 (1.0%)	14 (4.9%)	1 (0.3%)	288 (100.0%)
Total		927 (47.0%)	116 (5.9%)	129 (6.5%)	597 (30.2%)	33 (1.7%)	115 (5.8%)	57 (2.9%)	1974 (100.0%)

Table 5: Condition of the examined teeth by the type/brand of the fissure sealant material used

		Present tooth condition							Present tooth condition
		sound with good FS	Sound with partial FS	Sound with defected FS	Sound with no FS	Decayed with FS	Decayed with no FS	Filled	
FS material	Master-Dent™	145	14	17	161	2	18	3	360
		40.3%	3.9%	4.7%	44.7%	0.6%	5.0%	0.8%	100.0%
	Seal-Rite™	116	20	40	79	2	13	16	286
		40.6%	7.0%	14.0%	27.6%	0.7%	4.5%	5.6%	100.0%
	Embrace Wet-Bond™	119	14	8	83	4	30	6	264
		45.1%	5.3%	3.0%	31.4%	1.5%	11.4%	2.3%	100.0%
	Eco-S™	204	28	27	88	14	22	15	398
		51.3%	7.0%	6.8%	22.1%	3.5%	5.5%	3.8%	100.0%
	Seal-It™	142	25	14	157	9	16	5	368
		38.6%	6.8%	3.8%	42.7%	2.4%	4.3%	1.4%	100.0%
	Clinpro™	201	15	23	29	2	16	12	298
		67.4%	5.0%	7.7%	9.7%	0.7%	5.4%	4.0%	100.0%
Total		927	116	129	597	33	115	57	1974
		47.0%	5.9%	6.5%	30.2%	1.7%	5.8%	2.9%	100.0%

Table 6: Effects of all the studied variables on success rate of FS before and after adjustments

Variable		Tooth condition*		p-value before adjustments	OR*** (95% C.I)	*p*-value after adjustments
		Success**	Failure			
Age		6.86±0.86	6.71 ± 0.81	<0.001	0.849 (0.753-0.957)	0.007
Level of fluoride	High	55.2%	44.8%	<0.001	1	--
	Low/ optimal	41.4%	58.6%		0.45 (0.35-0.54)	<0.001
Type of area	Urban	49.3%	50.7%	<0.001	1	--
	Rural	44.1%	55.9%		2.14 (1.60-2.86)	<0.001
Existance of a chair-side assistant	Yes	56.5%	43.5%	<0.001	1	--
	No	38.4%	61.4%		0.44 (0.33-0.57)	<0.001
Child's sex	Girl	43.0%	57.0%	<0.001	1	--
	Boy	50.4%	49.6%		1.35 (1.11-1.64)	0.003
Jaw	Lower	41.0%	59%	<0.001	1	--
	Upper	53.4%	46.4%		1.71 (1.41-2.08)	<0.001
Caries free status	Yes	59.3%	40.7%	<0.001	1	--
	No	45.1%	54.9%		0.57 (0.43-0.77)	<0.001
Type of clinician	Dental Hygienist	32.6%	67.4%	<0.001	1	--
	Dentist in VT	45.8%	51.2%		1.47 (1.05-2.04)	0.024
	Dentist with <5y experience	64.0%	36.0%		2.41 (1.57-3.70)	<0.001
	Dentist with >5y experience	51.1%	48.9%		1.60 (1.04-2.44)	0.031
Type of FS material	Clinpro™	67.4%	32.6%	<0.001	1	--
	Masterdent™	40.3%	59.7%		0.30 (0.20-0.43)	<0.001
	Seal-Rite™	40.6%	59.4%		0.47 (0.32-0.69)	<0.001
	Wet-Bond™	45.1%	54.9%		0.45 (0.31-0.66)	<0.001
	Eco-S™	51.3%	48.7%		0.55 (0.39-0.79)	0.001
	Seal-It™	38.6%	61.4%		0.41 (0.29-0.59)	<0.001

*Tooth condition at the examination date (about one year after FS application). Age was described using mean±SD and categorical variables were described using rate(%)

"**Sound teeth with acceptable FS in place" was considered success. Other conditions were considered failure.

***Adjusted Odds Ratio using a logistic regression model.

adjust for other affecting variables such as the level of fluoride in the area's water, children's gender and age, rural or urban area of living, upper or lower jaw teeth, the type and experience of those who applied the FS, presence of a chair-side assistant, and if the children were caries-free at the time of fissure sealant application.

It was found that less than half (47.0%) of the teeth reported to have fissure sealant were sound and had intact or acceptable FS in place one year after application. It is better to say that these teeth "were sound" not "remained sound" at the time of examination, as we could not be sure if all of the examined teeth were sound at the time of fissure sealant teeth. Some clinicians might have applied fissure sealant to the teeth that were questionable or had dental caries in their initial phase either by mistake or with the hope that the FS could stop or postpone the caries progress [17].

Three main types of material are available for sealing pits and fissures: resins, glass-inomers and poly-acid modified resin composites (compomers), which are a combination of the first two. To date, the resin-based pit and fissure materials are still the most widely used material, which have also showed the highest effectiveness even in comparison with the newer types of material [5,18]. In the current study, six different materials were found being used for FS application, and all of them were resin-based.

One of the findings of this study was that when a wet bond system was used for FS application (Embrace Wet-Bond™ – Pulpdent- USA), a high number of decayed teeth with no FS were reported. This could be due to the inappropriate placement of FS, which in turn could be considered as a result of the applicant being unfamiliar with this system. Some other studies have also reported similar findings [19].

It was found that near five percent of the examined teeth were filled. That was just around one year after FS application. These were either filled during one year between FS application and the examination date which could be filled instead of FS application at the time of program, or were wrongly reported as having sealed while they were filled before. As this was a retrospective study, there was no way to distinguish between the three possibilities.

Many previous studies on FS reported much higher success rate [1,20]. A study by Ismail and Gagnon (1995) was one the first studies that evaluated an FS program in field. They reported that only 2.5% of the sealed teeth needed filling after one year [21]. However, in the current study 2.9% of the sealed teeth were already filled after one year; the other 7.5% of the teeth were found having caries and, therefore, should have been filled. In another study by Heller et al., 8% of the sealed teeth had or needed filling after five years of FS application [22]. This is almost equal to the percentage of the teeth which had or needed filling just one year after FS application in the current study.

One of the reasons for low success rate of FS reported in the current study could be the possibility of application of fluoride varnish right before FS application. Both fluoride therapy and FS were parts of the oral health reform program. Thus, it is assumed that some clinicians had possibly applied fluoride and FS in the same visit. It is argued that the reaction of fluoride with the enamel would add to the enamel's resistance to acids; and therefore, lowers the resin bond to the tooth surface [23,24]. Data on the possible concurrency of fluoride and FS therapies were not obtained in this study.

Another fact worth mentioning is the possibility of over-reporting the number of FS application by clinicians in the Iran's current program. False reporting could happen in any similar community program. However, the high rate of sound teeth with no FS in this study should ring the bells. A quality and quantity control would be necessary if the policy makers would really intend to continue this program and lower the DMFT in future. Even by considering all limitations of the FS program and limitations of this study, the results of Clinpro™ (3M ESPE – USA) were much better than the others; however, the difference could neither be ignored nor be related to the limitations.

Based on the findings of the current study, it seems that the teeth sealed in the oral health reform program in 2015 need to be reevaluated and either get filled or sealed again. Nevertheless, it is a global finding that repeating FS application would increase its success rate by both increasing the rate of the existence of a good FS on tooth surface after any specific period of time and decreasing the caries rate [25,26].

Conclusions

In this study, it was shown that several factors affect the success rate of a fissure sealant therapy program in schoolchildren. The type of material used in such program plays a vital role which is independent from other affecting factors. In this study, resin-based fissure sealant material made by 3M/ESPE, USA (Clinpro™) showed higher longevity and retention than other five materials.

Conflict of Interest: None declared.

References

1. Dennison JB, Straffon LH, Smith RC. Effectiveness of sealant treatment over five years in an insured population. J Am Dent Assoc. 2000;131:597-605.
2. Carvalho JC, Dige I, Machiulskiene V, *et al.* Occlusal Caries: Biological Approach for Its Diagnosis and Management. Caries Res. 2016;50:527-542.
3. Takeuchi M. Sealing of the pit and fissure with resin adhesive. 3. Outlines of its progress to the present time. Jpn Dent J. 1967;4:33-46.
4. Wright JT, Tampi MP, Graham L, *et al.* Sealants for Preventing and Arresting Pit-and-fissure Occlusal Caries in Primary and Permanent Molars. Pediatr Dent. 2016;38:282-308.
5. Hicks M, Flaitz CM. Fissure sealants and conservative adhesive restoration: Scientific and clinical rationale. In: Pinkham JR, Casamassimo PS, Fields HW, McTique DJ, Nowak A, editors. Pediatric dentistry: Infancy through adolescence. 4th Edition. St. Louis: WB Saunders; 2005. P. 522-576.
6. Griffin SO, Griffin PM, Gooch BF, *et al.* Comparing the costs of three sealant delivery strategies. J Dent Res. 2002;81:641-645.
7. Yeung CA. Sealant costs. Br Dent J. 2014;217:3.
8. Bahadori M, Ravangard R, Alimohammadzadeh K, *et al.* Plan and road map for health reform in Iran. BMJ. 2015;351:4407.
9. Editorial. Plan promises reform in oral healthcare system. Financial Tribune. 2015.
10. Wales. National A. NHS dental services : fissure sealant programme; health inequalities fund: Wales, National Assembly; 2001.
11. Deery C. Pit and fissure sealant retention. Evid Based Dent. 2012;13:9-10.
12. Azarpazhooh A, Main PA. Pit and fissure sealants in the prevention of dental caries in children and adolescents: a systematic review. J Can Dent Assoc. 2008;74:171-177.
13. Correr GM, Caldo-Teixeira AS, Alonso RC, *et al.* Effect of saliva contamination and re-etching time on the shear bond strength of a pit and fissure sealant. J Appl Oral Sci. 2004;12:200-204.
14. Castillo Dutra Borges B, Roger Pinho de Silva P, Catelan A, *et al.* Influence of the light curing tip distance and material opacity on selected physical properties of a pit and fissure sealant. Pediatr Dent. 2011;33:505-509.
15. Khalaj M. ‘ RouhaniCare’ set to give Iran president healthy boost in poll. Financial Times. 2016 5 September.
16. Editorial. The best and worst of worlds: Tehran’s public hospital wards. The Guardian. 2015 28 January.
17. Harris N. Primary Preventive Dentistry. 8th Edition: Pearson; 2013.
18. Goldman AS, Chen X, Fan M, *et al.* Cost-effectiveness, in a randomized trial, of glass-ionomer-based and resin sealant materials after 4 yr. Eur J Oral Sci. 2016;124:472-479.
19. Panigrahi A, Srilatha KT, Panigrahi RG, *et al.* Microtensile Bond Strength of Embrace Wetbond Hydrophilic Sealant in Different Moisture Contamination: An In-Vitro Study. J Clin Diagn Res. 2015;9:23-25.
20. Gooch BF, Griffin SO, Gray SK, , *et al.* Preventing dental caries through school-based sealant programs: updated recommendations and reviews of evidence. J Am Dent Assoc. 2009;140:1356-1365.
21. Ismail AI, King W, Clark DC. An evaluation of the Saskatchewan pit and fissure sealant program: a longitudinal followup. J Public Health Dent. 1989;49:206-211.
22. Bhuridej P, Damiano PC, Kuthy RA, *et al.* Natural history of treatment outcomes of permanent first molars: a study of sealant effectiveness. J Am Dent Assoc. 2005;136:1265-1272.
23. Koh SH, Chan JT, You C. Effects of topical fluoride treatment on tensile bond strength of pit and fissure sealants. Gen Dent. 1998;46:278-280.
24. Takahashi Y, Arakawa Y, Matsukubo T, *et al.* The effect of sodium fluoride in acid etching solution on sealant bond and fluoride uptake. J Dent Res. 1980;59:625-630.
25. Askarizadeh N, Norouzi N, Nemati S. The effect of bonding agents on the microleakage of sealant following contamination with saliva. J Indian Soc Pedod Prev Dent. 2008;26:64-66.
26. O’Reilly MT, De Jesús Viñas J, Hatch JP. Effectiveness of a sealant compared with no sealant in preventing enamel demineralization in patients with fixed orthodontic appliances: a prospective clinical trial. Am J Orthod Dentofacial Orthop. 2013;143:837-844.

10

The Effect of Different Polishing Methods and Storage Media on Discoloration of Resin Composites

Deljoo Z[a], Sadeghi M[a], Azar MR[b], Bagheri R[c]

[a]Shiraz Dental School, Shiraz University of Medical Sciences, Shiraz, Iran
[b] Department of Endodontics and Prevention of Oral and Dental Disease Research Center, School of Dentistry, Shiraz University of Medical Sciences, Shiraz, Iran
[c] Department of Dental Materials and Biomaterials Research Centre, School of Dentistry, Shiraz University of Medical Sciences, Shiraz, Iran

ARTICLE INFO

Key words:
Colour Change
Nanohybrid Composite
Microhybrid Composite
Storage Media

Corresponding Author:
Rafat Bagheri
Department of Dental Materials and Biomaterials Research Centre, Shiraz Dental School, Shiraz University of Medical Sciences, Shiraz, Iran
Email: bagherir@yahoo.com

Abstract

Statement of Problem: Accumulation of plaque and staining due to a rough surface, and penetration of colourant agents from food and beverages in to the resin composite results in an incomplete polymerization. There is a little information on the effect of finishing and polishing techniques on the discoloration of nanohybrid and microhybrid composites when exposed to staining solutions.

Objectives: To determine the degree of surface staining of nanohybrid and microhybrid composites after polishing and immersion in distilled water and two commonly used staining solutions.

Materials and Methods: A nanohybrid (Ice; SDI) and microhybrid (Gradis direct; GC) composites were used. Disc-shaped specimens were prepared and treated with either a matrix finish or polished using Sof-Lex discs (3M/ESPE) and Enhance point (Dentsply). After 24 h immersion in distilled water at 37°C the specimens were polished and colour coefficients (CIE L* a* b*) was measured by a spectrophotometer. All specimens were immersed in 37°C distilled water in an incubator for 7 days and colour coefficients were measured again. The colour change (ΔE) was calculated using the following formula: $\Delta E = [(\Delta a)^2+(\Delta b)^2+(\Delta L)^2]^{1/2}$. The data were analyzed using three-way ANOVA, one-way ANOVA/Tukey HSD and Student's *t*-test.

Results: There was a significant interaction between resin composites, polishing systems and staining solutions ($p < 0.05$). ANOVA and Tukey's tests showed that Ice had a significantly lesser colour change than Gradia direct and matrix finish revealed the smoothest surface followed by Sof-Lex discs and Enhance point. Distilled water and cola caused no perceptible colour change ($\Delta E < 3.3$). The effect of surface polish on staining was statistically significant ($p < 0.05$).

Conclusions: Sof-Lex discs in comparison to Enhance point stimulated greater staining resistance for both composites. The nanohybrid exhibited less colour change than microhybrid composite. Coffee was the only storage media that induced a perceptible colour change ($\Delta E > 3.3$) compared to cola and distilled water.

Introduction

The majority of patients desire that tooth-coloured materials used in their restorative to be long lasting, withstand harsh oral environments and hence have high colour stability. This is especially significant for the anterior teeth. New amendments in resin composites and bonding systems targeted a better aesthetics as well as function authorizing these materials to be used for anterior and posterior restorations [1,2].

To improve physical and mechanical properties of resin composites, the size of filler particles incorporated in the resin matrix has been gradually decreased over the years [3,4]. The most recent developed resin composites contain only nanoparticles called nanofill composites. However, most manufacturers produce nanohybrid composites which mostly contain nanaoscales particles and less pre-polymerized resin fillers. These materials are used for most anterior and posterior applications due to their combination of strength and polishability [5,6].

Colour change of aesthetic materials can be affected by several factors such as accumulation of plaque, penetration of staining agents (food and beverages), incomplete polymerization, water sorption, dietary and smoking habits, exposure to chemical, and surface smoothness of the restoration [1,2,7,8]. Heavy drinkers of alcohol and/or soft drinks with tooth-coloured restoratives predispose their restorations to discoloration affecting the clinical outcome and colour stability of the restorations. The effect of aging, beverages and food stimulating solutions on the colour stability of resin composites has been widely studied and various degrees of staining have been reported [9-13].

Additionally, surface characteristics and material's composition such as filler particles' shape and sizes may influence the discoloration of the composites [14]. Finishing and polishing techniques are reported to have a great influence on the discoloration of tooth-coloured restorative materials [15-17]. High finished and polished surface improves the aesthetics and the longevity of the restorations, while rough surfaces accumulate plaque and staining; hence, discoloration of the composite restoration occurs [18,19]. Therefore, the smooth surface contributes to aesthetics by prevention of staining and plaque retaining [20].

There are controversial reports on the effect of surface polish, foods and beverages on the colour change of the nanocomposites. Nasim *et al.* [2] found significant differences among microfill, microhybrid and nano composites after storage in tea, carbonated drink and distilled water for 30 days. Microfill composite exhibited the most colour change and microhybrid the least. Malhotra *et al.* [1] in their study on the effect of three indigenous food stains (tea, tobacco, and turmeric) on microhybrid, and nanofill composites revealed that all of the tested groups showed clinically perceptible colour change. Moreover, Gönülol and Yılmaz [16] studied the effect of finishing and polishing techniques on the colour stability of two nanohybrids (Grandio/Voco and Aelite/Bisco) and found a significant difference between colour change of these two materials. A recent study [21] found no significant difference in the colour stability of the nanofill composite after immersion in different media. They also reported that the finishing and polishing procedures did not have any influence on the colour stability of the nanofill composite [21] .

There are few published studies comparing colour change of microhybrid and nanohybrid composites subjected to different polishing systems exposed to daily used staining beverages. Therefore, the aim of this study was to compare the colour change of a microhybrid and a nanohybrid composite after polishing by Sof-Lex discs or Enhance point versus Mylar strip after immersion in distilled water, cola and coffee for 7 days. The null hypothesis is that there is no difference between microhybrid and nanohybrid composites after immersion in those staining solutions, and that the polished or unpolished surfaces do not affect the colour change of these materials differently.

Materials and Methods

Two types of resin composite were selected; Ice (nanohybrid, SDI, Australia) and Gradia direct (microhybrid, GC, Japan). Three surface finish/polishes (matrix finish, Sof-Lex discs / 3M ESPE, and Enhance point / Dentsply) and three storage media (distilled water, cola and coffee) were used. Fifty-four disc-shaped specimens for each composite were prepared using a polyethylene mould of 10 mm diameter and 1 mm thickness. Resin composite was placed into the mould and sandwiched between two Mylar strips and glass slabs with slight hand pressure in order to extrude the excess material. The specimen was cured over the Mylar strip using an LED curing unit [Radii plus LED, (wavelength of 440-480 nm/ output of 1500mW/cm^2, SDI, Bays water, Victoria, Australia). Thirty minute after curing, the specimen was removed from the mould and ground gently using 600 grit silicon carbide paper to make a smooth edges. All the specimens were stored in distilled water at 37°C for 24 h in an incubator.

The specimens were divided into three groups of 18; one group was designated 'matrix finish' and left without further polishing after removal of the Mylar strip. Specimens in the second group were polished using a sequence of four Sof-Lex (3M/ESPE, St Paul, MN, USA) discs (coarse, medium, fine and super fine) on a low speed hand piece. The third group was polished using Enhance Point (Dentsply, Detrey Gmbh, Konstanz,Germany). Each group of 18 was then divided into 3 subgroups of 6 and immersed in either distilled water, cola or coffee for another 7 days at 37°C. The staining solution was replaced with fresh solution every 24 h during the storage period.

After 24 h, when the polymerization completed, before polishing the baseline *L**, *a**, *b** (CIE system) values of all specimens were measured using a spectrophotometer (Vita Easyshade, Ivoclar Vivadent AG, Schaan, Liechtenstein). Each specimen was measured at three areas, and then the mean values were calculated. The spectrophotometer was recalibrated when required.

After 7 days of immersion in the solutions, colour measurement was recorded again for all groups with the same method mentioned above. Before colour measurement, the specimens were dried with paper towel slowly. The second measurement was served as the treatment for each specimen to enable the calculation of colour change (ΔE) using the following formula:

$\Delta E=[(\Delta a)^2+(\Delta b)^2+(\Delta L)^2]^{1/2}$, where $\Delta a^* = (a^*_1 - a^*_0)$, $\Delta b^* = (b^*_1 - b^*_0)$, and $\Delta L^* = (L^*_1 - L^*_0)$.

Zero represents the baseline reading, whereas 1 represents the colour reading after 7 days of immersion in the staining solutions or distilled water.

Statistical Analysis

Three-way ANOVA was used to assess the effect of different polishing methods, storage media and composites. Due to the significant interaction effects, subgroup analysis using one-way ANOVA/ Tukey HSD and Student's *t*-test were performed. SPSS version 18.0 (Chicago, IL, USA) was used for statistical analysis. A $p < 0.05$ was considered statistically significant.

Results

Results of Three-way ANOVA showed a significant interaction between two resin composites, storage media and polishing systems (all $p < 0.05$). Table 1 shows the statistical analysis within groups using one-way ANOVA and Tukey's test. Generally, Ice showed less colour change than Gradia direct in all storage media and all polishing systems (Figure 1). Matrix finish caused significantly less colour change than Sof-Lex discs and both less than Enhance point for both composites in all storage media. Among the storage media, coffee revealed significantly more colour change than cola and both more than distilled water for two tested composites and all polishing methods.

For both composites in all 3 polishing groups, mean values of ΔE was significantly different between

Table 1: Mean colour change (ΔE values) ± standard deviation of the materials for all polishing systems in all storage media

Composite	Storage Medi	Matrix finish	Sof-Lex	Enhance
Gradia direct	Distilled water	$1.8\pm0.58^{a,A}$	$2.5\pm0.63^{a,AB}$	$2.9\pm0.73^{a,B}$
	Cola	$2.2\pm0.48^{a,A}$	$2.9\pm0.57^{a,AB}$	$3.1\pm0.60^{a,B}$
	Coffee	$4.1\pm0.48^{b,A}$	$6.2\pm0.46^{b,B}$	$6.5\pm0.44^{b,B}$
Ice	Distilled water	$1.1\pm0.50^{a,A}$	$1.8\pm0.40^{a,AB}$	$2.1\pm0.56^{a,B}$
	Cola	$1.6\pm0.36^{a,A}$	$2.1\pm0.67^{a,A}$	$2.3\pm0.38^{a,A}$
	Coffee	$3.2\pm0.42^{b,A}$	$5.5\pm0.49^{b,B}$	$6.1\pm0.38^{b,B}$

Different upper case letters show significant differences in the colour change (ΔE) between different polishing systems (Tukey's HSD test)

Different lower case letters show significant differences in the color change (ΔE) between storage media (Tukey's HSD test)

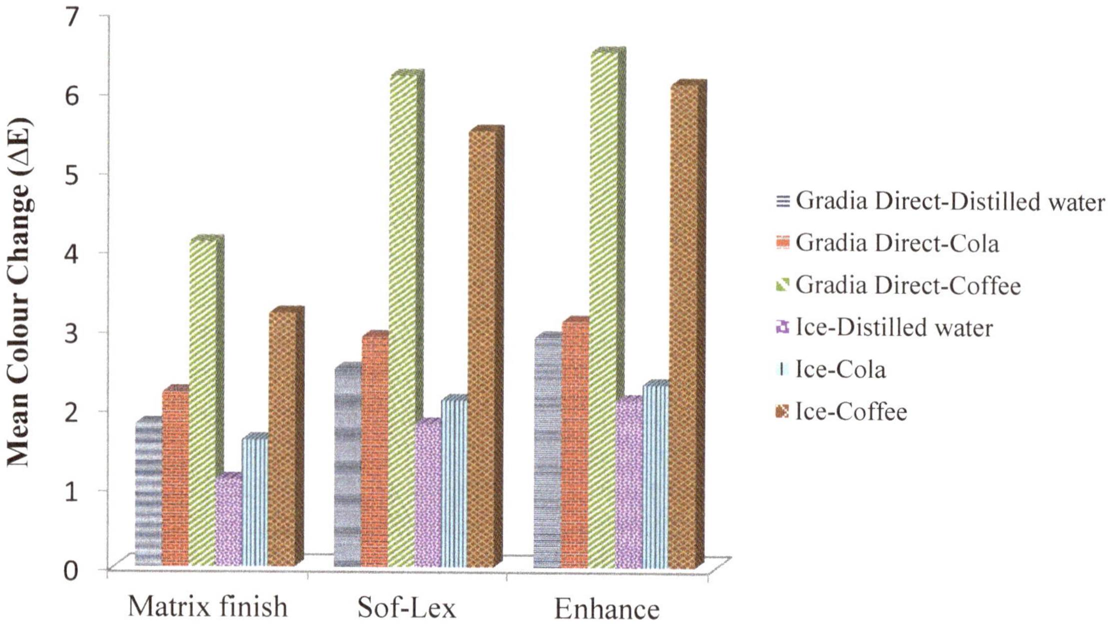

Figure 1: Mean colour change (ΔE values) of tested resin composites for all polishing systems in all storage media

coffee and distilled water or coffee and cola ($p < .05$), but no significant difference between distilled water and cola. Table 2 compares the differences between the ΔE values of all storage media for both composites. Only coffee produced clinically perceptible colour change (ΔE > 3.3).

Discussion

The results of this study showed that the null hypothesis was rejected, i.e. nanohybrid and microhybrid composite performed differently when subjected to different finishing and polishing procedures. Immersion in storage media also showed diverse effects on the colour change of the two tested materials. The microhybrid composite (Gradia direct) showed significantly greater colour change than the nanohybrid (Ice) in matrix finish and polished groups in all storage media (Table 1). This different performance of the two composites supports the effect of material's composition as intrinsic factors in their colour change. Ice with filler loading of 61vol% and particle sizes range of 0.04-3 μm contains UDMA/Bis-EMA/TEGDMA showed less discoloration than Gradia having 59 vol% and average particle sizes of 0.85μm contain mainly UDMA. The differences could be related to the resin phase of the composite [10] or filler volume, sizes or the porosity of the aggregated filler particles [22]. The degree of conversion has been mentioned as a prominent factor on the discoloration of resin composites.

Table 2: Comparison between two composites for each storage media in all polishing methods, using Student's *t*-test

Polishing Methods	Storage Media	*p* value
Matrix finish	Distilled water	0.051
	Cola	0.038*
	Coffee	0.007*
Sof-Lex	Distilled water	0.045*
	Cola	0.051
	Coffee	0.031*
Enhance	Distilled water	0.061
	Cola	0.022*
	Coffee	0.122

*:Significant difference ($p < 0.05$)

(Tukey's HSD test)

However, Al Kheraif *et al.* [23] examined th e effect of coffee, tea, cola and distilled water on colou r stability and degree of conversion of nanofill an d microhybrid composites. They found that nanofill composite with greater ΔE values when exposed to coffee despite having a higher degree of conversion compared to microhybrid composite [23].

Besides material composition, mechanical and chemical elements such as finishing and polishing procedures, and exposure to staining solutions might also result in surface roughness, thus high stainability [24,25]. In the present study, in contrast to distilled water (pH = 6.8) and cola (pH = 2.47), immersion in coffee (5.41) for both composites and two polished groups resulted in clinically perceptible colour change ($\Delta E > 3.3$). Results of other studies [9,23] on the effect of food colourants on the discoloration of resin composites showed results similar to ours. Although cola had the lowest pH that might damage the surface integrity of the materials, it did not produce as much discoloration as coffee which may be due to the lack of a yellow colourant in cola. It is concluded that discoloration by coffee might be due to adsorption and absorption of colourants by materials. This sorption of colourants into the organic phase of the materials was probably due to the porosity of polymer phase with the yellow colourants of coffee [9].

Another explanation for more discoloration due to immersion in coffee would be alteration in the surface hardness of the resin composite. Karaman *et al.* [26] studied the influence of cola and coffee on the colour stability of silorane and methacrylate-based composites. Immersion in coffee caused a significant discoloration for all the composites tested, showing a lower colour change in silorane-based than that of methacrylate-based composite. Immersion in coffee caused the most changes in the surface hardness of methacrylate-based composite [26].

In the current study, the specimens polymerized under Mylar strip without receiving further polishing treatment (matrix finish group) had the lowest ΔE values followed by Sof-Lex discs. Enhance point showed the most colour change in both nanohybrid and microhybrid composites that could be due to the defect and scratches created by the polishing procedure on the surface of the materials make them more disposed to staining [27]. Previous studies [28-30] also reported similar results that the roughest surface is generated by using Enhance polishing systems in comparison with Mylar strip and Sof-Lex discs. A current study investigated the effect of polishing systems on stain susceptibility and surface roughness of nanocomposites, reporting that staining susceptibility depends mainly on material composition and on the polishing procedures. It has been shown that polishing improved the staining resistance of the resin composites; and nanocomposites exhibited similar staining resistance or surface roughness to microhybrid composite [31]. However, it is shown that the smoothest surface was not necessarily the most stain resistant [32], which may support the hypothesis that discoloration is not exclusively dependent on the surface roughness but exposure to the staining media may change the surface quality and predispose the materials to discoloration [9]. In our study, coffee and cola were used as colourant agents, due to their frequent intake in daily life and having different pH levels. The results indicated that coffee induced the most colour change in both materials in matrix finish and two other polished groups, which is in agreement with other studies [12,23,33].

Conclusions

Within the limitations of this in vitro study, the following conclusions were drawn. Multiple-step polishing technique (Sof-Lex discs) in comparison to one-step (Enhance Point) stimulated greater staining resistance for both composites. The nanohybrid exhibited less colour change than microhybrid composite. Stain susceptibility altered not only due to the composition of the material, but also the polishing techniques and storage media. Therefore, the practitioners should try to minimize discoloration of the composite restorations by adopting excellent polishing techniques and educating patients on the staining effects and erosive potential of the soft drinks if consumed heavily.

Acknowledgments

The authors thank the Vice-Chancellor of Shiraz University of Medical Sciences for supporting this research which is based on the thesis by Dr. Zahra Deljoo (Grant#9250). The authors also thank Dr Mehrdad Vossoughi Statistician in Shiraz Dental School for his help with the statistical analysis, and SDI and GC for providing the materials used in this study.

Conflict of Interest: None declared.

References

1. Malhotra N, Shenoy RP, Acharya S, *et al.* Effect of Three Indigenous Food Stains on Resin-Based, Microhybrid and Nanocomposites. J Esthet Restor Dent. 2011;23:250-257.
2. Nasim I, Neelakantan P, Sujeer R, *et al.* Color stability of microfilled, microhybrid and nanocomposite resins—an in vitro study. J Dent. 2010;38:e137-e142.
3. Ilie N, Hickel R. Resin composite restorative materials. Aust Dental J. 2011;56:59-66.

4. Ferracane JL. Resin composite—state of the art. Dent Mater. 2011;27:29-38.
5. Ilie N, Hickel R. Investigations on mechanical behaviour of dental composites. Clin Oral investig. 2009;13:427-438.
6. Sarrett DC. Restorative Materials. ADA Professional Product Review. 2010;5(2).
7. Patel SB, Gordan VV, Barrett AA, *et al.* The effect of surface finishing and storage solutions on the color stability of resin-based composites. J Am Dent Assoc. 2004;135:587-594.
8. Türkün Ls, Türkün M. Effect of bleaching and repolishing procedures on coffee and tea stain removal from three anterior composite veneering materials. J Esthet Restor Dent. 2004;16:290-301.
9. Bagheri R, Burrow M, Tyas M. Influence of food-simulating solutions and surface finish on susceptibility to staining of aesthetic restorative materials. J Dent. 2005;33:389-398.
10. Villalta P, Lu H, Okte Z, *et al.* Effects of staining and bleaching on color change of dental composite resins. J Prosthet Dent. 2006;95:137-142.
11. Türker S, Koçak A, Aktepe E. Effect of five staining solutions on the colour stability of two acrylics and three composite resins based provisional restorations. Eur J Prosthodont Restor Dent. 2006;14:121-125.
12. Fontes ST, Fernández MR, de Moura CM, *et al.* Color stability of a nanofill composite: effect of different immersion media. J Appl Oral Sci. 2009;17:388-391.
13. Al-Dharrab A. Effect of energy drinks on the color stability of nanofilled composite resin. J Contemp Dent Pract. 2013;14:704-711.
14. Mundim FM, Garcia L da F, Pires-de-Souza Fde C. Effect of staining solutions and repolishing on color stability of direct composites. J Appl Oral Sci. 2010;18:249-254.
15. Turkun L, Turkun M. The effect of one-step polishing system on the surface roughness of three esthetic resin composite materials. Oper Dent. 2004;29:203-211.
16. Gönülol N, Yılmaz F. The effects of finishing and polishing techniques on surface roughness and color stability of nanocomposites. J Dent. 2012;40:64-70.
17. Baseren M. Surface roughness of nanofill and nanohybrid composite resin and ormocer-based tooth-colored restorative materials after several finishing and polishing procedures. J Biomater Appl. 2004;19:121-134.
18. Lopes GC, Vieira LC, Araujo E. Direct composite resin restorations: a review of some clinical procedures to achieve predictable results in posterior teeth. J Esthet Restor Dent. 2004;16:19-31.
19. Yalcin F, Korkmaz Y, Baseren M. The effect of two different polishing techniques on microleakage of new composites in Class V restorations. J Contemp Dent Pract. 2006;7:18-25.
20. Alawjali S, Lui J. Effect of one-step polishing system on the color stability of nanocomposites. J Dent. 2013;41:53-61.
21. Oliveira AL, lorenzetti CC, Garcia PP, *et al.* Effect of finishing and polishing on color stability of a nanofilled resin immersed in different media. Revista de Odontologia da UNESP. 2014;43:338-342.
22. Lazzetti G, Burgess JO, Gardiner D, *et al.* Color stability of fluoride containing restorative materials. Oper Dent. 2000;25:520-525.
23. Al Kheraif AA, Qasim SS, Ramakrishnaiah R, *et al.* Effect of different beverages on the color stability and degree of conversion of nano and microhybrid composites. Dent Mater J. 2013;32:326-331.
24. Sarafianou A, Iosifidou S, Papadopoulos T, *et al.* Color stability and degree of cure of direct composite restoratives after accelerated aging. Oper Dent. 2007;32:406-411.
25. Hachiya Y, Iwaku M, Hosoda H, *et al.* Relation of finish to discoloration of composite resins. J Prosthet Dent. 1984;52:811–814.
26. Karaman E, Tuncer D, Firat E, *et al.* Influence of Different Staining Beverages on Color Stability, Surface Roughness and Microhardness of Silorane and Methacrylate-based Composite Resins. J Contemp Dent Pract. 2014;15:319-325.
27. Reis AF, Giannini M, Lovadino JR, *et al.* Effects of various finishing systems on the surface roughness and staining susceptibility of packable composite resins. Dent Mater. 2003;19:12-18.
28. Can Say E, Yurdaguven H, Yaman BC, *et al.* Surface roughness and morphology of resin composites polished with two-step polishing systems. Dent Mater J. 2014;33:332-342.
29. Vieira AC, Oliveira MC, Lima EM, *et al.* Evaluation of the Surface Roughness in Dental Ceramics Submitted to Different Finishing and Polishing Methods. J Indian Prosthodont Soc.

2013;13:290-295.

30. Barakah HM, Taher NM. Effect of polishing systems on stain susceptibility and surface roughness of nanocomposite resin material. J Prosthet Dent. 2014;112:625-631.
31. Sadeghi M, Deljoo Z, Bagheri R. The infulence of Surface Polish and Beverages on the Roughness of Nanohybrid and Microhybrid Resin Composite. J Dent Biomater. 2016;3:177-185
32. Tjan AH, Chan CA. The polishability of posterior composites. J Prosthet Dent. 1989;61:138-146.
33. Ertas E, Guler AU, Yucel AC, *et al.* Color stability of resin composites after immersion indifferent drinks. Dent Mater J. 2006;25:371–376.

11

Evaluating the Accuracy of Kvaal's Method for Age Estimation in a Selected Iranian Population

Haghnegahdar AA[a]; Vossoughi M[b]*; Teymoorienik Z[c]; Khojastepour L[a]

[a]Department of Oral and Maxillofacial Radiology, School of Dentistry, Shiraz University of Medical Sciences, Shiraz, Iran
[b]Oral and Dental Disease Research Center, Department of Dental Public Health, School of Dentistry, Shiraz University of Medical Sciences, Shiraz, Iran
[c]Student Research Committee, Shiraz University of Medical Sciences, Shiraz, Iran

ARTICLE INFO

Key words:
Dental age estimation Kvaal's method
Adults
Accuracy
Iranian population

Corresponding Author:
Mehrdad Vossoughi
Oral and Dental Disease Research Center, Department of Dental Public Health, School of Dentistry, Shiraz University of Medical Sciences, Shiraz, Iran.
Email: vossoughim@sums.ac.ir

Abstract

Objectives: This study aimed to evaluate the efficacy of Kvaal et al.'s method (1995) for dental age estimation of adult individuals in a sample of Iranian population. For this purpose, the accuracy of the regression formulas and M and W-L variables were studied.

Materials and methods: Pulp and tooth lengths and widths were measured on 100 digital panoramic radiographs. Then Kvaal's M and W-L variables were computed and substituted in Kvaal's formulas to evaluate their accuracies. The efficacy of these two variables in our population was assessed using a k-fold cross-validation technique for regression analysis. Principle component analysis was also performed to develop population-specific dental variables.

Results: Applying Kvaal's regression formulas on multiple teeth in different jaws resulted in highly insensible estimations. In contrast, developing regression formulas based on Kvaal's M and W-L variables yielded reasonable and sensible estimates especially for younger individuals; standard error of estimate (SEE) values ranged from 6.36-6.80 years. The models based on multiple teeth in different jaws performed similar.

Conclusions: For young adults, the M and W-L variables anticipated accuracy rates lower than those of Kvaal's reference study which were within an acceptable threshold for forensic application (SEE<10 years). Therefore, the two variables and not formulas are proper measurements for forensic age estimation in Iranian young adults. However, underestimation was predominant for the middle age and old age participants.

Introduction

Scientific techniques for age estimation play critically important roles in forensic and legal medicine [1]. It is especially a very clarifying principal in identifying the cadavers and body remains. Moreover, it is widely used in many instances of social activities such as school attendance, employment, and marriage as well, all planning some hormonal therapies in pediatric endocrinology for persons with no valid proof of the date of birth. Chronological age, as the most popular scale for age determination, may be lost or hidden and sometimes it does not show the exact developmental course of an individual. There are two main biological age defined according to the development occurred in the skeleton or skeletal maturation, usually detected by X-ray examinations, which can be used more reliably regarding the development. Many researchers have studied skeletal development especially using hand-wrist X-ray for forensic age estimation and as an aid to evaluate the growth disorders. Skeletal radiology has remained historically the most widespread method for age estimation of living individuals [2, 3]. There are two main methods for employing teeth in age estimation; tooth emergence analysis and tooth developmental stage analysis. Tooth emergence is a feeling event of a short duration and difficult to determine which can be affected by nutrition and local factors such as apace limitations [4,5]. On the contrary, tooth development is fundamentally influenced by genetic factors rather than environmental ones. Therefore, there is an increasing tendency to apply dental development as an age estimation tool. Demirjian *et al.* [2] proposed one of the most recognized techniques for age estimation. This method is based on radiographic evaluations of developmental stage of the teeth in the left mandibular quadrant, extracted from a French population. Although several studies verified its generalization to other populations [4], some authors have reported the overestimation of chronological age and incompatibility of the scoring system for their populations [5,6]. The time-limitation for application is another problem with Demirjian's technique. As the tooth development is generally completed about puberty, this method can be only used in childhood. Although Demirjian's stages have been extended to the wisdom teeth [7-9], the third molar development for age estimation is limited to late adolescence and early adulthood, i.e. the age range of 14-22 or up to 24 years [10-12]. Kvaal *et al.* [3] proposed a new technique for age estimation of adult individuals. This method is based on size of the pulp of the teeth. It had been proved that the size of pulps in the incisor teeth is considerably different between 10-year age groups [13]. It is because of continuous deposition of reparative dentin in the teeth, which decreases the pulp size through the life. The pulp size of six teeth (3 mandibular and 3 maxillary) was measured in different points to establish some specific ratios on the periapical views of individuals. Then, a regression model was used to develop a formula for age estimation. Rösing and Kvaal [14] stated that regression estimates with a standard error greater than 5-7 years are not suitable for routine forensic application as they provide wide confidence intervals [15]. Some studies reported a wider acceptable range for standard error of estimate (SEE) in forensic field (<10 years) [16-18]. Multiple studies have been performed to evaluate the accuracy of Kvaal's method in other populations [16, 19-26]. Research on Kvaal's method has revealed a great deal of variation among different populations with respect to accuracy level. The most amount of variation may be attributable to "age mimicry" bias [27-31], i.e. the bias of estimates by the age structure of reference sample. This research has two main objectives in order to study the worthiness of Kvaal's method. First, the accuracy of Kvaal's regression formulas is evaluated in a selected Iranian population. Second, the efficiency of Kvaal's M and W-L variables in age estimations is studied to insure whether they can be extended to our population.

Methods and materials

Kvaal's method for age estimation

Kvaal *et al.* [3] proposed a technique for age estimation based on indicators of reduction in the size of the dental pulp cavity. Their study has been conducted on 100 dental patients who had attended the clinics of Dental Faculty in Oslo. The radiographs of six types of teeth from each jaw were measured: maxillary central, lateral incisors and second premolars; and mandibular lateral incisors, canines and first premolars.

The following measurements were performed on the radiographs of each tooth: T: maximum tooth length; R: root length on the mesial surface; P: maximum pulp length; A: root and pulp width at the enamel-cementum junction (ECJ or level A); B: root and pulp width midway between measurement levels A and C; and C: root and pulp width midway between apex and ECJ. Six ratios between the tooth and pulp measurements were computed; P: ratio between the length of the pulp and root; T: ratio between the length of the tooth and root; R: ratio between the length of the pulp and tooth; A: ratio between the width of the pulp and root at enamel-cementum junction (level A); B: ratio between the width of the pulp and root at midpoint between level C and A (level B); and C: ratio between the width of the pulp and root at mid-root level (level C). In order to reduce the number of variables, principal component analysis was performed on the 6 ratios and it demonstrated that the following combinations were the best subsets to account for the variability of ratios: M: mean value of P, R, A, B, and C (all the ratios except for T); and W-L: mean value of width ratios from levels B and C (W) minus mean value of the length ratios P and R (L). Finally, M and W-L variables were used as predictor variables in a multiple linear regression model when chronological age was considered as dependent variable. Kvaal's regression formulas for age estimation are presented in the Results section.

Population and sample size

A total of 100 digital panoramic radiographs were collected from the records of the Department of Dental Radiology, School of Dentistry, Shiraz University of Medical Sciences, Shiraz, Iran. The radiographs were from 56 males and 44 females, with acceptable quality and presence of the teeth: central, lateral, and second premolar in the maxilla and lateral, canine, and first premolar in mandible at the right and left sides. A written informed consent form from all participants was acquired. The written consent form is a standard form, which has been developed in full accordance with World Medical Association Declaration of Helsinki by Ethical committee of Shiraz University of Medical Sciences. The mean age of the individuals was 28.44±6.68 years with a range of 19.25 to 55.17 years. Table 1 shows age group distribution of the individuals. Panoramic views containing rotated teeth or dental anomalies, such as dens invagination and dentin dysplasia or amelogenesis imperfecta, were excluded from the study. Exposure parameters were prepared according to the patient size. The radiographs were viewed over a monitor in standard viewing conditions. The observer was blind to the age and gender of the individual. The six ratio parameters (P, T, R, A, B, and C) were calculated using digital calipers. We also computed M and W-L variables proposed by Kvaal from these ratio parameters.

Statistical analysis

Qualitative variables were described using frequency (and percentage) and quantitative variables were described using mean and standard deviation (SD.). For assessing the accuracy of Kvaal's formulas, some accuracy indices such as standard error of estimate (SEE.) and mean of absolute differences (MAD.) were used. K-fold cross-validation technique (with k=2) for linear regression was used to assess the efficacy of the variables that had been proposed by Kvaal (M and W-L) for age estimation in our population. In this method, first, the original data were randomly divided into two sub-samples with equal sample sizes (here, n1=n2=50). Then, in each step, one of the sub-samples was used for developing a regression model (training data) using the proposed variables and the other one (testing or hold-out data) for assessing how the resulting model will predict it. Moreover, principal component analysis (PCA) was employed to evaluate the reliability of the variables and propose new population-specific variables for age estimations based on our dataset. PASW SPSS software for Windows version 18.0 (SPSS Inc., Chicago, IL, USA) was used for data analysis. Throughout this study, the significant level was considered 0.05.

Table 1: Age and sex distribution of the 100 individuals included in the study

Age group (year)	Sex		Total
	Male	Female	
19-30	35	22	57
30-40	16	15	31
40-50	2	6	8
50-60	3	1	4
Total	56	44	100

Table 2: Mean (±SD) Kvaal's components for different age groups

Teeth	Age	P	T	R	A	B	C	W	L	Kvaal's variables M	Kvaal's variables W-L
3 maxillary	<30	0.78±0.09	1.47±0.11	0.53±.06	0.29±0.05	0.26±0.05	0.21±0.05	0.24±0.04	0.65±0.08	0.41±0.04	0.42±0.08
	30-40	0.75±0.09	1.49±0.13	0.51±0.07	0.27±0.04	0.24±0.05	0.21±0.05	0.22±0.04	0.63±0.08	0.40±0.04	0.40±0.08
	>40	0.67±0.13	1.46±0.09	0.46±0.10	0.39±0.38	0.20±0.05	0.16±0.03	0.18±0.04	0.56±0.11	0.38±0.05	0.39±0.10
3 mandibular	<30	0.77±0.73	1.28±0.08	0.60±0.06	0.24±0.04	0.25±0.04	0.24±0.05	0.25±0.04	0.69±0.06	0.42±0.08	0.44±0.08
	30-40	0.77±0.05	1.27±0.08	0.61±0.05	0.22±0.04	0.22±0.04	0.22±0.05	0.22±0.04	0.69±0.05	0.41±0.03	0.46±0.06
	>40	0.77±0.10	1.31±0.12	0.59±0.07	0.17±0.03	0.19±0.05	0.17±0.04	0.18±0.04	0.68±0.08	0.38±0.05	0.50±0.07
6 teeth	<30	0.77±0.06	1.38±0.07	0.57±0.05	0.26±0.03	0.26±0.03	0.23±0.04	0.24±0.03	0.67±0.05	0.42±0.03	0.43±0.06
	30-40	0.76±0.06	1.38±0.08	0.56±0.05	0.24±0.04	0.23±0.04	0.21±0.04	0.22±0.04	0.66±0.05	0.40±0.03	0.43±0.05
	>40	0.72±0.08	1.38±0.06	0.52±0.07	0.28±0.19	0.20±0.04	0.17±0.02	0.18±0.03	0.62±0.07	0.38±0.02	0.44±0.07

P, ratio between length of pulp and root; T, ratio between length of tooth and root; R, ratio between length of pulp and tooth; A, ratio between width of pulp and root at enamel-cementum junction (levelA); B, ratio between width of pulp and root at midpoint between level C and A (level B); C, ratio betweenwidth of pulp and root at mid-root level (level C); W, meanvalue of width ratios from levels B and C; L, mean value of the length ratios P and R;M,mean value of all ratios (first Kvaal'spredictor); W-L, differencebetween W and L (secondKvaal's predictor).

Results

This study comprised 100 individuals, 56 males, and 44 females. The individuals' age ranged from 19.25 to 55.17 years (mean age 28.44±7.13 years). Descriptive statistics for Kvaal's components from dental radiographs for different age groups are reported in Table 2.

Kvaal's regression formulas are presented in Table 4. Surprisingly, almost all age estimates were negative, especially when the teeth in mandibular and both jaws were used; 59%, 100%, and 98% of the individuals using 3 maxillary, 3 mandibular and all teeth, respectively. Age estimation using the 3 maxillary, 3 mandibular and all 6 teeth resulted in extremely large SEE and MAD values. Applying

Table 3: Correlation coefficients between tooth ratios and chronological age

									Kvaal's variables	
Teeth	P	T	R	A	B	C	W	L	M	W-L
3 maxillary	-0.34*	-0.07	-0.30*	0.10	-0.38*	-0.30*	-0.38*	-0.34*	-0.35*	-0.14
3 mandibular	0.08	0.04	-0.87*	-0.40	-0.37*	-0.37*	-0.41*	-0.09	-0.36*	-0.17
6 teeth	-0.30*	-0.03	-0.26*	-0.03	-0.41*	-0.41*	-0.48*	-0.30*	-0.44*	0.02

*Statistically significant at α=0.05.

The correlation between Kvaal's dental components and chronological age for each tooth is reported in Table 3. There was no significant relationship between T, A, and W-L with age in the maxillary, mandibular, and all six teeth (all P>0.05). There was a negative significant relationship between P and L with age only in the maxillary and six teeth.

Kvaal's formulas yielded SEE (and MAD) values of 34.35 (31.84), 79.52 (78.18), and 58.66 (57.58) years for 3 maxillary, 3 mandibular and all teeth, respectively. Although, the formula based on 3 maxillary teeth attained smaller accuracy indices, its estimates still highly deviated from the chronological ages and obtained insensibly

Table 4: Accuracy indices for age estimations using Kvaal's regression formulas

Teeth	Kvaal's formula	Kvaal's SEE*	SEE	MAD	SD	Min	Max
3 maxillary	Age=120-256.6(M)-45.3(W-L)	8.9	34.35	31.84	12.94	0.16	60.03
3 mandibular	Age=135.3-356.8(M)-82.5(W-L)	9.4	79.52	78.18	14.59	40.68	120.50
6 teeth	Age=129.8-316.4(M)-66.8(W-L)	8.6	58.66	57.58	11.23	22.10	85.12

*: Accuracy values that had been reported by Kvaal et al.

However, R, B, C, and W had negative significant correlations with age in all positions.

The SEE values of age estimates using Kvaal's regression formulas, the mean, SD, minimum and maximum values of absolute differences between the chronological and the estimates using applying

negative estimations. Kvaal's formula based on 3 mandibular teeth performed the worst.

Table 5 shows the results of multiple linear regression models using Kvaal's M and W-L variables on training dataset in each step and accuracy indices for combined testing datasets

Table 5: The results of K-fold cross-validation technique for assessing the accuracy of Kvaal's variables

Teeth	Regression Formula†	R^2*	SEE	MAD	%(2)	%(4)	%(6)	%(10)
3 maxillary	34.75-23.67(M)+7.15(W-L) 54.85-55.91(M)-7.61(W-L)	0.09	6.74	5.11	78.6	48.0	30.6	9.2
3 mandibular	71.20-121.15(M)+15.99(W-L) 38.97-50.17(M)+24.23(W-L)	0.27	6.36	5.01	76.5	51.0	36.7	9.2
6 teeth	61.04-102.53(M)+21.03(W-L) 60.77-89.44(M)+11.37(W-L)	0.19	6.08	4.72	74.5	50.0	30.6	8.2

†: Each model has two formula because the dataset divided into two sub-datasets and a regression model developed based on one of them and the accuracy was evaluated using the other one in each step.
*: R^2 values which presented here were averaged over the two sub-samples.
Note: %(n) is the percentage of subjects whose estimation deviated more than n years (n = 2, 5, 10).

(cross-validation method). In contrast to applying Kvaal's formula directly, developing a new formula based on Kvaal's variables resulted in positive and sensible estimates. The values of SEE (and MAD) were 6.74 (5.11), 6.36 (5.01) and 6.08 (4.72) years for the 3 maxillary, 3 mandibular and all teeth, respectively. Interestingly, the indices showed estimates that are more accurate in younger participants. About 25%, 50%, 75% and 91% of all participants were estimated up to 2, 4, 6 and 10 years deviated from their chronological ages, respectively.

Table 6 shows the accuracy indices for Kvaal's variables based on 6 teeth in different age groups. In order to avoid redundancy, the results for different jaws were not presented. The variables performed accurately for those aged <30 and 30-40 years old (SEE=4.68 and 5.42, respectively). SEE value was insensibly high in the age group over 40 years. Underestimation was predominant for the two higher age groups in comparison with the first. The results of principal component analysis for the two second premolar (15/25) are presented in Table 7. The coefficients yielded in this study and

Table 6: The accuracy indices for assessing Kvaal's variable on the 6 teeth for different age groups

Age group	SEE	%UE	%(2)	%(4)	%(6)	%(10)
<30	4.68	26.3	66.7	43.9	22.8	00.0
30-40	5.42	90.3	87.1	54.8	35.5	00.0
≥40	15.39	100	100	100	100	83.3

Note: %(n) is the percentage of subjects whose estimation deviated more than n years (n = 2, 5, 10).
Because the number of subjects in 40-50 and 50-60 year old groups were small, the two groups were aggregated.

Table 7: The two first principal components (PCs) for the ratios from the two second premolar (15/25)

			*Kvaal's results	
Ratio	1st PC	2nd PC	1st PC	2nd PC
P	0.88	0.32	0.43	0.51
R	0.87	0.34	0.42	0.51
A	-0.46	-0.41	0.50	-0.03
B	0.58	0.67	0.44	-0.51
C	0.66	0.58	0.42	-0.46

*: Coefficients that had been reported by Kvaal et al.

those of Kvaal's study were highly divergent. The two first principal components explained 71.3% of the total variance of age. Although small values of regression R^2 and principal component coefficients implied inefficiency of Kvaal's variables for explanation of age variation in our population, the estimation accuracy was reasonable for the forensic field.

Discussion

Techniques for age estimation are increasingly applied to various scientific, medical, and legal conflict cases. Kvaal *et al.* [3] asserted that age could be estimated based on the degree of calcification in the pulp of teeth since this calcification is mild and continuously occurring in teeth throughout lifetime. Regarding the widespread need for age estimation in adults, this study was performed to evaluate the accuracy of Kvaal's formulas and variables in a selected Iranian population.

Kanchan-Talreja *et al.* [23] assessed the accuracy of Kvaal's formulas on digital radiographs of 100 Indians. Although the SEEs were not reported, the mean differences between estimated and chronological ages were high, 18-21 years for different combination of teeth. When population-specific regression formulas were applied, the errors were reduced to 11-14 years. For Indian formula, the SEE values were highly greater than those values achieved in Kvaal's study (8.6-9.4 years) and our study. The differences may be due to several reasons. First, environmental, and genetic factors can possibly affect the secondary dental deposition. Second, in developing the Indian regression formulas, Kvaal's M and W-L variables were not used directly, whereas one main goal of our study was set to assess the accuracy of these two variables in age estimation. Finally, the percentage of individuals aged >50 years was greater in their study when compared to Kvaal's (36%) and our study (4%); hence, the results might have highly influenced by age mimicry bias.

Bosmans *et al.* [20] studied 197 participants in Belgium, 18 (9%) of whom were aged <50 years, and directly applied the Kvaal's formulas for age estimation. The SEEs were 9.2-9.9 years for the teeth in the three positions. The values were relatively similar to those obtained by Kvaal (8.6-9.4 years) and were remarkably smaller than values yielded by present study for direct application of the Kvaal's formulas, 34.35-74.52 years. They found out that the estimations were more precise when 3 mandibular or all 6 teeth were examined. In contrast, the relatively more precise estimates were obtained when the 3 maxillary teeth were examined in our study.

Meinl *et al.* [25] assessed the reliability of some age estimation techniques on young individuals, 44 Austrians aged 13 to 24 years, and reported a consistent underestimation for Kvaal's formulas.

Chandramala *et al.* [21] studied the reliability of M and W-L variables in regression analyses. Although it did not report SEE values, the coefficients of determinations (R^2) were as low as our study. The reported R^2s were 0.076, 0.049, and 0.017 for the upper 3 teeth, lower 3 teeth and all the 6 teeth, respectively. It was concluded that these two variables were not able to explain the amount of variation in age. However, no significant differences were found between mean estimated and chronological ages in the three tooth positions. Similar small R^2s but acceptable estimations in terms of SEEs were yielded in our study.

In a study by Erbudak *et al.* [22] on 123 digital radiographs in Turkey, neither M and W-L and not the three teeth positions were directly entered in regression models. Regression models were developed based on ratios that predict age in the best way. I all of the models, M variable was excluded. They achieved a large SEEs with a range of 12.7-25.10 years.

Mittal *et al.* [26] examined 152 participants with a few number of individuals (5) older than 50 years old. Regression equations for age were derived based on M and W-L variables. Although the greater R^2 values were obtained for the teeth in the three positions (ranged 0.28-0.45) than those of our study (ranged 0.09-0.27), the SEE values for three maxillary teeth (8.59), three mandibular teeth (7.51) and all 6 teeth (7.97) were greater. Nevertheless, the values did not exceed the acceptable limit of age estimation in forensic medicine (SEE<10 years).

Similar to the present study, Karkhanis *et al.* [24] applied a cross-validation technique on M and W-L variables and similar findings were reported. The SEE values were 9, 8.36, and 9.61 years for the

3 maxillary teeth, 3 mandibular teeth and all 6 teeth, respectively. Like our findings, even though, their study yielded small R^2 values, the accuracy indices were acceptable. Compared to our study, they studied a larger sample size (n=279) and 50 individuals from the total sample size were considered as holdout data.

Marroquin Penaloza *et al.* [16] applied Kvaal's method on 101 CBCT images from a Malaysian population. Instead of M and W-L variables, several regression formulas were built based on different combinations of Kvaal's pulp/root measurements and ratios on the sagittal and coronal views. The accuracy was outside the acceptable range for forensic application; all SEE values were greater than 10 years. However, the number of individuals aged >50 (20) was lower than that of Kvaal's study. The larger SEE in some mentioned studies and our study on elderly individuals may be attributable to the tendency of regression techniques to underestimate the age of old individuals, *"Attraction of the middle"* bias [27, 29, 30, 32, 33], and age mimicry bias. The reference study comprised more individuals aged >50 years than the present study. Nevertheless, two studies [20, 26] with an age group distribution similar to our study yielded remarkably smaller SEE values for Kvaal's regression formulas. Other possible factors that might explain the variation are genetic differences and environmental parameters. Genetic and environmental factors can change the pattern and speed of dentin deposition in the teeth, causing discrepancy in results.

The variation in results across the studies with the similar age structure may encourage the researchers to build population-specific regression formulas based on Kvaal's variables independently in the age groups < 40, 40-50, and >50 years. However, it requires studies with larger sample sizes in all age groups and validation of new formulas.

Conclusions

Direct application of Kvaal's regression formulas for age estimation yielded insensible results in the Iranian sample examined in this study. Developing regression models based on Kvaal's M and W-L variables provided sensible estimation accuracy rates for young adults (aged <40 years) which were noticeably lower than the acceptable threshold for forensic application (SEE<10 years). However, underestimation was predominant for the middle age and old age participants whose SEE values were large. Conflict of interests: The authors declare that they have no competing interest. All authors listed on the title page have read the manuscript, attest to the validity and legitimacy of the data, and agree to its submission to the journal.

Acknowledgements

The present article was extracted from the thesis written by Dr. Zahra Teymoorienik. The authors would like to thank the Vice-Chancellery of Shiraz University of Medical Sciences for supporting this research (Grant number 10837). We would also like to thank Dr Shahram Hamedani, Dr. Nasrin Shokrpour and Center for Development of Clinical Research of Nemazee Hospital for editorial assistance.

Conflict of Interest: None declared.

References

1. Williams G. A review of the most commonly used dental age estimation techniques. J Forensic Odontostomatol. 2001;19:9-17.
2. Demirjian A, Goldstein H, Tanner JM. A new system of dental age assessment. Hum Biol. 1973;45:211-27.
3. Kvaal SI, Kolltveit KM, Thomsen IO,*et al.* Age estimation of adults from dental radiographs. Forensic Sci Int. 1995;74:175-85.
4. Hegde RJ, Sood PB. Dental maturity as an indicator of chronological age: radiographic evaluation of dental age in 6 to 13 years children of Belgaum using Demirjian methods. J Indian Soc Pedod Prev Dent. 2002;20:132-8.
5. Tunc ES, Koyuturk AE. Dental age assessment using Demirjian's method on northern Turkish children. Forensic Sci Int. 2008;175:23-6.
6. Nik-Hussein NN, Kee KM, Gan P. Validity of Demirjian and Willems methods for dental age estimation for Malaysian children aged 5-15 years old. Forensic Sci Int. 2011;204:208. e1-6.

7. Lewis AJ, Boaz K, Nagesh KR, *et al.* Demirjian's method in the estimation of age: A study on human third molars. J Forensic Dent Sci. 2015;7:153-7.
8. Streckbein P, Reichert I, Verhoff MA, Bodeker RH, Kahling C, Wilbrand JF, *et al.* Estimation of legal age using calcification stages of third molars in living individuals. Sci Justice. 2014;54:447-50.
9. Zandi M, Shokri A, Malekzadeh H, *et al.* Evaluation of third molar development and its relation to chronological age: a panoramic radiographic study. Oral Maxillofac Surg. 2015;19:183-9.
10. Mincer HH, Harris EF, Berryman HE. The ABFO study of third molar development and its use as an estimator of chronological age. J Forensic Sci. 1993;38:379-90.
11. Ritz-Timme S, Cattaneo C, Collins MJ, *et al.* Age estimation: the state of the art in relation to the specific demands of forensic practise. Int J Legal Med. 2000;113:129-36.
12. Solari AC, Abramovitch K. The accuracy and precision of third molar development as an indicator of chronological age in Hispanics. J Forensic Sci. 2001;47:531-5.
13. Morse DR, Esposito JV, Schoor RS. A radiographic study of aging changes of the dental pulp and dentin in normal teeth. Quintessence Int. 1993;24:329-33.
14. Rösing FW, Kvaal SI. Dental age in adults—a review of estimation methods. Dental Anthropology: Springer; 1998.p.443-68.
15. Giles E, Klepinger LL. Confidence intervals for estimates based on linear regression in forensic anthropology. J Forensic Sci. 1988;33:1218-22.
16. Marroquin Penaloza TY, Karkhanis S, Kvaal SI, *et al.* Application of the Kvaal method for adult dental age estimation using Cone Beam Computed Tomography (CBCT). J Forensic Leg Med. 2016;44:178-82.
17. Marroquin Penaloza TY, Karkhanis S, Kvaal SI, *et al.* Age estimation in adults by dental imaging assessment systematic review. Forensic Sci Int. 2017;275:203-11.
18. Willems G, Moulin-Romsee C, Solheim T. Non-destructive dental-age calculation methods in adults: intra-and inter-observer effects. Forensic Sci Int. 2002;126:221-6.
19. Ardakani F, Bashardoust N, Sheikhha M. The accuracy of dental panoramic radiography as an indicator of chronological age in Iranian individuals.J Forensic Odontostomatol. 2007:25:30-5.
20. Bosmans N, Ann P, Aly M, *et al.* The application of Kvaal's dental age calculation technique on panoramic dental radiographs. Forensic Sci Int. 2005;153:208-12.
21. Chandramala R, Sharma R, Khan M, Srivastava A. Application of Kvaal's Technique of Age Estimation on Digital Panoramic Radiographs. Dentistry. 2012;2(6):1-5.
22. Erbudak HÖ, Özbek M, Uysal S, Karabulut E. Application of Kvaal *et al.*'s age estimation method to panoramic radiographs from Turkish individuals. Forensic science international. 2012;219(1):141-6.
23. Kanchan-Talreja P, Acharya AB, Naikmasur VG. An assessment of the versatility of Kvaal's method of adult dental age estimation in Indians. Archives of oral biology. 2012;57(3):277-84.
24. Karkhanis S, Mack P, Franklin D. Age estimation standards for a Western Australian population using the dental age estimation technique developed by Kvaal *et al.* Forensic science international. 2014;235:104. e1-. e6.
25. Meinl A, Tangl S, Pernicka E, Fenes C, Watzek G. On the applicability of secondary dentin formation to radiological age estimation in young adults. Journal of forensic sciences. 2007;52(2):438-41.
26. Mittal S, Nagendrareddy SG, Sharma ML, Agnihotri P, Chaudhary S, Dhillon M. Age estimation based on Kvaal's technique using digital panoramic radiographs. Journal of forensic dental sciences. 2016;8(2):115.
27. Aykroyd RG, Lucy D, Pollard AM. AM and Solheim, T.(1997) Technical Note: Regression Analysis in adult age estimation. Am J Physical Anthropol.104:259-65.
28. Bocquet-Appel J-P, Masset C. Farewell to paleodemography. Journal of Human Evolution. 1982;11(4):321-33.
29. Konigsberg LW, Frankenberg SR. Estimation of age structure in anthropological demography. American Journal of Physical Anthropology. 1992;89(2):235-56.

30. Konigsberg LW, Frankenberg SR, Walker RB. Regress what on what? Paleodemographic age estimation as a calibration problem. Integrating archaeological demography: Multidisciplinary approaches to prehistoric population. 1997:64-88.
31. Masset C. Age estimation on the basis of cranial sutures. Age markers in the human skeleton. 1989:71-103.
32. Aykroyd RG, Lucy D, Pollard AM, Roberts CA. Nasty, brutish, but not necessarily short: a reconsideration of the statistical methods used to calculate age at death from adult human skeletal and dental age indicators. American antiquity. 1999;64(1):55-70.
33. Prince DA, Konigsberg LW. New Formulae for Estimating Age-at-Death in the Balkans Utilizing Lamendin's Dental Technique and Bayesian Analysis. Journal of forensic sciences. 2008;53(3):578-87.

A Comparison of Push-Out Bond Strength of Two Endodontic Sealers to Root Canal Dentin: An In Vitro Study

Adl A[a], Sobhnamayan F[b], Sadat Shojaee N[b], Azizi Sh[c]

[a]Department of Endodontics, Biomaterial Research Center, School of Dentistry, Shiraz University of Medical Sciences, Shiraz, Iran

[b]Department of Endodontics, School of Dentistry, Shiraz University of Medical Sciences, Shiraz, Iran

[c]Dentist

ARTICLE INFO

Key words:
Endodontic Sealers
MTA
Push-out Bond Strength

Corresponding Author:
Fereshte Sobhnamayan,
Department of Endodontics,
School of Dentistry, Shiraz
University of Medical
Sciences, Shiraz, Iran

E-mail: sobhf@sums.ac.ir

Abstract

Statement of Problem: Adhesion to root canal dentin is one of the necessary characteristics of endodontic sealers. MTA Fillapex (Angelus, Londria, PR, Brazil) is one of the recently introduced MTA-based sealer. Only a limited number of studies have evaluated the bonding of this sealer to the dentin, with conflicting results.

Objectives: The purpose of this study was to evaluate the bond strength of MTA Fillapex sealer) to root canal dentin compared to an epoxy resin-based sealer (AH26 sealer).

Materials and Methods: Twenty root blocks (6mm length) were acquired from the middle part of the extracted single-rooted central or lateral maxillary incisor roots and their lumens were enlarged to achieve a diameter of 1.3 mm. MTA Fillapex and AH26 were placed in the lumens of root blocks ($n = 10$). The specimens were kept in an incubator for 7 days, the roots were sectioned perpendicular to their long axis to achieve slices with thickness of 1 mm and the push-out test was carried out by a universal testing machine.

Results: The mean value of bond strength was 1.84 ± 0.7 Mpa for AH26 and 0.19 ± 0.1 Mpa for MTA Fillapex. The difference between the two groups was statistically significant ($p < 0.001$).

Conclusions: With in the limitation of this study, AH 26 showed significantly higher bond strength in comparison to MTA Fillapex.

Introduction

Apical periodontitis is predominantly caused by microorganisms and their by-products [1]. Successful endodontic treatment depends on the complete debridement of the root canal system, elimination of pathogenic microorganisms, and complete filling of the canal space to prevent ingress of the bacteria from the oral environment and its spread to the periradicular tissues [2]. The physical properties for achieving a complete sealing include adaptation and adhesion of the filling material to the root canal wall [3]. The use of a root canal sealer with a core filling material is considered as a standard procedure in endodontic obturation. Because gutta percha, as the core material, does not directly bond to the dentin surface, the sealer should be capable of filling the gaps between gutta percah cones and also present bond strength to root dentin [3,4]. It has been suggested that the ability of the root canal sealers to adhere to the core material and to the dentin may result in better sealing ability and reduction of the coronal and apical leakage [5].

Several types of sealer have been used in endodontics, including those based on zinc oxide eugenol, glass-ionomer cement, calcium hydroxide and a range of resins. However, the absence of an ideal endodontic sealer has encouraged the development of new materials.

Mineral trioxide aggregate (MTA) is a material consisting of tricalcium oxide, tricalcium silicate and silicate oxide [6]. Biocompatibility, low toxicity, low microleakage, antimicrobial properties and its ability to set in the presence of moisture or blood are among the advantages of this material [7]. Because of these properties, MTA has been used for several clinical applications such as root repair material, root-end filling, and pulp capping [8]. However, because of its working time, setting time, and difficult handling, MTA does not exhibit the physical characteristics needed to be used as an endodontic sealer [9].

In order to use this material as endodontic sealers, the original formulation has been modified to improve the characteristics such as setting time, flow and adhesion [10-12]. MTA Fillapex (Angelus, Londria, PR, Brazil) is one of the recently introduced MTA-based sealers which is presented in a paste/paste system. Its composition after mixing is basically MTA, salicylate resin, natural resin, bismuth oxide, and silica. It has been shown that this sealer has acceptable physicochemical properties, such as good radiopacity, flow, and alkaline pH [7]. Another study showed that MTA Fillapex has a suitable flow, working and setting times, solubility and water sorption [13].

Only a limited number of studies have evaluated the bonding of this sealer to the dentin, with conflicting results. Two studies have shown that MTA Fillapex sealer has a lower bond strength to the root dentin compared to the epoxy resin –based sealer AH Plus (Dentsply-De Trey, Konstanz, Germany) [14,15]. On the other hand, on the basis of another study, MTA Fillapex presented acceptable resistance to dislodgment, which was similar to that of AH Plus sealer [16].

Therefore, the aim of the present study was to evaluate the push out bond strength of MTA Fillapex to root canal dentin compared with the epoxy resin-based sealer AH 26 (Dentsply-De Trey, Konstanz, Germany).

Materials and Methods

Twenty extracted human maxillary incisors with similar morphologies were selected for this study. All the teeth had mature apices and intact roots, and no cracks were seen on them under light electron microscope. Very long or very short teeth, curved roots, and teeth with any sign of internal root resorption, calcification or previous endodontic treatment were excluded from the study. Apical and coronal parts of the roots were sectioned so that root blocks with 6 mm in length were obtained. In order to standardize the internal diameter of all root blocks, the lumens were instrumented with Gates Glidden burs (Many, Tochigi, Japan), size 2 to 5, to achieve a standardized diameter of 1.3 mm. In order to remove the smear layer, the sections were immersed in 5.25% sodium hypocholorite (Glorang, Iran) followed by 17%EDTA (Ariadent Tehran, Iran), each for five minutes. The samples were then immediately washed with distilled water and dried. The apical ends of all blocks were sealed with waxed resin. Root blocks were then randomly allocated in two groups (n = 10) and the root canal sealers were filled: Group I, MTA Fillapex (Angelus, Londria, PR, Brazil); and Group II, AH 26 (Dentsply-De Trey, Konstanz, Germany). All specimens were filled with the sealers without core material. The sealers were prepared according to the manufacturer's instructions and introduced into the root canals using a lentulo spiral (Sevenska Dentorama, Solna, Sweden) ≠ 40. The specimens were stored in an incubator at 37° C and 100% humidity in the vertical position. After 7 days, all the root blocks were sectioned transversally into 1 ± 0.2 mm thick slices. The slices were then examined under a light microscope (dine –lite Taiwan) at ×20 magnification for the roundness of the lumens and presence of any voids in the samples (Figure 1). Slices with any observable voids in the sealer mass or in the sealer dentin interface were excluded from the study. Finally, 20 slices for each sealer were obtained from the dentin blocks.

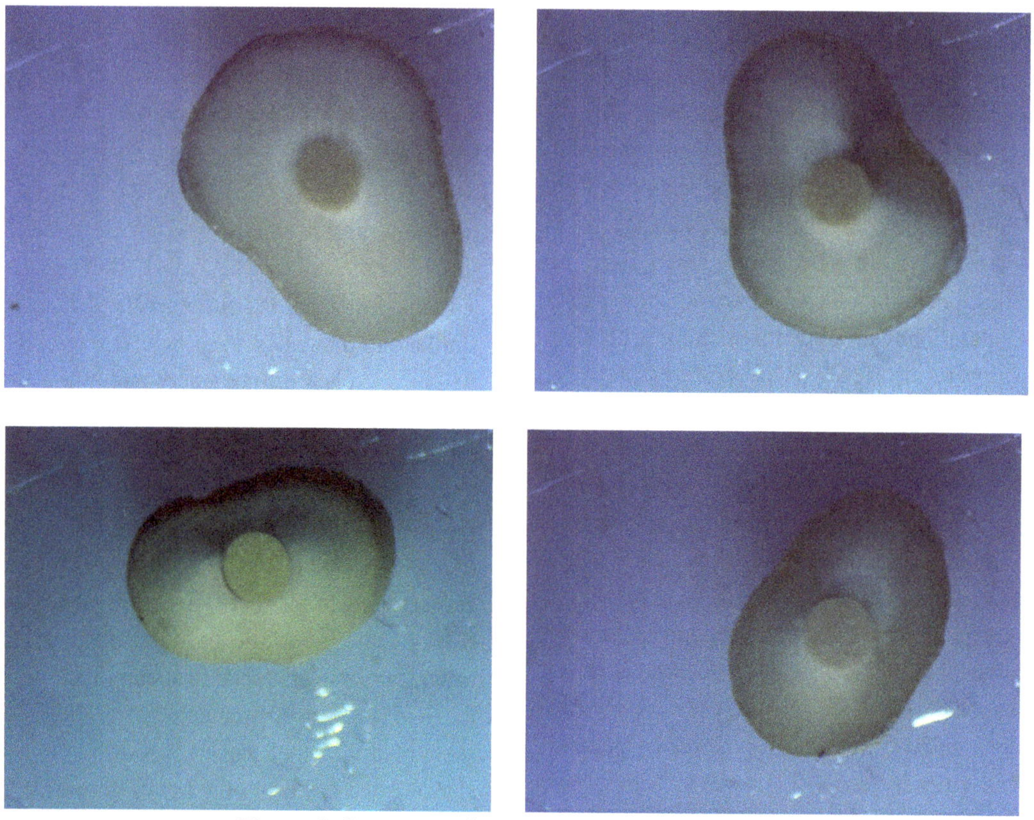

Figure 1: Some root slices selected for push-out test

The samples were subjected to Push-Out bond strength test by using a universal testing machine (Zo20; Zwick/Roell/ Germany). The samples were placed on a metal slab with a central hole to allow the free motion of the plunger. The compressive load was applied by exerting a downward pressure on the surface of the materials using a 0.7 mm diameter cylindrical stainless steel plunger at a speed of 1 mm/ min. The maximum load applied to the materials was recorded in newtons (N) at the time of dislodgment by a computer. In order to express the bond strength in Mpa, the following formula was used: Mpa = N/2πrh, where N = the maximum load for each specimen, r = root canal radius in mm, h = the thickness of the root dentin slice in millimeters, and π = 3.14.

The values of the bond strength were analyzed using independent T-test. Statistical analysis was performed by using SPSS software version 17 for windows (SPSS Inc, Chicago, IL) and the significant level was set at .001.

Results

The mean push out bond strength for AH26 was 1.84 ± 0.7 Mpa whereas it was 0.19 ± 0.1Mpa for MTA Fillapex. AH26 sealer showed a statistically significant higher bond strength compared with MTA Fillapex ($p < 0.001$).

Discussion

Adhesion to the root canal dentin is one of the necessary characteristics of endodontic sealers for two reasons: the superior seal which in turn results in less leakage [5], and prevention of the dislodgment of the filling material during restorative procedures [17].

Different methods including microtensile, shear-bond strength, pull-out and push-out tests have been used to evaluate the bond strength [18]. Among these methods, microtensile and push-out tests are able to evaluate the bond strength in different parts of the root canal. However, preparing the samples for microtensile test is very difficult and they may fracture before the test. On the other hand, the push-out test does not have the limitation of microtensile test; therefore, the results are more accurate and reliable [19].

In some studies that have investigated the bond between sealers and the canal wall, the samples have been filled with a sealer in association with a core material [4,14,16] while in some studies the canals were filled only with sealer [4,20]. When canals are filled with sealer and core material, the sealer is generally present as a thin layer, with two interfaces: between the dentin and sealer and between the sealer and the main cone. On the other hand, when the canal is filled only with sealer, like the present study, only one interface (sealer and dentin) is present, making it possible to only evaluate the bond strength between the sealer and dentin [4]. Moreover, the absence of a core material allows the root canal sealer to achieve its full expansion without being affected by the weak interface between the sealer and core material.

In this study, all root blocks were prepared with the same 1.3 mm-diameter gates glidden drill, making sure to avoid the influence of anatomical variation over the results.

As the presence of smear layer may affect the bond strength of the materials to root canal dentin, in the present study the smear layer was removed from all samples before the application of sealers. Based on the majority of studies, irrespective of the type of the sealer, the bond strength to dentin is decreased in the presence of the smear layer [21-23].

The results of the present study showed that AH 26 sealer had significantly higher bond strength to dentin, compared with MTA Fillapex. This result is in agreement with the results of the study conducted by Sagsen *et al.* [14] and Amin *et al.* [15]. Previous studies have explained the higher bond strength obtained with the epoxy resin–based sealers by the ability to form a covalent bond by an open epoxide ring to any exposed amino groups in collagen, long-term dimensional stability, and low polymerization stress [24-26].

MTA is one of the ingredients of MTA Fillapex, and it has been suggested that the release of calcium and hydroxyl ions from the set MTA will result in the formation of apatites as the material comes into contact with phosphate-containing fluids [27]. Reyes-Carmona *et al.* reported that the apatite formed by MTAis deposited within collagen fibrils, promoting controlled mineral nucleation on the dentin, seen as the formation of tag-like structures [28]. The reason for the low bond strength of MTA Fillapex to the dentin has been attributed to low adhesion capacity of these tag-like structures.

Conclusions

On the basis of the findings of this study, AH 26 had higher bond strength to dentin in comparison to MTA Fillapex.

Acknowledgment

This manuscript is based on the thesis by Dr. Shahabaldin Azizi.

References

1. Kakehashi S, Stanley HR, Fitzgerald RJ. The effects of surgical exposures of dentalpulps in germ-free and conventional laboratory rats. Oral Surg Oral Med Oral Pathol.1965;20:340–349.
2. Sundqvist G, Figdor D, Persson S, *et al.* Microbiological analysis of teeth withfailed endodontic treatment and the outcome of conservative retreatment. Oral Surg Oral Med Oral Pathol. 1998;85:86–93.
3. Skinner RL, Himel VT. The sealing ability of injectionmoldedthermoplasticized gutta-percha with and without the use of sealers. J Endod.

1987;13:315–317.

4. Jainaen A, Palamara JEA, Messer HH. Push-out bond strengths of the dentine-sealer interface with and without a main cone. Int Endod J. 2007;40:882-890.
5. Saleh IM, Ruyter IE, Haapasalo MP, *et al.* Adhesion of endodontic sealers: scanning electron microscopy and energy dispersive spectroscopy. J Endod. 2003;29:595-601.
6. Parirokh M, Torabinejad M. Mineral triocide aggregate: a comprehensive literature review-part I: chemical, physical, and antibacterial properties. J Endod. 2010;36:16-27.
7. Silva EJ, Rosa TP, Herrera DR, *et al.* Evaluation of cytotoxicity and physicochemical properties of calcium silicate-based endodontic sealer MTA Fillapex. J Endod. 2013;39:274-277.
8. Parirokh M, Torabinejad M. Mineral triocide aggregate: a comprehensive literature review-part III: clinical applications, drawbacks, and mechanism of action. J Endod. 2010;36:400-413.
9. Roberts HW, Toth JM, Berzins DW, *et al.* Mineral trioxide aggregate materialuse inendodontic treatment: a review of the literature. Dent Mater. 2008;24:149–164.
10. Scarparo RK, Haddad D, Acasigua GA, *et al.* Mineraltrioxide aggregate–based sealer: analysis of tissue reactions to a new endodonticmaterial. J Endod. 2010;36:1174–1178.
11. Camilleri J. Modification of MTA: physical and mechanical properties. Int Endod J. 2008;41:843–849.
12. Camilleri J. Evaluation of selected properties of mineral trioxide aggregate sealercement. J Endod. 2009;35:1412–1417.
13. Vitti RP, Parti C, Silva EJ, *et al.* Physical properties of MTA Fillapex sealer. J Endod. 2013;39:915-918.
14. Sagsen B, Ustun Y, Demirbuga S, *et al.* Push-out bond strength of two new calcium silicatebased endodontic sealers to root canal dentin. Int Endod J. 2011;44:1088-1091.
15. Amin SA, SeyamRS, EL-Samman MA. The effect of prior calcium hydroxide intracanalplacement in the bond strength of two calcium silicate-based and an epoxy resin-based endodontic sealer. J Endod. 2012;38:696-699.
16. Assmann E, Scarparo RK, Bottcher DE, *et al.* Dentin bond strength of two mineral trioxideaggregate-based and one epoxy resin-based sealers. J Endod. 2012; 38:219-221.
17. Haffman BP, Mai S, Pinna L, *et al.* Dislocation resistance of ProRoot Endo Sealer, a calciumsilicate-based root canal sealer, from radicular dentin. Int Endod J. 2009;42:34-46.
18. Teixeira CS, Alfredo E, Thome LH, *et al.* Adhesion of an endodontic sealer to dentin andgutta-percha: shear and push-out bond strength measurement and SEM analysis. J Appl Oral Sci. 2009;17:129-135.
19. Goracci C, Tavares AU, Fabianelli A, *et al.* The adhesion between fiber posts and root canalwall: comparison between microtensile and push-out bond strength measurements. Eur J Oral Sci. 2004;112:353-361.
20. Barbizam JVB, Trope M, Tanomaru-Filho M, *et al.* Bond strength of different endodonticsealers to dentin: push-out test. J Appl Oral Sci. 2011;19:644-647.
21. Rocha AW, de Andrade CD, Leitune VC, *et al.* Influence of endodontic irrigants on resinsealer bond strength to radicular dentin. Bull Tokyo Dent Coll. 2012;53:1-7.
22. Gettleman BH, Messer HH, El Deeb ME. Adhesion of sealer cements to dentin with andwithout the smear layer. J Endod. 1991;17:15-20.
23. Eldeniz AU, Erdemir A, Belli S. Shear bond strength of three resin based sealers to dentinwith and without the smear layer. J Endod. 2005;31:293-296.
24. Vilanova WV, Carvalho-Junior JR, Alfredo E, *et al.* Effect of intracanal irrigants on thebond strength of epoxy resin-based and methacrylate resin-based sealers to root canal walls. Int Endod J. 2012;45;42–48.
25. Lee KW, Williams MC, Camps JJ, *et al.* Adhesion of endodontic sealers to dentin and guttapercha. J Endod. 2002;28:684–688.
26. Fisher MA, Berzins DW, Bahcall JK. An in vitro comparison of bond strength of variousobturation materials to root canal dentine using a push-out

test design. J Endod. 2007;33;856–858.

27. Sarkar NK, Caicedo R, Ritwik P, *et al*. Physicochemical basis of the biologic properties ofmineral trioxide aggregate. J Endod. 2005;31:97-100.

28. Reyes-Carmona JF, Felippe MS, Felippe WT. Biomineralization ability and interaction of mineral trioxide aggregate and white portland cement with dentin in a phosphate containingfluid. J Endod. 2009;35:731–736.

Factors Affecting Oral Hygiene and Tooth Brushing in Preschool Children, Shiraz/Iran

Shaghaghian S[a], Zeraatkar M[b*]

[a]Department of Dental Public Heath, School of Dentistry, Non-communicable Diseases Research Center, Shiraz University of Medical Sciences, Shiraz, Iran
[b]Department of Dental Public Health, School of Dentistry, Shiraz University of Medical Sciences, Shiraz, Iran

ARTICLE INFO

Key words:
Child
Inadequate Tooth Brushing
Oral Hygiene
Oral Hygiene Index
Risk Factors

Corresponding Author:
Maryam Zeraatkar
Department of Dental Public Health, School of Dentistry, Shiraz University of Medical Sciences, Shiraz, Iran
E-mail: zeraatkarm@sums.ac.ir

Abstract

***Statement of Problem*:** Inadequate tooth brushing and inappropriate oral hygiene can lead to dental caries, the most common chronic diseases of childhood with several side effects.

***Objectives*:** To evaluate factors affecting on preschool children's oral hygiene and tooth brushing in Shiraz, Iran

***Materials and Methods*:** In this cross-sectional study, we selected 453 children registered in Shiraz kindergartens in 2013 by randomized cluster sampling. The children's tooth brushing and oral hygiene were assessed using a reliable and valid questionnaire and Simplified Debris Index (DI-S), respectively. A dental student examined all the children in each kindergarten to determine their DI-S. The relationship between the children's demographic variables and their oral hygiene and tooth brushing status were evaluated.

***Results*:** Tooth brushing for 272 children (71.2%) had been started after the age of 2 years. The teeth in 96 children (24.2%) had been brushed lower than once daily. The mean of the children's DI-S was 1.19 ± (0.77). The DI-S of only 126 children (31.8%) was found to be good and very good. After controlling the effect of confounding factors, we found that the children's tooth brushing frequency was significantly associated with the number of children in the family and mothers' employment status. The age at which tooth brushing had been started was significantly associated with the fathers' education. Furthermore, the DI-S was associated with children's age, number of the children in the family, and their mothers' education.

***Conclusions*:** Oral hygiene and tooth brushing of the preschool children were not in a desirable status. Interventional procedures, especially educational programs, are recommended for children and their parents. These programs seem to be more necessary for older children, low socioeconomic families, and families with more than one child.

Introduction

Oral hygiene is careful mechanical cleaning of the teeth that disrupts the bacterial plaque, the main predisposing factor of dental caries. Therefore, it produces a clean enamel surface and prevents dental caries and periodontal disease [1]. Dental caries is a preventable infectious disease and one of the most common chronic diseases of childhood. It can cause pain, high treatment costs, reduced growth and development, speech disorders, and premature tooth loss that lead to chewing problems, loss of self-confidence, and harm to the permanent dentition [2].

For appropriate oral hygiene, dental flossing, tooth brushing [1], regular dental visits, and preventive dental procedures such as fissure sealant and fluoride therapy [3] are recommended. It is suggested that parents brush their children's teeth twice daily with a soft toothbrush of age-appropriate size and fluoridated toothpaste. It should be started early in life as soon as the first primary tooth erupts [4]. For assessing the oral hygiene, several methods have been established. Greene and Vermillion created one of the most useful methods, Simplified Oral Hygiene Index. It consists of two parts: Simplified Calculus Index and Simplified Debris Index (DI-S) which measures the amount of calculus and debris found on the tooth surfaces, respectively [5].

To enhance the children's oral hygiene, authorities need to know the factors affecting it. Previous studies showed the relationship between children's oral hygiene and some of their demographic factors such as parents' educational and occupational status [6], number of sibling in family [7], and family structure (one or two parents family) [8]. However, to the best of our knowledge, no study has assessed the impact of all important children's demographic factors on their oral hygiene in Shiraz.

Because basic information about the present oral status of the children is necessary to implement strategies to improve it, this study was designed to determine factors affecting on preschool children's oral hygiene and tooth brushing in Shiraz, Iran in 2013. The results of this study will help authorities to establish effective and appropriate interventional programs in this regard.

Materials and Methods

Setting and sampling

Participants of this cross-sectional study were the children registered in kindergartens in Shiraz, Iran in 2013. By randomized cluster sampling, 10 out of 147 Shiraz kindergartens were selected and all the children aged 3-6 years in the kindergartens in 2013 (453 children) were enrolled in the study. However, the children who were uncooperative or absent at the examination day, did not have any teeth, or did not have parental consent were excluded from the study.

Instruments

The children's tooth brushing and oral hygiene were assessed using a self-made questionnaire, and Simplified Debris Index (DI-S), debris component of Simplified Oral Hygiene Index, respectively [5]. The self-made questionnaire was prepared by evaluating and incorporating the questionnaires of previous studies [9,10]. The content validity of the questionnaire was approved by three faculty members of dental school of Shiraz University of Medical Sciences. To approve its reliability, we conducted a pilot study on 30 children's parents. The parents filled out the questionnaire twice, two weeks apart. The test-retest reliability was calculated using Spearman correlation. The coefficient values were all acceptable and highly significant (range: 0.572-0.833). The questionnaire included two parts evaluated the child's demographic information, and their tooth brushing and oral hygiene status. The first part consisted of seven questions about the child's sex and age, number of children in the family, father's job and education, and mother's employment status and education. The second part consisted of six questions as following:

Frequency of children's tooth brushing either by themselves or by their parents

- The age tooth brushing had been started for the children by their parents
- Use of preventive dental procedures such as fissure sealant and fluoride therapy for the children
- The children's previous dental visits
- Parents' satisfaction of their children's dental cleaning
- Parents' evaluation of their children's oral health status

To determine the children's DI-S, the researcher examined four labial and two lingual surfaces of six different teeth in each child. Each tooth was scored from zero to three based on the inciso/occlusocervical extent of the visible debris on its surface. The DI-S of each child was recorded as the mean scores for the 6 teeth. These scores which were from zero to three were further categorized as very good (0-0.2), good (0.3-0.6), fair (0.7-1.8), and poor (1.9-3.0) [11].

Data collection

The study protocol was approved by the Research Ethics Committee of Shiraz University of Medical Sciences (Application # 8615). After obtaining informed consent from the children's parents, a dental student examined the children in each kindergarten using a probe, a disposable dental mirror, and a headlight to determine the children's DI-S. The probe was placed on each tooth and moved along the surface to detect the inciso/occlusocervical extent of the debris. He also asked the parents to complete the questionnaires.

Data analysis

The collected data were analyzed using SPSS software version 18.0 (SPSS Inc., Chicago, IL, USA. Pearson Chi-square, one way ANOVA (with Tukey Post Hoc test), and Student`s *t*-test were used to assess the relationship between the children's demographic variables and their oral hygiene. The effect of possible confounding factors was assessed using multiple logistic regression and multiple linear regression models. An alpha level of 0.05 was considered as statistical significance.

Results

Description of the participants

87% of the invited parents (396 out of 453) participated in the study. Although more than half of the mothers (236 mothers) had university degrees, more than two-thirds of them (289) were housewives. 162 families (40.9%) had only one child and 234 (59.1%) had more than one child. The participating children were about 36-72 months old with a median age of 64 months and almost half of them (194) were girls.

Children's oral hygiene and tooth brushing

Tooth brushing for more than two-thirds of the children had been started by their parents after the age 2 years. The teeth in one-fourth of the children had been brushed fewer than once a day. About half of the children had a prior dental visit; however, most of them were visited because of the child's dental pain or other dental problems and only 77 (19.4%) were visited for check-up. Similarly, preventive dental procedures such as fissure sealant or fluoride therapy were performed only for a few children (12.9%). About half of the parents evaluated their children's oral health status as good and very good and nearly the same percentage were satisfied with the cleanness of their children's teeth (Table 1). According to our dental examination, the mean of the children's DI-S

Table 1: Oral hygiene of the studied children (N=396)

Oral health status	Frequency	Percentage
Frequency of tooth brushing		
Once a day or more	300	75.8
Lower than Once a day	96	24.2
Never	0	0
The age tooth brushing had been started		
2 years old or younger	114	28.8
After 2 years old	282	71.2
Preventive dental procedures		
Yes	51	12.9
No	345	87.1
Previous dental visits		
No previous dental visits	189	47.7
Dental visits for check-up	77	19.4
Dental visits for pain and other oral problems	130	32.8
Parents' satisfaction of their children's dental cleaning		
Yes	226	57.1
No	103	26.0
Don't know	67	16.9
Parents' evaluation of their children's oral health status		
Very good	55	13.9
Good	164	41.4
Moderate	85	21.5
Bad	61	15.4
Very bad	26	6.6
Don't know	5	1.3

was 1.19 (± 0.77) and it varied from zero to three. The DI-S of 126 children (31.8%) was considered as very good and good; that of 270 children (68.2%) was regarded as fair and poor.

Impact of children's demographic factors on their tooth brushing and oral hygiene

The factors relating to children's tooth brushing frequency

Univariate analysis showed that the children's tooth brushing frequency was significantly associated with the number of children in the family ($p = 0.002$), father's job ($p = 0.005$), mother's employment status ($p < 0.001$), fathers' education ($p = 0.003$), and mothers' education ($p < 0.001$). According to this analysis, a higher percentage of the mothers and fathers with university degree, employed mothers, employee fathers and parents with only one child brushed for their children once or more per day. However, in multivariate analysis, the only variables that showed significant associations with the children's tooth brushing frequency were the number of children in the family ($p = 0.001$) and mother's employment status ($p = 0.037$). The employed mothers were about two times more likely to brush their children's teeth daily or more than the housewives (OR=2.24, 95%CI: 1.05-4.77). Moreover, odds ratio of daily tooth brushing for the parents with one child in comparison to those with more than one child was 2.44 (95%CI: 1.43-4.15, Table 2).

The factors relating to the age tooth brushing had been started for the children by their parents

In univariate analysis, most factors showing impact on the children's tooth brushing frequency had a significant relationship with the age tooth brushing had been started, as well. For instance, a higher percentage of the employed fathers ($p = 0.001$), employed mothers ($p < 0.001$) and mothers ($p < 0.001$) and fathers ($p < 0.001$) with university degrees had started tooth brushing for their children in age less than 2 years old. However, multivariate analysis

Table 2: Univariate and regression analyses regarding the impact of children's demographic factors on their tooth brushing frequency (N=396)

Children's demographic factors	Total	Children's tooth brushing frequency				
		Univariate analysis*			Regression analysis**	
		≥Once a day N(%)	<Once a day N(%)	*p* value	OR	*p* value
Child's sex				0.486		0.268
Boy	202(51)	156(77.6)	46(22.8)		1.32	
Girl	194(49)	144(74.2)	50(25.8)		1	
Child's age				0.856		
36-47 months old	49(12.4)	38(77.6)	11(22.4)		1.04	0.924
48-59 months old	84(21.2)	65(77.4)	19(22.6)		0.94	0.851
60-72 months old	263(66.4)	197(74.9)	66(25.1)		1	
Number of children in the family				0.002		0.001
One child	162(40.9)	136(84.0)	26(16.0)		2.44	
More than one child	234(59.1)	164(70.1)	70(29.9)		1	
Father's job				0.005		0.142
Self-employed	258(65.2)	184(71.3)	74(28.7)		1	
Employee	138(34.8)	116(84.1)	22(15.9)		1.58	
Mother's employment status				<0.001		0.037
Employed	107(27)	95(88.8)	12(11.2)		2.24	
Homemaker	289(73)	205(70.9)	84(29.1)		1	
Fathers' education				0.003		0.430
High school or less	171(43.2)	158(70.2)	67(29.8)		1	
University degree	225(56.8)	142(83.0)	29(17.0)		1.29	
Mothers' education				<0.001		0.497
High school or less	160(40.4)	164(69.5)	72(30.5)		1	
University degree	236(59.6)	136(85.0)	24(15.0)		1.26	

* Pearson's chi square N= Number

**Logistic regression OR= Odds Ratio

only showed a significant association between the age teeth brushing had been started and the fathers' education. The fathers with university degree were almost two times more likely to start tooth brushing for their children under two years old than the fathers without the degree (OR=1.91, 95%CI:1.08-3.41, Table 3).

The factors relating to the children's DI-S

According to univariate analysis, there was a significant association between the children's DI-S and the following variables: the children's age (p = 0.007), number of children in the family (p < 0.001), mother's employment status (p = 0.013), and mothers' education (p < 0.001). Moreover, multivariate analysis showed that the children's DI-S was statistically related to the children's age, number of the children in the family, and mothers' education. A lower DI-S (better oral hygiene) was found in the younger children, single child in the family, and children whose mother had a university degree (Table 4).

Discussion

This cross-sectional study assessed factors affecting on preschool children's oral hygiene and tooth brushing. . Although two-thirds of the children had brushed their teeth once a day or more, most of them had been started to brush after the age of 2 years old. Only 20% and 13% of the children had a dental check-up and preventive dental procedures, respectively. Although most of the parents were satisfied about their child's dental cleaning and evaluated their child's oral health status as good and very good, more than two thirds of the children were considered as fair to poor oral hygiene in our clinical examination. Parent's employment status and educational level, number of children in the family, and child's age had a significant association with the child's oral hygiene.

Although American Academy of Pediatric Dentistry (AAPD) recommended that tooth brushing should be performed for children twice daily [4], only 75% of those in our study had brushed their teeth

Table 3: Univariate and multivariate analyses regarding the impact of the children's demographic factors on the age tooth brushing had been started for them (N=396)

Children's demographic factors	Total	Age tooth brushing had been started for children				
		Univariate analysis*			Regression analysis**	
		≤2 years old N(%)	>2 years old N(%)	*p*-value	OR	*p*-value
Child's sex				0.682		0.615
Boy	202(51)	60(29.7)	142(70.3)		1.12	
Girl	194(49)	54(27.8)	140(72.2)		1	
Child's age				0.926		
36-47 months old	49(12.4)	13(26.5)	36(73.5)		0.67	0.277
48-59 months old	84(21.2)	24(28.6)	60(71.4)		0.90	0.736
60-72 months old	263(66.4)	77(29.3)	186(70.7)		1	
Number of children in the family				0.134		0.144
One child	162(40.9)	40(24.7)	122(75.3)		0.70	
More than one child	234(59.1)	74(31.6)	160(68.4)		1	
Father's job				0.001		0.358
Self-employed	258(65.2)	60(23.3)	198(76.7)		1	
Employee	138(34.8)	54(39.1)	84(60.9)		1.28	
Mother's employment status				<0.001		0.290
Employed	107(27)	45(42.1)	62(57.9)		1.37	
Housewife	289(73)	69(23.9)	220(76.1)		1	
Fathers' education				<0.001		0.027
High school or less	171(43.2)	44(19.6)	181(80.4)		1	
University degree	225(56.8)	70(40.9)	101(59.1)		1.91	
Mothers' education				<0.001		0.231
High school or less	160(40.4)	50(21.2)	186(78.8)		1	
University degree	236(59.6)	64(40.0)	96(60)		1.45	

*Pearson's chi square N= Number

**Logistic regression OR= Odds Ratio

Table 4: Univariate and multivariate analyses regarding the impact of the children's demographic factors on their DI-S (N=396)

Children's demographic factors	Total number	Children's DI-S			
		Univariate analysis		Regression analysis ***	
		Mean ± SD	*p* value	B (SE)	*p* value
Child's sex			0.629*		
Boy	202(51)	1.21 ± 0.75		0.01 (0.07)	0.895
Girl	194(49)	1.17 ± 0.80		1	
Child's age			0.007**		
36-47 months old	49(12.4)	1.05 ± 0.72[ab¶]		-0.25 (0.12)	0.031
48-59 months old	84(21.2)	1.00 ± 0.73[a]		-0.22 (0.09)	0.019
60-72 months old	263(66.4)	1.27 ± 0.79[b]		1	
Number of children in the family			<0.001*		
One child	162(40.9)	0.98 ± 0.70		-0.32 (0.08)	<0.001
More than one child	234(59.1)	1.34 ± 0.79		1	
Father's job			0.477*		
Self-employed	258(65.2)	1.21 ± 0.77		0.01 (0.09)	0.886
Employee	138(34.8)	1.15 ± 0.78		1	
Mother's employment status			0.013*		
Employed	107(27)	1.03 ± 0.72		-0.08 (0.10)	0.447
housewife	289(73)	1.25 ± 0.79		1	
Fathers' education			0.263*		
High school or less	171(43.2)	1.23 ± 0.78		1	
University degree	225(56.8)	1.14 ± 0.76		0.07 (0.10)	0.486
Mothers' education			<0.001*		
High school or less	160(40.4)	1.30 ± 0.78		1	
University degree	236(59.6)	1.02 ± 0.74		-0.24 (0.10)	0.019

DI-S: Simplified Debris Index SD: Standard Deviation SE: Standard Error
*Student's *t*-test
**One way ANOVA
***Multiple linear regression
¶Note: The result of Tukey test was shown using letters in superscript. There was a statistically significant difference between groups without a common letter.

once a day or more. This finding was similar to those reported from other developing countries. About, 76% of Indian [12] and 44% of Hong Kong [13] preschool children had brushed their teeth once daily. Results from developed countries were similar, as well. Only 90% of 5-year-old American children were brushing their teeth once a day or more [14]. Also, in a Norwegian study, 61% of 3-year-old children and 76% of 5-year-old children had brushed their teeth twice daily [15].

Although AAPD suggested that tooth brushing should be started as soon as the first primary tooth erupted [4], only 29% of the children in our study had started tooth brushing at 2 years of age or younger. Similarly, 25% of Indian [12] and 29% of Mexican children began brushing their teeth before the age of two years [16]. Nevertheless, 86% of Hong Kong children [13] and most of Norwegian children [15] started tooth brushing before the mentioned age. The children's oral hygiene has an important effect on their oral health related quality of life and is a major predictor of adult oral health [16]. Therefore, parents should be informed about the importance of the deciduous teeth and tooth brushing at the early years of their children's life.

Through clinical examination, we found that oral hygiene status of the children in our study, similar to other developing countries, was much worse than that of the children in developed countries. Less than one-third of the children in our study were found to have very good and good oral hygiene. Mean DI-S of the children in our study was 1.19. Similarly, in a study conducted in Kuwait, the DI-S means for girls and boys were 1.5 and 1.6, respectively [17]. However, the mean DI-S in children in a Canadian study was 0.87 [18]. The results emphasize the importance of interventional programs for improving the children's oral hygiene.

AAPD recommended that children should be visited by a dentist at the time of the eruption of the first primary tooth [3]. However, about 48% of the children in our study had not been visited by a dentist previously and just 20% of them had a dental visit for check-up. Similarly, about 50% of African Immigrants' children in a Canadian study had never visited a dentist previously [19]. Also, only 25% of the children in a Hong Kong study [13] had visited a dentist for check-up. Likewise, studies showed that a large percentage of children in developed countries had never seen a dentist when they registered in the kindergarten [20,21]. This might be due to the fact that parents do not believe in the importance of regular dental visit.

In our study, preventive dental procedures had been performed for only a few children. Similarly, a study on immigrant population in San Francisco [22] and an Indian study [12] showed that there was low utilization of preventive dental services by the preschool children. This may be due to lack of parental belief in the importance of the primary teeth. Therefore, the parents' effective attention to primary teeth is an important issue to improve the children's oral hygiene, and educational interventions in this regard are recommended.

About half of the parents were satisfied with their child's dental cleaning and the same percentage of them evaluated their child's oral health status as good and very good, while more than two-thirds of the children were considered as fair to poor oral hygiene in our clinical exam. Other studies had also documented the caregivers' tendency to rate their children's dental status positively [23,24]. Amin *et al.*'s study showed that in Canada, parents rated the dental status of 44% of children as good; however, 56% of them had dental decay [19]. They were unrealistically optimistic probably because their children had not still suffered from the severe consequences of caries or parents were afraid of being judged for their carelessness [24].

Our study, similar to other researches, revealed a significant association between some of the children's demographic factors and their oral hygiene. However, there were some differences between our results and those of other studies. Although previous studies showed that the frequency of tooth brushing increased by increasing the child's age [7,25,26], our study did not show a significant difference in tooth brushing frequency of children in different ages. However, our clinical examination, similar to the studies conducted in England and Belgium [27,28] showed better oral hygiene in smaller children. The parents brush their small child's teeth; however, as the child grows up, he/she brushes his/her teeth. Children younger than 3 years of age are not developmentally ready to brush their teeth independently. Although they should be encouraged to brush their own teeth, parents are expected to perform brushing and support them in this procedure until age 6 [29]. According to this result, if parents do not do so, this preventive procedure may not be adequately efficient. Previous studies also revealed that girls brushed more frequently [15,25,27] and had a better oral hygiene status than boys [27,28]. However, our research, similar to a Mexican study [30], did not show any differences between tooth brushing frequency of boys and girls. In addition, we could not show a difference between boys and girls in DI-S and the age tooth brushing had been started. Therefore, interventional programs for improving oral health status are similarly necessary for boys and girls.

In our study, the children who were the only child of a family had better oral health. Similarly, in a Spanish and a Norwegian study, a lower tooth brushing frequency was detected in children with larger family size [7,26]. Therefore, education about the child's tooth brushing and oral health is more necessary for parents having several children. In our study, similar to previous studies, parents with higher educational level [7,25,26] and better occupational status [25,26] brushed their child's teeth more frequently and had better child's oral hygiene [6]. The findings confirm the fact that families in low socioeconomic status need more educational programs about their child's oral health.

Small children's oral hygiene has a significant impact on their oral and consequently on other systemic diseases throughout their life[31]. Therefore, it is highly recommended that authorities implement interventional programs to enhance the children's oral hygiene. It is necessary that the children be educated about the tooth, tooth brushing and consequence of disregarding oral hygiene in their kindergartens. This education needs methods compatible to their age that adequately influence not only their knowledge but also their attitude and practice. Appropriate methods of tooth brushing should be demonstrated for them; afterwards, they should brush their teeth under observance of their instructors. Appropriate and age-compatible booklet and brochure should be designed for preschool children. Preschool teachers should be trained so that they believe in the importance of oral hygiene and educate the children in this regard. In addition, some media such as television, which are the children's favorite, should participate in children's education. As parents have an important role in their preschool child's oral hygiene, it would be better to involve them in planning and implementing the programs and policies that address oral health promotion for children.

Parents should be adequately educated about correct methods of tooth brushing and other home-based preventive procedures. In addition, the importance of routine dental visits and office-based preventive procedures such as fluoride therapy and fissure sealant should be explained to them. These interventions are more necessary for low socioeconomic parents and parents with more than one child. Moreover, older preschool children need the educational programs more than younger ones.

Our study had some limitations, the most important of which being the study type which was cross-sectional. This study type has several limitations; therefore, in order to determine the factors affecting the oral hygiene of preschool children more accurately, other study types, especially a cohort one, are recommended. In addition, in this study, we relied on the parents' statements about their child's oral hygiene habits. It should be considered that these statements might be different from actual ones. However, we also evaluated the children's oral hygiene by clinical examination. Furthermore, our participants were the children attending the kindergartens, including the majority of, but not all, the 3-6-year-old children in Shiraz. For better evaluation, a community-based study is recommended.

Conclusions

Comparing our results to AAPD recommendations, we concluded that tooth brushing habits of the studied preschool children was not desirable. Furthermore, although most parents believed that their children's oral hygiene was good, Our clinical exam did not show so. To enhance the oral hygiene, interventional procedures are necessary not only for children but also for their parents. These programs are more recommended for older children, low socioeconomic families and families with more than one child.

Acknowledgments

The authors would like to thank the Vice Chancellery for Research Affairs of Shiraz University of Medical Sciences for financial support of the research (Grant#8615).

Conflict of Interest: None declared.

References

1. Heyman H, Swift EJ, Ritter AV. Art and Science of Operative Dentistry. 6th Edition. St.Louis: Elsevier; 2013. p. 41-50.
2. Kagihara LE, Niederhauser VP, Stark M. Assessment, management, and prevention of early childhood caries. J Am Acad Nurse Pract. 2009;21:1-10.
3. American Academy of Pediatric Dentistry. Guideline on periodicity of examination, preventive dental services, anticipatory guidance/counseling, and oral treatment for infants, children, and adolescents. Pediatr Dent. 2013;37:123-130.
4. American Academy of Pedodontics, the American Academy of Pediatrics. Policy on early childhood caries (ECC): classifications, consequences, and preventive strategies. Pediatr Dent. 2014;37:50-52.
5. Greene JC, Vermillion JR. The simplified oral hygiene index. J Am Dent Assoc. 1964;68:7-13.
6. Abiola Adeniyi A, Eyitope Ogunbodede O, Sonny Jeboda O, *et al.* Do maternal factors influence the dental health status of Nigerian pre-school children? Int J Paediatr Dent. 2009;19:448-454.
7. Wigen TI, Wang NJ. Caries and background factors in Norwegian and immigrant 5-year-old children. Community Dent Oral Epidemiol. 2010;38:19-28.
8. Demers M, Brodeur J, Mouton C, *et al.* A multivariate model to predict caries increment in Montreal children aged 5 years. Community Dent Health. 1992;9:273-281.
9. Hallett K, O'Rourke P. Social and behavioural determinants of early childhood caries. Aust Den J. 2003;48:27-33.
10. Begzati A, Berisha M, Meqa K. Early childhood caries in preschool children of Kosovo-a serious public health problem. BMC Public Health. 2010;10:788.
11. De Almeida CM, Petersen PE, André SJ, *et al.* Changing oral health status of 6-and 12-year-old schoolchildren in Portugal. Community Dent Health. 2003;20:211-216.
12. Chhabra N, Chhabra A. Parental knowledge, attitudes and cultural beliefs regarding oral health and dental care of preschool. Eur Arch Paediatr Dent. 2012;13:76-82.
13. Chan S, Tsai J, King N. Feeding and oral hygiene habits of preschool children in Hong Kong and their caregivers' dental knowledge and attitudes. Int J Paediatr Dent. 2002;12:322-331.
14. Franzman MR, Levy SM, Warren JJ, *et al.* Tooth-brushing and dentifrice use among children ages 6 to 60 months. Pediatr Dent. 2004;26:87-92.
15. Wigen TI, Wang NJ. Tooth brushing frequency and use of fluoride lozenges in children from

1.5 to 5 years of age: a longitudinal study. Community Dent Oral Epidemiol. 2014;42:395–403.

16. Leroy R, Bogaerts K, Lesaffre E, *et al.* Effect of caries experience in primary molars on cavity formation in the adjacent permanent first molar. Caries Res. 2005; 39:342-349.
17. Al-Mutawa S, Shyama M, Al-Duwairi Y, *et al.* Oral hygiene status of Kuwaiti schoolchildren. East Mediterr Health J. 2011;17:387-391.
18. Schroth RJ, Moore P, Brothwell DJ. Prevalence of early childhood caries in 4 Manitoba communities. J Can Dent Assoc. 2005;71:567.
19. Amin MS, Perez A, Nyachhyon P. Parental Awareness and Dental Attendance of Children Among African Immigrants. J Immigr Minor Health. 2015;17:132-138.
20. Kanellis MJ, Damiano P, Momany E. Utilization of dental services by Iowa Medicaid-enrolled children younger than 6 years old. Pediatr Dent. 1997;19:310-314.
21. Waldman HB. Preschool children. Need and use of dental services. Dent Clin North Am. 1995;39:887-896.
22. Hilton IV, Stephen S, Barker JC, *et al.* Cultural factors and children's oral health care: a qualitative study of carers of young children. Community Dent Oral Epidemiol. 2007;35:429-438.
23. Talekar BS, Rozier RG, Slade GD, *et al.* Parental perceptions of their preschool-aged children's oral health. J Am Dent Assoc. 2005;136:364-372.
24. Sohn W, Taichman SL, Ismail AI, *et al.* Caregiver's perception of child's oral health status among low-income African Americans. Pediatr Dent. 2008;30:480-487.
25. Maes L, Vereecken C, Vanobbergen J, *et al.* Tooth brushing and social characteristics of families in 32 countries. Int Dent J. 2006;56:159-167.
26. Herrera Mdel S, Lucas-Rincon SE, Medina-Solis CE, *et al.* Socioeconomic inequalities in oral health: factors associated with tooth brushing frequency among Nicaraguan schoolchildren. Rev Invest Clin. 2009;61:489-496.
27. Martens L, Leroy R, Jara A, *et al.* Variables associated with longitudinally registered plaque accumulation in a cohort of Flemish schoolchildren. Quintessence Int. 2007;38:555-564.
28. Martens L, Vanobbergen J, Leroy R, *et al.* Variables associated with oral hygiene levels in 7-year-olds in Belgium. Community Dent Health. 2004;21:4-10.
29. Canadian Dental Association. Cleaning teeth. Available at: http://www.cda-adc.ca/en/oral_health/cfyt/dental_care_children/cleaning.asp
30. Casanova-Rosado JF, Vallejos-Sanchez AA, Minaya-Sanchez M, *et al.* Frequency of tooth brushing and associated factors in Mexican schoolchildren six to nine years of age. West Indian Med J. 2013;62:68-72.
31. Li X, Kolltveit KM, Tronstad L, Olsen I. Systemic diseases caused by oral infection. Clin Microbiol Rev. 2000; 13: 547-558.

14

Analysis of Ground Water Fluoride Content and its Association with Prevalence of Fluorosis in Zarand/ Kerman: (Using GIS)

Malek Mohammadi T[a], Derakhshani R[b], Tavallaie M[c*], Raoof M[d], Hasheminejad N[e], Haghdoost AA[f]

[a]Social Determinants of Health Research Center, Institute for Futures Studies in Health, Department of Dental Public Health, Kerman University of Medical Sciences, Kerman, Iran
[b]Department of Geology, Shahid Bahonar University, Kerman, Iran
[c]Oral and Dental Diseases Research Center and Kerman Social Determinants on Oral Health Research Center, Kerman University of Medical Sciences, Kerman, Iran
[d]Department of Endodontic, School of Dentistry, Kerman University of Medical Sciences, Kerman, Iran
[e]Oral and Dental Diseases Research Center and Kerman Social Determinants on Oral Health Research Center, Kerman University of Medical Sciences, Kerman, Iran
[f]Modeling in Health Research Center, Institute for Futures Studies in Health, Kerman University of Medical Sciences, Kerman, Iran

ARTICLE INFO

Key words:
Fluoride
Fluorosis
Geographic Information System
Zarand/Kerman/Iran

Corresponding Author:
Morteza Tavallaie
Oral and Dental Diseases Research Center and Kerman Social Determinants on Oral Health Research Center, Kerman University of Medical Sciences, Kerman, Iran
Email: morteza_tavallaie@yahoo.com

Abstract

***Statement of Problem*:** The concentration of fluoride in water is usually higher in areas around the coal mines. Zarand region in the south-east of Iran is known for its coal mines. Some studies have shown the high prevalence of fluorosis and some studies reported high levels of fluoride in the region.
***Objectives*:** This study aimed to use Geographic Information System (GIS) to assess the relationship between water fluoride content and the prevalence of fluorosis and its spatial distribution in Zarand region.
***Materials and Methods*:** This cross-sectional study aimed to recruit 550 people aged 7-40 years in Zarand. Dental examination for fluorosis was conducted based on the Dean's Index. The level of fluoride in the water was determined in samples of water taken from 35 areas. Information on fluorosis and fluoride content was mapped on GIS.
***Results*:** Most participants lived in rural areas (87.25%) and had an educational status of high school level (66%). About 23% of the examined people had normal teeth, 10% had severe and 67% had mild to moderate fluorosis. Distribution of severe fluorosis was higher in areas with higher levels of fluoride in the water according to GIS map.
***Conclusions*:** GIS map clearly showed a positive relationship between the prevalence and severity of fluorosis with the level of fluoride in water in Zarand. The GIS analysis may be useful in the analysis of other oral conditions.

Introduction

Fluoride is considered to be among the top ten chemicals which are a concern for public health [1]. Based on exposure levels, it can provide both protective and harmful effects on the teeth. Exposure to optimum levels of fluoride has an anti-cariogenic and anti-bacterial effect whereas long-term exposure to higher levels of fluoride, during age periods in which the teeth crowns are formed, is associated with dental fluorosis [2-5]. Adults are not at risk of dental fluorosis, although bone fluorosis and poisoning may occur rarely in extreme fluoride intake in all ages [1, 6].

Ground water is the main source of drinking water and, therefore, is the main source of fluoride ingestion [7]. A concentration of more than 1.5 ppm increases the risk of fluorosis [8,9]. Several factors contribute to environmental and natural factors associated with high fluoride levels in the ground waters. Coal industries are among the ways in which humans add fluoride into the environment [5]. Coal mine districts in Kerman (the largest province in the southeast of Iran) are areas with major concern. Among them are Zarand city and its surrounding villages [4]. Until now it has not received enough attention for this problem. Therefore, the aim of this study was to assess the fluoride content and fluorosis prevalence in Zarand in details using geographical soft wares.

A geographic information system (GIS) is a computer system designed to present spatial or geographic data on maps. It is used for better visualization and interpretation of data. In this system, maps related to different datasets are combined, overlaid and presented as one final diagram. This diagram illustrates the alteration of different variables on a geographic map and enables the lay people to understand and interpret the relationships easier. This would give a new, more precise and attractive view of the problem which could motivate the policy makers to present a final solution for the problem. Therefore, geographic information system (GIS) was used to assess the relationship between the water fluoride content and prevalence of fluorosis and its spatial distribution on GIS.

Materials and Methods

This cross-sectional study was conducted on 7- to 40-year-old people (the population with permanent dentition) living in Zarand, in the south east of Iran. This study was approved by Kerman University of Medical Science research committee. Based on previously reported prevalence of fluoride in the region and considering a power of 90%, a sample size of 550 people was recruited for the study using a multi-stage random sampling method (city district/village, street, family, and person). Before data collection, a written and informed consent was obtained from the participants or their parents.

Demographic data (age, gender, and education level), place of living before 12 years of age (rural or urban areas), duration of residency and their past and present drinking water source were recorded.A trained and calibrated dentist carried out all dental examinations using disposable mirrors and probes and a head light. The participants' fluorosis status was recorded using the Dean's Index (Table 1)[10].

All participants should have been residents in the region for the first six years of their life (the time period in which dental fluorosis may affect the permanent teeth). People with severe systemic disease, those who had lost more than six of their anterior teeth or covered them with crowns/veneers, and those under orthodontic treatment were excluded from the study. All 35 main ground water sources of Zarand were chosen in a consensus method for water sampling. One liter plastic containers were acid washed and sterilized before sampling. Each container was flushed with the sample water three times and then filled in. After final filling, the samples were sent to Kerman geology research lab on the same day. Ion chromatography was used to assess the fluoride concentration of water samples. Detailed data related to water sampling and each regions' fluoride content were presented in a previously published paper [7]. Data on prevalence of fluorosis and severity of cases, and also on fluoride content of water were adjusted and recorded using GIS Arc and Map 10 software.

Results

In the present study, 549 eligible subjects were examined. Among them, 231 (42%) were men and 318 (58%) women. The majority of the participants (22.4%) were in the 25-35 age groups. Most participants (87.25%) lived in rural areas and had an education level of high school level (66%).

Figure 1 shows the alteration of Fluoride content in different regions of Zarand on a GIS map. Motahar-abad had the highest fluoride level with 3.51 ppm and Sang village had the lowest level of fluoride (0.33

Table 1: Dean's Index for study of dental fluorosi

Classification	Code	Criteria – description of enamel
Normal Fluorosis	0	The enamel represents the usual translucent semivitriform (glass-like) type of structure. The surface is smooth, glossy and usually of pale creamy white color
Questionable Fluorosis	1	The enamel discloses slight aberrations from the translucency of normal enamel, ranging from a few white flecks to occasional white spots. This classification is utilised in those instances where a definite diagnosis is not warranted and a classification of 'normal' not justified
Very Mild Fluorosis	2	Small, opaque, paper white areas scattered irregularly over the tooth but not involving as much as approximately 25% of the tooth surface. Frequently included in this classification are teeth showing no more than about 1 – 2mm of white opacity at the tip of the summit of the cusps, of the bicuspids or second molars.
Mild Fluorosis	3	The white opaque areas in the enamel of the teeth are more extensive but do involve as much as 50% of the tooth.
Moderate Fluorosis	4	All enamel surfaces of the teeth are affected and surfaces subject to attrition show wear. Brown stain is frequently a disfiguring feature
Severe Fluorosis	5	All enamel surfaces are affected and hypoplasia is so marked that the general form of the tooth may be affected. The major diagnostic sign of this classification is discrete or confluent pitting. Brown stains are widespread and teeth often present a corroded-like appearance.

ppm). As illustrated in Figure 1, the regions located in the west, southwest and to a little extent north-east of Zarand had a water fluoride content of lower optimum level whereas central areas through east and southeast had a water fluoride content which was higher than the optimum level.

Regarding dental fluorosis, about 23% of people had normal teeth, 10% had severe and 67% had mild

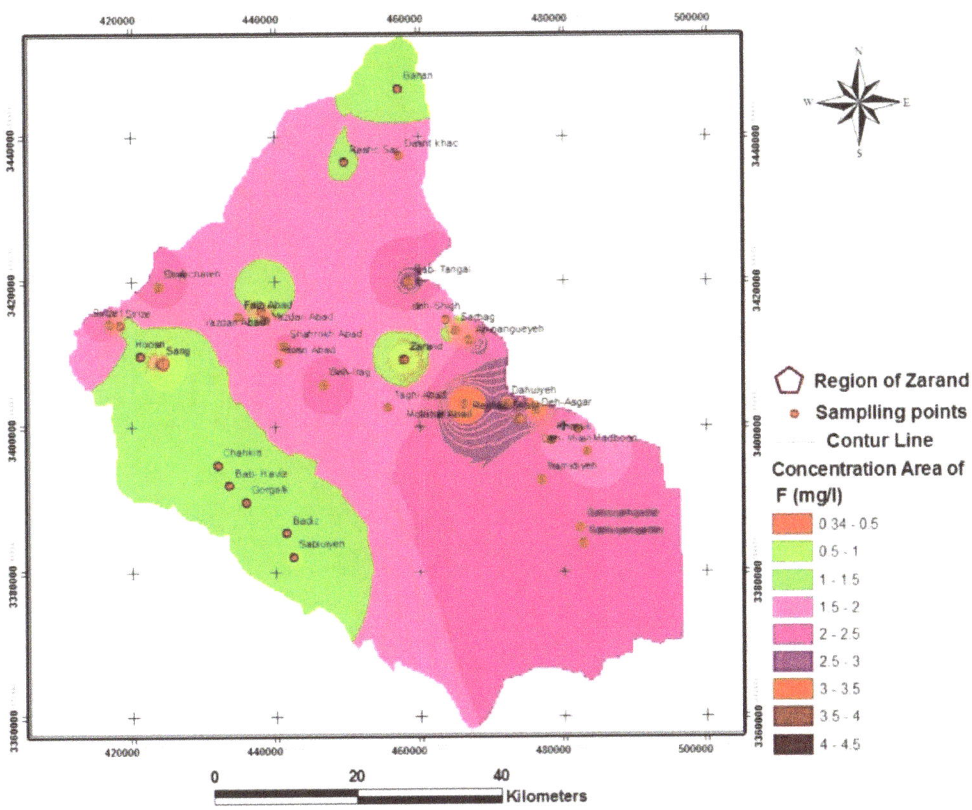

Figure 1: The alteration of Fluoride content in different regions of Zarand on a GIS map

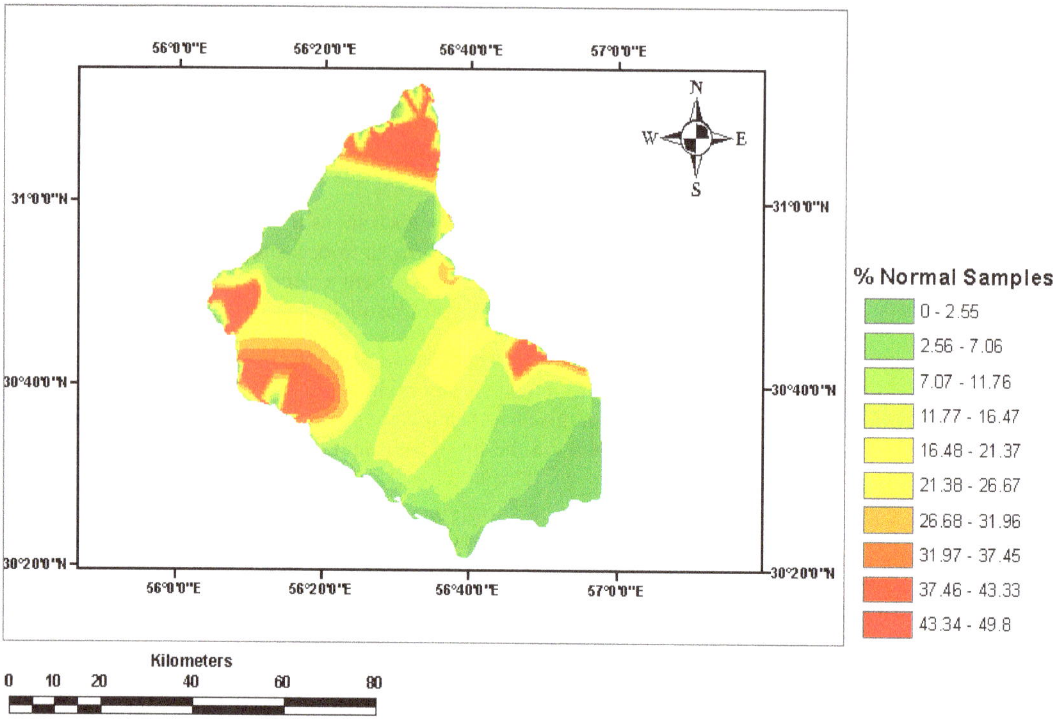

Figure2: Prevalence of "no fluorosis" in different regions of Zarand

to moderate fluorosis. The highest prevalence of severe fluorosis (45%) was seen in two villages of Gorgak and Ab-pangueyeh. Figures 2 to 6 illustrate the prevalence of fluorosis according to its severity in different regions of Zarand. Figure 7 shows the integrated prevalence of fluorosis and fluoride concentration of water in Zarand regions on one map. It is clear that those residing in the east and south-east areas with high fluoride in the ground water had a higher prevalence of severe fluorosis. Also, it is not a problem in western areas which have fluoride lower than the optimum level.

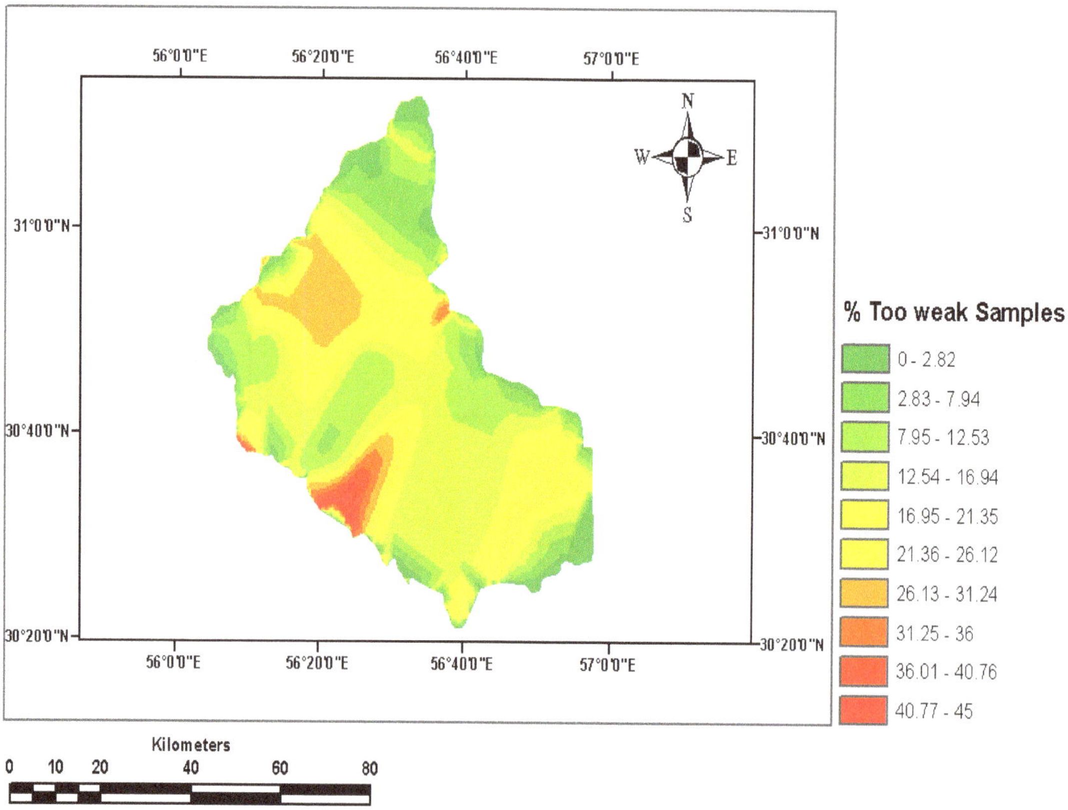

Figure3: Prevalence of "very mild fluorosis" in different regions of Zarand

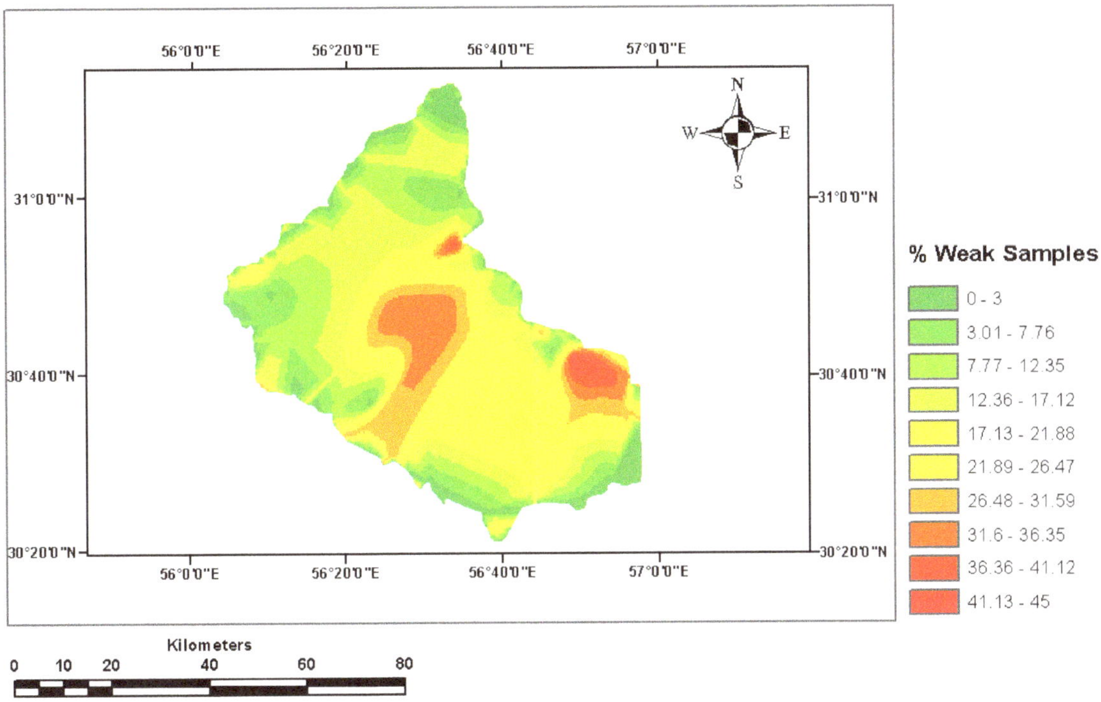

Figure 4: Prevalence of "mild fluorosis" in different regions of Zarand

Discussion

The aim of the study was to illustrate the fluorosis status and fluoride content of water on GIS maps and to integrate maps in order to give a clearer picture of the relationship between them. According to the GIS map, it is clear that regions with higher fluoride concentration in their ground water had higher levels of fluorosis. Zarand City had a fluoride concentration of 0.53ppm which was under the optimum level. Among the surrounding villages, Motahar-abad, Deh-asgar, Ab-pangueyeh and Dehuiyeh had the highest levels of ground water fluoride, respectively. It was also prevalent in these areas especially in Ab-pangueyeh with a 44.4% prevalence of severe dental fluorosis. This is possibly due to the environmental

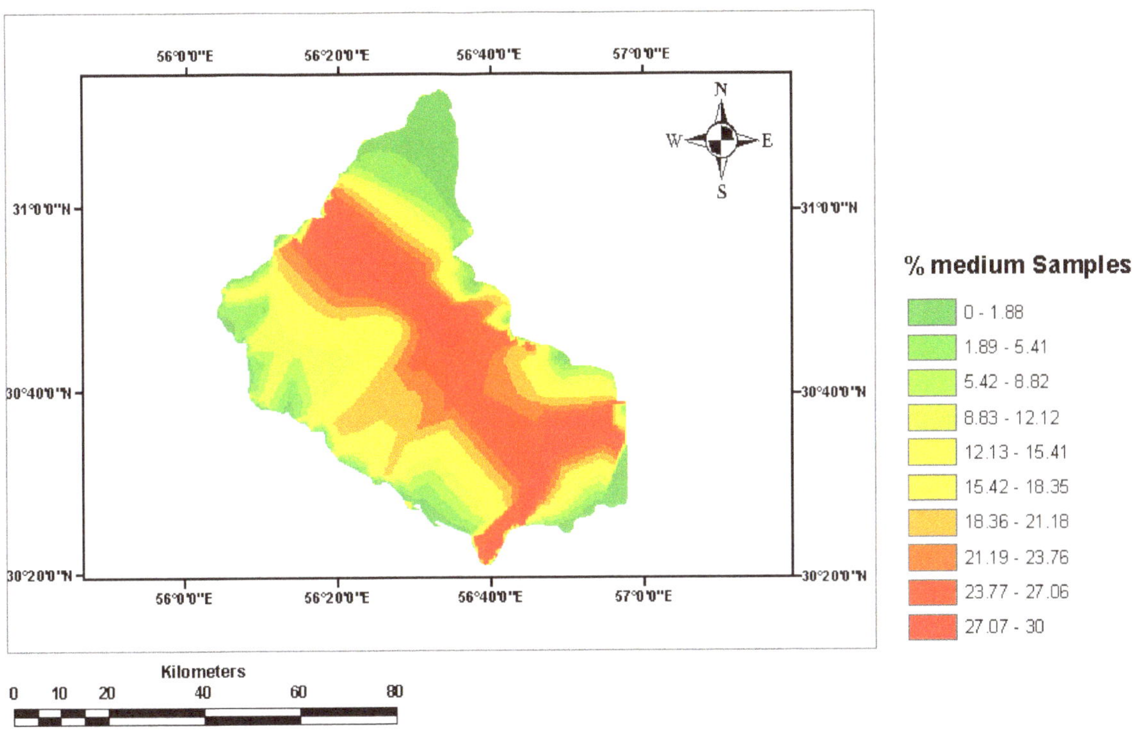

Figure5: Prevalence of "moderate fluorosis" in different regions of Zarand.

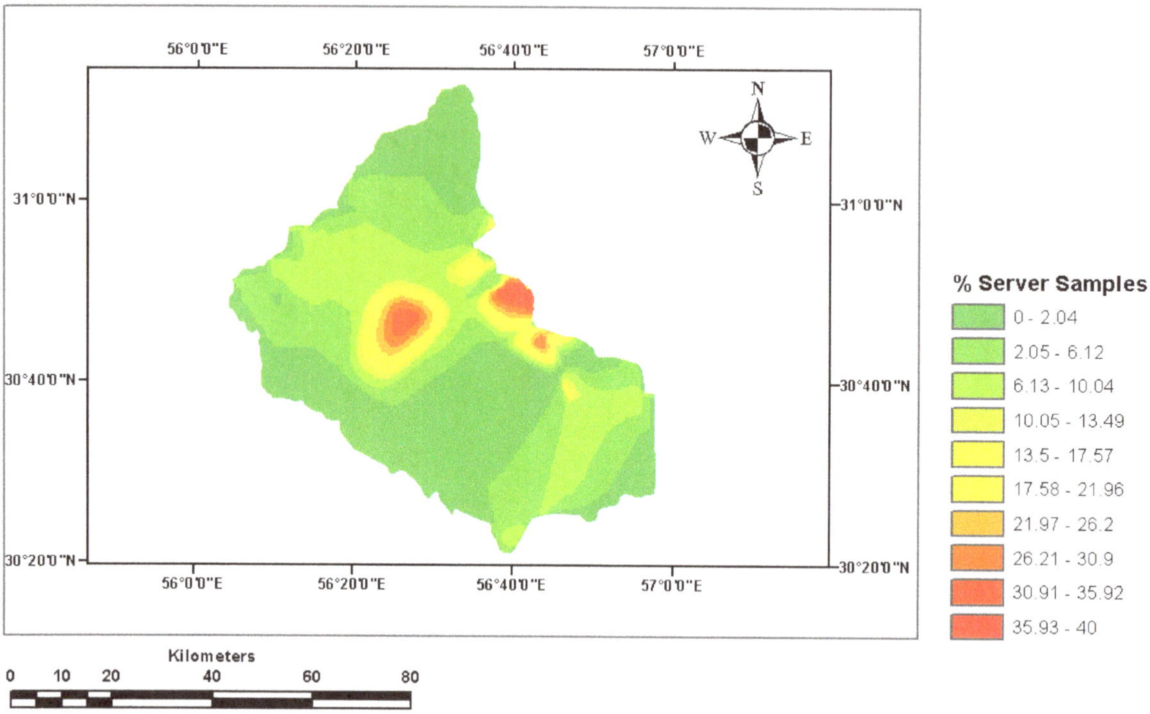

Figure 6: Prevalence of "severe fluorosis" in different regions of Zarand

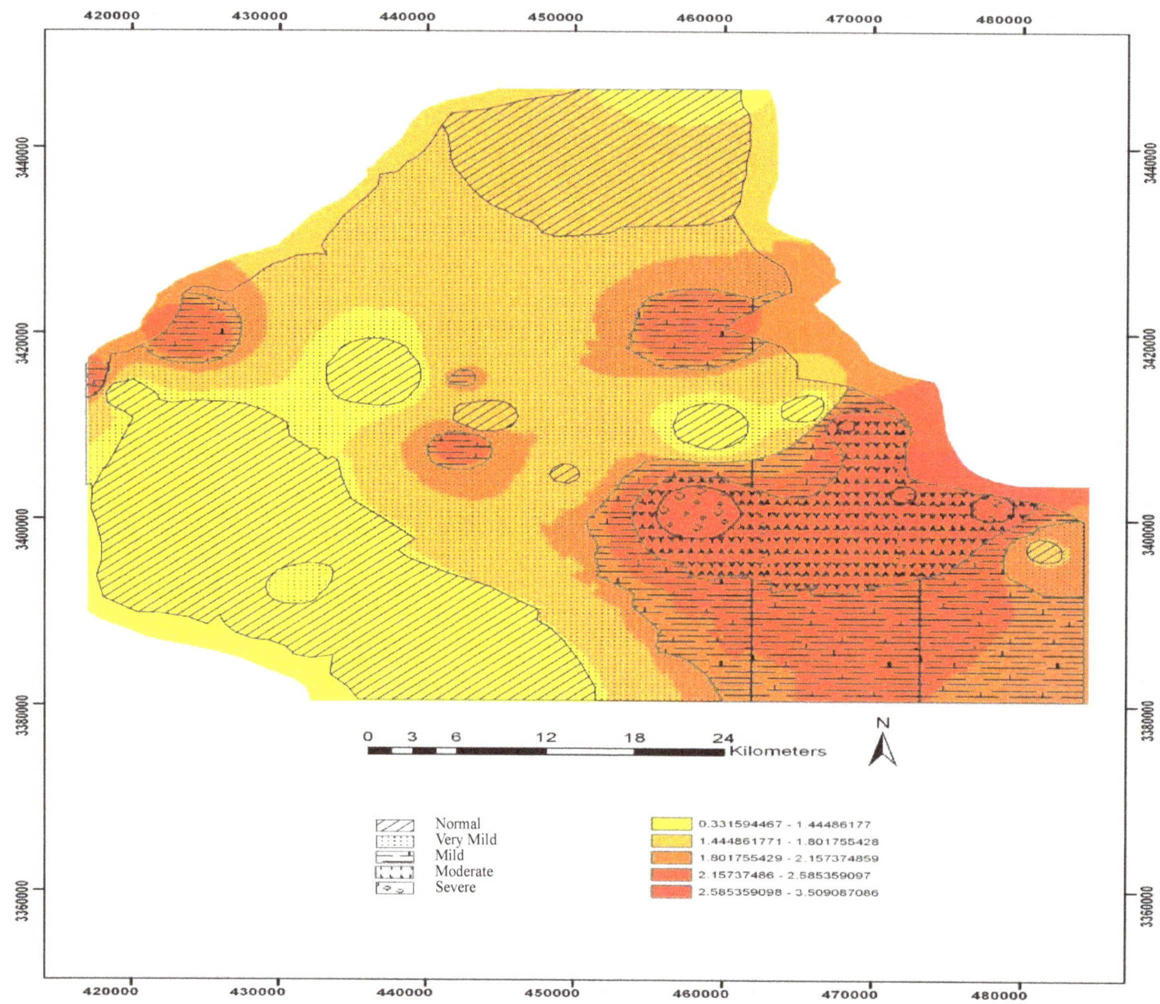

Figure 7: Lowest Prevalence of fluorosis, Low P of F, Medium P of F, High P of F, Highest P of F

and geologic characteristics of the region. Presence of Scheelite structures containing layers of coal and Alluvial deposits due to weathering is the main cause of fluoride increase in the ground water of these regions.

Other studies have also found a positive relationship between fluoride concentrations and severity [11-16]. In another study, the main cities of Kerman were assessed regarding their water fluoride content. Although Zarand city had the highest fluoride content (0.92 ppm) and Rafsanjan had the lowest fluoride concentration (0.13 ppm) in their drinking water, the fluorosis status was not significantly different between these two cities. In this study, Zarand city was investigated (not the villages and towns around Zarand, as in our study) and its fluoride content was still under the optimum level. This is why fluorosis status was not prominent [4].

Fluorine is the lightest halogen element which can be found as the fluoride ion in nature [17]. It is prevalent in rocks where it can replace the hydroxide ion. In Zarand, weathering of sandstones, Claystones and Siltstones with inlayers of coal, dolomite, lime and Scheelite results in the replacement of hydroxide by fluoride. Fluoride dissolves in the surrounding water passing through the rocks and, therefore, it enters the ground water. When the water PH is acidic, fluorine is absorbed into kaolinite clay minerals, but in Zarand due to alkaline PH, the water is left enriched with fluorine elements.

Studies have shown that GIS is a powerful tool for investigating different characteristics of the ground water [18]. GIS map shows that the ground water fluoride level is higher than optimum in a large area of Zarand region which poses a health risk to people residing there. Although drinking water fluoride is the main source of the ingested fluoride in one's diet, other foods which are high in fluoride and have a prominent role in fluoride uptake [19,20] should also be carefully consumed, especially in young children. Black tea is among the popular drinks in the diet of Iranians and contributes to a high daily intake of fluoride [21]. However this study had some difficulties because of the wide geographic area and hard access to people for examination, but it could be a good start to propose oral diseases on GIS maps for all the country.

Conclusions

GIS was a very good tool to determine relationship between severities of fluorosis with fluoride content of the drinking water in Zarand region. In the east and southeast of Zarand region, the level of fluoride was higher than optimum. Higher prevalence of fluoride in these areas indicates the need for continuous monitoring of the ground water before being it is piped into residential areas. Also, west and southwest regions had ground water fluoride levels lower than optimum; this could be a risk factor for dental caries. Therefore, regular dental visits and the use of professionally applied fluoride or education regarding the use of fluoride mouthwashes is essential for residents of these areas.

Acknowledgments

The authors wish to sincere thanks to all participants of the study and also many thanks to vice chancellor of research of Kerman University of Medical Science for financial support of the study.

Conflict of Interest: None declared.

References

1. Rango T, Vengosh A, Jeuland M, *et al.* Biomarkers of chronic fluoride exposure in groundwater in a highly exposed population. Sci Total Environ. 2017;596:1-11.
2. Petersen PE, Lennon MA. Effective use of fluorides for the prevention of dental caries in the 21st century: the WHO approach. Community Dent Oral Epidemiol. 2004;32:319-321.
3. Guissouma W, Hakami O, Al-Rajab AJ, *et al.* Risk assessment of fluoride exposure in drinking water of Tunisia. Chemosphere. 2017;177:102-108.
4. Ramezani G, Valaie N, Rakhshan V. The effect of water fluoride concentration on dental caries and in five Iran provinces: A multi-center two-phase study. Dent Res J. 2015;12:31-37.
5. Fordyce FM, Vrana K, Zhovinsky E, *et al.* A health risk assessment for fluoride in Central Europe. Environ Geochem Health. 2007;29:83-102.
6. Molina-Frechero N, Nevarez-Rascón M, Nevarez-Rascón A, *et al.* Impact of Dental Fluorosis, Socioeconomic Status and Self-Perception in Adolescents Exposed to a High Level of Fluoride in Water. Int J Environ Res Public Health. 2017;14:73.
7. Derakhshani R, Tavallaie M, Raoof M, *et*

al. Occurrence of fluoride in groundwater of Zarand region, Kerman province, Iran. Fluoride. 2014;47:133-138.

8. Chowdhury CR, Shahnawaz K, Kumari D, *et al.* Spatial distribution mapping of drinking water fluoride levels in Karnataka, India: fluoride-related health effects. Perspect Public Health. 2016;136:353-360.
9. Naik RG, Dodamani AS, Vishwakarma P, *et al.* Level of Fluoride in Soil, Grain and Water in Jalgaon District, Maharashtra, India. J Clin Diagn Res. 2017;11:ZC05-ZC07.
10. Malek Mohammadi T, Hajizamani A. Indexes for Measuring Health and Diseases in Dentistry.1st Edition. Kerman: Darkoob; 2011. p. 98-101.
11. Chen H, Yan M, Yang X, *et al.* Spatial distribution and temporal variation of high fluoride contents in groundwater and prevalence of in humans in Yuanmou County, Southwest China. J Hazard Mater. 2012;235-236:201-209.
12. Mandinic Z, Curcic M, Antonijevic B, Lekic CP, Carevic M. Relationship between fluoride intake in Serbian children living in two areas with different natural levels of fluorides and occurrence of dental fluorosis. Food Chem Toxicol. 2009;47:1080-1084.
13. Shitumbanuma V, Tembo F, Tembo JM, *et al.* Dental associated with drinking water from hot springs in Choma district in southern province, Zambia. Environ Geochem Health. 2007;29:51-58.
14. Kantharaja DC, Lakkundi TK, Basavanna M, *et al.* Spatial analysis of fluoride concentration in groundwaters of Shivani watershed area, Karnataka state, South India, through geospatial information system. Environ Earth Sci. 2012;65:67-76.
15. Kumar KD. Patterns and Distribution of Dental Caries and Dental Fluorosis in Areas with Varying Degrees of Fluoride Ion Concentration in Drinking Water. J Oral Hyg Health. 2013; 1:108.
16. Ruan JP, Yang ZQ, Wang ZL, *et al.* Dental fluorosis and dental caries in permanent teeth: Rural schoolchildren in high-fluoride areas in the Shaanxi province, China. Acta Odontol Scand. 2005;63:258-265.
17. Everett ET. Fluoride's Effects on the Formation of Teeth and Bones, and the Influence of Genetics. J Dent Res. 2011;90:552–560.
18. Shomar B, Abu Fakher S, Yahya A. Assessment of groundwater quality in the Gaza Strip, Palestine using GIS mapping. J Water Resource Prot. 2010;2:93-114.
19. Newbrun E. Water fluoridation and dietary fluoride ingestion. West J Med. 1975;122;437-442.
20. Ekstrand J, Ziegler EE, Nelson SE, *et al.* Absorption and retention of dietary and supplemental fluoride by infants. Adv Dent Res. 1994;8:175-180.
21. Simpson A, Shaw L, Smith AJ. The bio-availability of fluoride from black tea. J Dent. 2001; 29:15-21.

15

Gingival Retraction Methods for Fabrication of Fixed Partial Denture

Safari S[a], Vossoghi Sheshkalani Ma[a], Vossoghi Sheshkalani Mi[b], Hoseini Ghavam F[a], Hamedi M[a]

[a]Department of Prosthodontics, School of Dentistry, Kerman University of Medical Sciences, Kerman, Iran
[b]Department of Endodontics, School of Dentistry, Ilam University of Medical Sciences, Ilam, Iran

ARTICLE INFO

Key words:
Impression Making
Gingival Retraction
Cordless Retraction
Implant

Corresponding Author:
Maryam Vossoghi sheshkalani, Department of Prosthodontics, School of Dentistry, Kerman University of Medical Sciences, Kerman, Iran.
Email: mvossoghis@gmail.com

Abstract

Fixed dental prosthesis success requires appropriate impression taking of the prepared finish line. This is critical in either tooth supported fixed prosthesis (crown and bridge) or implant supported fixed prosthesis (solid abutment). If the prepared finish line is adjacent to the gingival sulcus, gingival retraction techniques should be used to decrease the marginal discrepancy among the restoration and the prepared abutment. Accurate marginal positioning of the restoration in the prepared finish line of the abutment is required for therapeutic, preventive and aesthetic purposes. In this article, conventional and modern methods of gingival retraction in the fixed tooth supported prosthesis and fixed implant supported prosthesis are expressed. PubMed and Google Scholar databases were searched manually for studies on gingival tissue managements prior to impression making in fixed dental prosthesis since 1975. Conclusions were extracted and summarized. Keywords were impression making, gingival retraction, cordless retraction, and implant. Gingival retraction techniques can be classified as mechanical, chemical or surgical. In this article, different gingival management techniques are discussed.

Introduction

Several factors affect the success and durability of restorations. In general, the type of impression making, setting accuracy, material flow, temperature, humidity, mixing, disinfection and pouring time have effects on the final accuracy of the indirect restorations. Supra-gingival margins are effective in periodontal health maintenance, but do not provide optimal aesthetics. So in most cases especially in aesthetics zone, the margin of the restoration is placed sub-gingivally. In tooth supported and implant supported fixed prosthesis, impression making requires accurate record of the prepared finish line area, especially in cases where the prepared finish line is located at same level of gingiva or sub-gingiva [1-3]. The gingival margin should be clean and available during impression making, allowing adequate flow of the impression material on it. Gingival sulcus must also be wide enough. Accurate impression is usually achieved with the sulcular width of 0.15 to 0.20 mm. If the sulcus width is less than this value, impression material is unable to resist against the rupture and deformation, thereupon the impression marginal accuracy is reduced. The primary factor in defective record of marginal details is due to the inefficacy of the gingival displacement technique [2]. In the present study, articles involving various gingival displacement techniques, recording accurate finish line and its effect on impression procedure are discussed.

Search strategy

Related articles on gingival management methods before impression making of the fixed prosthesis were obtained by manual searching from databases as Pub Med and Google Scholar from 1975 to 2015, then summarized and analyzed. Keywords included impression making, gingival retraction and cordless retraction.

Ideally, the retraction technique choice must be simple, quick, and inexpensive and should not cause damage to periodontal tissues. There are a variety of retraction methods including retraction cords with and without medication, rotary curettage, copper band, rubber dam, electro surgery, laser and some types of polymeric and plastic materials [4,5].

Discussion

Gingival displacement comprises bending the gingival margin far from the tooth surface which provides adequate horizontal and vertical space between the prepared finish line and gingiva to inject sufficient amounts of impression material [1,6-10].

Four forces such as retraction, relapse, collapse and displacement have a role in displacing the periodontal tissue [5,11]. Elasticity of the gingival cuff and rebound of the adjacent attached gingiva are effective in the relapse [1,12]. During retraction in the natural teeth, well differentiated periodontal fibers support the gingival fibers and partially reduce the tissue collapse after removing the retraction agent [5,12]. After preparing the finish line of the abutment tooth, the marginal gingiva is displaced to control the bleeding, gingival fluid flow and more penetration of the impression material. There are three general methods for gingival displacement including mechanical, chemical and surgical methods which can be used separately or in combination [2,5,12]. Gingival displacing (retraction) agents must have the following characteristics:

A-Effectiveness: It causes significant horizontal and vertical gingival recession and controls bleeding and gingival fluid flow. B-Retraction: The agents applied do not make up certain permanent damage in adjacent tissues. Any manipulation and chemical tissue treatment result in damage to some extent. However, this damage must be reversible and recover within 2 weeks clinically and histologically. Maximum apical recession following the gingival retraction should not exceed 0.10 mm. C-Absorption of the retraction agents into the surrounding tissues must not cause systemic effects. The amount of reabsorbed material depends on the type of retraction agents, tissue ulceration and the amount of prepared tooth abutments [13].

This study aims to express all the mentioned methods in tooth supported and implant supported fixed prosthesis.

Gingival retraction in the fixed partial dentures

Mechanical retraction

The most common method in gingival retraction which is fast, simple and inexpensive is cord packing that can be used separately or in combination with hemostatic agents in two techniques: single cord or dual cord [14]. Retraction cord penetration depth is influenced by the sulcus depth and periodontal status. In dual cord technique, two knitted cords with different diameters are used. The apical cord is thinner and is kept in place during impression making. Thus a trough is made around the preparation area and gingival cuff recoil is delayed [15]. However, using the mentioned method is limited in supra-gingival preparation margins [16]. Unpredictable tissue resorption and patient's discomfort are problematic issues associated with Dual Cord technique [5,15]. One cord is used in Single Cord method which is removed before impression making. If the preparation finish line is deep at the sulcus, the soft tissue collapse prevents accurate impression making [15,16].

Feng *et al.* revealed that tumor necrosis factor alpha (TNF-α) level increases followed by cord packing causes Sulcular epithelium and connective tissue attachment damage; however, complete clinical improvement occurs within 2 weeks [17]. Cord filament remnants and improper cord packing force may be associated with the sulcular inflammation and marginal gingiva contraction [18]. Retraction cords require high technical sensitivity and clinical skill [3]. Non-medicated Simple cords are safe but it is not a proper option to control bleeding. Cord pressure cannot stop the gingival bleeding by itself [19] and in more than 50% of cases bleeding occurs after removing the cord [5]. A simple way to reduce bleeding is moisturizing the cord [5]. To prevent the rupture and deformation of silicon impression materials, the sulcus width must be at least 0.2 mm, so the retraction agent is needed to be located in the sulcus for at least 4 minutes [5,7,9].

Serrated round end cord packing instruments are generally used with braided cord since small indentations in the instrument's head sink in the cord and prevent the instrument slippage and further trauma to the epithelial attachment. Non-serrated flat end instruments are applied in twisted cords with sliding motion [5,14]. It is suggested that one kind of copper reinforced retraction has easier placement [20].

Chemical retraction

There are three types of chemical retraction.

a-Vasoconstrictive agents, b-Hemostatic agents, c-Astringent agents

Great Britain Pharmacology Research Center explains these agents as follows: [21,22]

-Vasoconstrictive agents are not coagulated like epinephrine but act out constricting and reducing the blood vessels' diameter. Impregnated cord with racemic epinephrine has no advantage over other retraction agents, due to increased blood pressure and heart rate [22,23].

-Hemostatic agents control severe bleeding from arterioles and cut vessels [22].

-Astringent agents such as alum, aluminum chloride and zinc chloride are metal salts that inhibit plasma proteins' inter-capillary immigration, decrease cell permeability, control the moisture in the peripheral tissues through protein precipitation on the superficial layer, and increase the mechanical strength of the mucosa. Thus, protein precipitation has hemostatic effects under physiological condition. For example, ferrous chloride and ferric sulfate are concentrated astringents which make superficial and topical coagulation. However, it should be noted that denatured proteins can be involved in topical tissue destruction [2,24,25]. Aluminum chloride and ferrous sulfate are the preferred astringents in dentistry owing to minimal tissue irritation, ease of use and satisfactory results [22,26]. Chemical agents without mechanical retraction have less efficiency in the pockets deeper than 2 mm [2,27].

Epinephrine and Sympathomimetic agents

It is a common retraction agent that provides good hemostasis and vasoconstriction. It has localized hemodynamic effects [28] and causes tissue ischemia by activating sympathetic peripheral vascular $\alpha 1$ receptors. Localized vasoconstriction produces temporary gingival retraction [25,29]. However, its side effects limit its use. Maximal permissible dose of epinephrine in healthy ones is 0.2 mg and in patients with cardiovascular disease is 0.04 mg; this is equivalent to the epinephrine that is in two local anesthesia cartridges containing epinephrine 1/100000 [13,30].

Epinephrine absorption depends on the gingival health. Kellam *et al.* reported that epinephrine absorption from the retraction cord is 64% to 94% [31]. Also, Madrid *et al.* reported that intact epithelium is an effective barrier against epinephrine binding to the plasma proteins [32]. Epinephrine use as a retraction agent aggravates the risk of overdose because a soaked thread contains 0.2 - 1 mg epinephrine depending on its diameter and length which is 2.5 times higher than the permissible dose for healthy subjects and 12 times higher than the permissible dose for patients suffering from cardiovascular disease [25].

Epinephrine is contraindicated in patients using β-blocker and antihypertensive drugs [29]. Epinephrine syndrome occurs in 33% of people and produces clinical symptoms like tachycardia, tachypnea, hyperventilation, hypertension, fatigue, anxiety and depression. Epinephrine is a myocardial stimulator, so its overdose can cause ventricular tachycardia, fibrillation, angina, and heart and brain infarction. Epinephrine should not be used as a retraction agent in patients suffering from hypertension, depression and are treated with mono amine oxidase (MAO) inhibitors [33]. Epinephrine absorption can increase the blood glucose level in diabetic patients [13].

Sudden increase in the epinephrine level after a stressful dentistry session can be seen even in healthy people. If the local anesthesia containing vasoconstrictor and retraction agent containing epinephrine are used simultaneously, additive effects occurs. In general, it is recommended that epinephrine use as a retraction agent should be restricted. The only advantage of epinephrine compared to astringents is its ability to control bleeding [2,30].

The preferred vasoconstrictive material has sufficient efficiency without systemic and local side effects [34]. Systemic reaction is rare in some of the alpha agonists' vasoconstrictor materials such as tetrahydrozoline and oxymetazoline that are often used as eye and nose decongestants drops. Therefore, a lower dose of the maximum allowed rate can be used in the gingival retraction. The study of Bowles *et al.* showed that tetrahydrozoline is a strong retraction agent without any systemic side effects. The study of Tardy *et al.* showed that tetrahydrozoline is better than epinephrine in gingival retraction [2,24].

Ferrous sulfate

It has a concentrated solution to coagulate bleeding finish line and can act as an effective astringent. Within a few days (1-2 days), it can cause temporary gingival discoloration yellowish brown and black [35]. Utilization of this compound has been controversial in implants, because it can delay the setting time of the polyether and polyvinyl siloxane impression material [36]. Complete rinse out with copious water is recommended to remove the excess material. Conrad *et al*. reported that in the case of using ferric sulfate retraction agent in the ceramic translucent restoration, black internal dentin discoloration and patient dissatisfaction occur [37].

An in vitro study showed that dentinal exposure with a strong acidic ferric sulfate can remove the smear layer during 30 seconds [38]. This material has a negative effect on bonding the self-etch adhesives, thereupon marginal discoloration by microleakage is justified [5,39]. Acidic compounds of ferric sulfate 15% can make severe tissue irritation and postoperative hypersensitivity. Usually, homeostasis is achieved within 1-3 minutes [40] and opens the sulcus wide for at least 30 minutes [21]. Ferric sulfate tissue irritation is much more than aluminum chloride [41]. Nowakowska *et al.* compared the cytotoxicity of the astringent retraction agents and expressed that ferric sulfate, aluminum chloride, and aluminum sulfate have the least toxic effects on human gingival fibroblasts, respectively [42].

Ferric sub-sulfate

Also called Monsel solution develops the gingival retraction within 3 minutes [43]. Greater gingival displacement and favorable tissue recovery is achieved compared to epinephrine. Soft and hard tissues discoloration may occur to acidic and corrosive properties of ferrous salts [22].

Zinc chloride (bitartrate)

It has a burning effect and may cause soft and probably hard tissues scar; as a result, both 8% and 40% concentrations are not recommended [22,43].

Tannic Acid

The recommended time is 10 minutes. It has less hemostatic effects Compared to epinephrine, but tissue recovery is better [22].

Negatol Solution

It is a strong acidic substance, a mixture of 45% metacresol sulfonic acid and formaldehyde that may decalcify the tooth structure [22].

Aluminum sulfate and aluminum potassium sulfate (alum)

They are both hemostatic agents that inhibit inter-capillary plasma proteins immigration and disrupt bleeding through vasoconstriction and precipitation of tissue proteins on the superficial layer of the mucosa [23]. Postoperative inflammation is slightly low in concentrations to the extent of treatment levels. Aluminum potassium sulfate at high concentrations can cause severe inflammation and tissue necrosis [5]. Its tissue contraction in a concentration of 100% is less than epinephrine in a slight difference. It has limited effect on the gingival retracting, but as an alternative to epinephrine it is safe and effective. The important thing is that sulfate compounds may inhibit or delay the polymerization reaction of the additive silicone impression materials [22].

Aluminum chloride

It is an astringent that acts by precipitation of tissue proteins and vascular constriction. Its vasoconstrictor effects are less than epinephrine [24]. Among the medical impregnated cords, it creates the least irritation [17]. It has been usually used in 5. 25% concentrations and has little systemic effects [22]. Its fundamental flaw is inhibition of polyether and polyvinyl siloxan material [36]. After removing the cord, it keeps the sulcus open longer and acts more effective than epinephrine (50% of the sulcus width is closed after removal of the cord impregnated with epinephrine at the same time while the sulcus which are retracted by the cord impregnated with aluminum chloride, 80% of the its first width will remain open after 12 minutes [9]. Before impression making, remnants of aluminum chloride must be well rinsed up not to interfere with the perfect setting of polyvinyl siloxane [43].

Chemicomechanical retraction

It is the most common method used by almost 80% of dentists. To prevent bleeding during cord packing and impression making, hemostatic agents can be used simultaneously [30]. Epinephrine, aluminum chloride and ferric sulfate are usually used as pre-treated retraction cord or impregnating simple cord [44]. The use of aluminum chloride is more common than epinephrine. In one study, 33% of the participants showed side effects to epinephrine and 24% had side effects to other retraction agents [14]. Removing aluminum chloride and ferrous sulfate impregnated cords causes bleeding due to hyperemia, but epinephrine provides optimal homeostasis by long-term constricting gingival capillaries [44].

However, epinephrine has the risk of drug interactions in cardiovascular disease patients [27]. Comparing two cordless retraction techniques" Expasyl and Korlex GR" with Ultrapak cords showed similar gingival deflection, but Ultrapak cords were more painful and made more gingival recession [45]. In 2014, Sarmento *et al.* evaluated the cordless and cord retraction techniques. Both methods are similar in terms of pain and increasing the periodontal index; just psychological stress is less in cordless retraction methods. Also, fewer inflammatory cytokines are released in cordless methods compared to cord packing methods [41]. In 2012, Bennani *et al.* compared the pressure generated from cordless methods to Knitted cords. Expasyl injection generated the least pressure and its pressure will be less in reuse [46].

Polymers and pastes

Recently, polymers and pastes have been introduced in gingival retraction. Two millimeters prepared spongy tapes made from polymeric materials are swelled in contact with moisture and slowly provide enough space between the gingival sulcus and prepared finish line. Gingival recovery happens slowly within 24 hours [47]. For example, Merocyl strip is effective in gingival tissue expansion to expose the prepared finish line [48]. The strength of epithelial attachment is 1 N / mm. Very low 0.01 N / mm pressure will cause the sulcus to open and quick recovery happens. Pressure of 0.1 N / mm makes the sulcus open at 1.5 mm limit and delays the recovery to 2 minutes per 0.5 mm opening. Paste infusion into the gingival sulcus provides constant and non-destructive pressure of 0.1 N / mm. If the paste remains in place for 1 minute, enough pressure to open the sulcus 0.5 mm will be achieved within 2 minutes [49].

Expasyl paste material provides high hemostasis and a little gingival retraction and is a chemical agent in an injectable matrix that may be applied in impression making and delivery of indirect restorations. It must be isolated to the saliva during application. Expasyl paste contains aluminum chloride 15% as a hemostatic agent and White Clay for consistency and is injected directly into the gingival sulcus [4,5]. Moreover, it can be compressed into the gingival sulcus via a plastic instrument or cotton pellet. If the soft tissue biotype is thin, the paste remains in place for 1-2 minutes and if it is thick, it remains for 3-4 minutes. Retraction effects remain 4 minutes after thorough rinsing with air and water. Disadvantages are greater cost, inhibiting polymerization of polyether and polyvinyl siloxane impression materials. It is also less effective in sub-gingival positioned deep margins [5]. But it is a simple, fast and painless method which doesn't create any chemical reaction, tissue inflammation and trauma. Compared to traditional methods, possible risk of tissue trauma to the epithelial attachment, gingival recession and bone loss is avoided [50].

Gingi Trac paste is an astringent agent, generally used in hemostasis and gingival retraction. To increase the width of the retraction, a cap for single unit prepared tooth or a stock tray containing the matrix of firm paste for multiple unit prepared teeth can be used for 3-5 minutes [5].

Inert Matrix Poly Vinyl Siloxane system introduced Magic Foam Cord paste material for gingival retraction which contains expandable polyvinyl siloxane. Setting expansion of the material against gingival sulcus wall is achieved by hydrogen dioxide release [4]. It provides some amount of homeostasis, but prior to injection it is essential to use hemostatic agents separately. Increasing the width of the retraction is recommended to bite on a cap about 5 minutes to compress more paste into the sulcus. This is a simple, fast and painless system which has no chemical reaction, inflammation, and tissue trauma. However, it is less effective in sub-gingival margins [5]. Expasyl and Magic Foam Cord resulted in less tissue destruction compared to other methods [22]. In 2009, a study conducted by Beier US *et al.* revealed that Magic Foam Cord is effective in epi-gingival and sub-gingival prepared margins less than 2 mm; however, in bevel and sub-gingival prepared margins, single cord is much more efficient to Magic Foam Cord [27]. In 2013, Gupta *et al.* evaluated horizontal and vertical retraction characteristics of Stay put cord, Magic Foam Cord and Expasyl and reported that Magic Foam Cord material had the greatest effect [20].

Matrix impression making

In 1983, Livaditis introduced a system that required impression using three different viscosities of the material [11]. In this method, at first an occlusal matrix of elastomeric material (semi rigid consistency) is provided from the prepared teeth and trimmed in certain dimensions; then, cord packing is done as the usual way. After removing the cord, final impression is done using high viscose matrix of the preparation; in other words, gingival retraction is achieved from precise placement of the high viscosity matrix material. Maintaining the matrix impression in place, full arch pick-up impression is done using a stock tray containing medium viscosity material. This technique can control four forces affecting the gingiva during sub-gingival impression. Sulcular debris is removed. Matrix design prevents the collapse of the gingival margin and tearing of the impression material by pressing high viscosity material into the sulcus. The only problem with this method is the increase in chair side time [5].

Surgical Retraction

Rotary curettage

A trough is prepared with a diamond bur in the gingival sulcus adjacent to the finishing line area, following the administration of local anesthesia. The height of the marginal gingiva is approximately preserved but the sulcus gets deeper. This method can be used only if adequate keratinized gingiva is available. Trauma to the epithelial attachment may cause gingival recession due to exacerbated inflammatory response [5,51].

Electrosurgery

Following local anesthesia, passing the electric current through a thin wire can prepare a trough in the gingival sulcus adjacent to the finishing line; also, hemostasis is achieved. Moving a small J-Shaped electrode parallel to the tooth long axis can increase the sulcus width [52]. Comparison of the electro-surgery with rotary curettage showed no difference in tissue response within 4-12 weeks [53]. The sulcular volume of the impression material was greater in electro surgery compared to the rotary curettage [53]. Electro surgery is contraindicated in patients with cardiac pacemakers. It has a high risk if used with Nitrous oxide [5,52,53].

Laser

Laser can be used for gingival retraction in either direct or indirect restorative treatments. Laser characteristics depend on the wavelength and waveforms. Laser is a high powered focused beam which causes tissue vaporization in 100°C -150°C [54]. Laser induced tissue retraction is a kind of trough allowing to make precise impression with biological width preservation. It provides great homeostasis and can be applied without any localized anesthesia. It has minimum postoperative pain and discomfort [5,15].

Er-based and Nd: YAG lasers energy is absorbed into the superficial and deep tissue layers, respectively [55]. Usually in natural dentition, retraction is done by diode laser as it has less bleeding and gingival recession [15]. YSGG Laser (Water lase) is useful in either soft or hard tissue surgical interventions [56]. Co2 laser has greater hemostatic effect than Er: YAG laser, but it does not make any tactile feedback; therefore, junctional epithelium injury is possible [54]. Unlike Dual cord technique, lasers prevent tissue recession . Comparison of the Pulsed Nd: YAG lasers to retraction cord impregnated with ferric sulfate or aluminum chloride revealed that bleeding and tissue inflammation are lower, but healing rate is greater [15].

Gingival retraction in implant supported prosthesis

The use of implant-related treatment modality has increased recently. Cement retained restorations are preferred to screw the retained restorations. Custom abutments with subgingival margins are useful in aesthetic regions and minimal inter-arch space [57]. Emergence profile of the abutment prevents pickup impression in the cement retained prostheses, but the resemblance of impression copings to the manufactured final abutment in screw retained implant allows the operator to make pick up impression [4].

Tissue support of the implant is not similar to the periodontal structure, so tissue collapse is not restricted following gingival retraction. In implants, the poorly adherent, permeable junctional epithelium has low regenerative capacity. The gingival fibers are parallel to implant collar and biologic width is 2.5

± 0.5 mm [4]. Collagen fiber orientation is parallel or parallel-oblique [58]. Soft tissue biotype is also effective, i.e. thin fragile periodontal biotypes should be managed gently to prevent recession while more often a pocket is formed in thick fibrotic biotypes [5,59].

Mechanical retraction
Mechanical retraction techniques may be contraindicated around the implants, except for shallow sulcus depth and a thick periodontal biotype [4]. Microscopic scratches on the implant collar and then biofilm aggregation might occur to traumatic application of packing instruments [5,60].

Injectable matrix
The retraction force is limited due to high viscosity of the matrix, preventing the sulcus from trauma, but efficient retraction is not obtained especially when the relapsing and collapsing forces are important. Biologic width is greater in dental implants compared to natural teeth, i.e. in aesthetics region the implants are deeply placed [5].

Rotary curettage, Electrosurgery, Laser
Rotary curettage has a high risk to scratch the implant surface and exposure of implant threads. Electro-surgery is contraindicated in implants (arcing happens). Unlike other lasers, prime chromphore for CO2 laser is water. Therefore, it reflects off metal surfaces. CO2 lasers absorb little energy near the metallic implant surfaces and temperature increases less than 3°C. Also, these lasers do not alter the implant surface properties. Lasers expose the implant margins by creating a trough. Therefore, its application around the deep implants creates large defects. Indeed, it is questionable in anterior, aesthetics regions [5,61].

G- Cuff
There are challenging techniques to record subgingival contour of the abutment. Comparison of the implants to the teeth showed that there was not a special technique to retract the gingiva before impression making. Chang *et al.* [62] evaluated the effects of cordless retraction material (Expasyl) on the implant surface and found that minimal changes occurred. Wide healing caps or temporary abutments which are used in some kinds of implant systems (e.g. Bicon) have not predictable results due to various tissue rebound. G-Cuff™ is an impression device that is claimed taking an accurate registration of a dental implant abutment.

The main purpose of G-Cuff is to support the soft tissue that surrounds the implant abutment. So it retracts the gingiva to allow the impression material or digital intra-oral scanner recording the implant abutment, so the final restoration can be accomplished within two visits. The instructor claimed that the restoration using G cuff is more accurate than open tray and close tray impression techniques [4]. It is helpful for unidentified dental implants and eliminates the need to transfer the copings and analogs. It is not traumatic for the soft tissue unlike retraction cord [63]. However, more studies are recommended to verify its efficiency. Further research is recommended, especially on abutment level impressions.

Conclusions

Gingival retraction techniques can be classified as mechanical, chemical or surgical. In this article, different gingival management techniques comprising non-medicated cords, medicated cord, cordless techniques, astringent hemostatic agents, gingival retraction paste, vasoconstrictive agents, lasers, rotary curettage, electrosurgery were discussed. Also, gingival retraction in dental implants and digital impression were discussed.

Conflict of Interest
None to declare.

References

1. Al Hamad KQ, Azar WZ, Alwaeli HA, *et al.* A clinical study on the effects of cordless and conventional retraction techniques on the gingival and periodontal health. J Clin Periodontol. 2008;35:1053-1058.
2. Kostić I, Najman S, Kostić M, *et al.* Comparative review of gingival retraction agents. Acta medica Medianae. 2012;51:81-83.
3. Rosenstiel SF, Land MF, Fujimoto J. Contemporary fixed prosthodontics: Elsevier Health Sciences;2006.
4. Bennani V, Schwass D, Chandler N. Gingival retraction techniques for implants versus teeth: current status. J Am Dent Assoc. 2008;139:1354-1363.
5. Prasad KD, Hegde C, Agrawal G, *et al.* Gingival displacement in prosthodontics: A critical review of existing methods. J Interdiscip Dentistry.

2011;1:80-86.
6. Baharav H, Kupershmidt I, Laufer B-Z, *et al.* The effect of sulcular width on the linear accuracy of impression materials in the presence of an undercut. Int J Prosthodont. 2004;17:585-589.
7. Donovan TE, Chee WW. Current concepts in gingival displacement. Dent Clin North Am. 2004;48:433-444.
8. Lampe I, Marton S, Hegedüs C. Effect of mixing technique on shrinkage rate of one polyether and two polyvinyl siloxane impression materials. Int J Prosthodont. 2004;17:590.
9. Laufer BZ, Baharav H, Langer Y, *et al.* The closure of the gingival crevice following gingival retraction for impression making. J Oral Rehabil. 1997;24:629-635.
10. Laufer BZ, Baharav H, Ganor Y, *et al.* The effect of marginal thickness on the distortion of different impression materials. J Prosthet Dent. 1996;76:466-471.
11. Livaditis GJ. The matrix impression system for fixed prosthodontics. J Prosthet Dent. 1998;79:208-216.
12. Livaditis GJ. Comparison of the new matrix system with traditional fixed prosthodontic impression procedures. J Prosthet Dent. 1998;79:200-207.
13. Kumbuloglu O, User A, Toksavul S, *et al.* Clinical evaluation of different gingival retraction cords. Quintessence Int. 2007;38:92-98.
14. Hansen PA, Tira DE, Barlow J. Current Methods of Finish-Line Exposure by Practicing Prosthodontists. J Prosthodont. 1999;8:163-170.
15. Scott A. Use of an erbium laser in lieu of retraction cord: a modern technique. Gen Dent. 2005;53:116-119.
16. Cloyd S, Puri S. Using the double-cord packing technique of tissue retraction for making crown impressions. Dent Today. 1999;18:54-59.
17. Feng J, Aboyoussef H, Weiner S, *et al.* The effect of gingival retraction procedures on periodontal indices and crevicular fluid cytokine levels: a pilot study. J Prosthodont. 2006;15:108-112.
18. De Gennaro G, Landesman H, Calhoun J, *et al.* A comparison of gingival inflammation related to retraction cords. J Prosthet Dent. 1982;47:384-386.
19. Ruel J, Schuessler PJ, Malament K, *et al.* Effect of retraction procedures on the periodontium in humans. J Prosthet Dent. 1980;44:508-515.
20. Gupta A, Prithviraj D, Gupta D, *et al.* Clinical evaluation of three new gingival retraction systems: A research report. J Indian Prosthodont Soc. 2013;13:36-42.
21. Mohan M, Gupta A, Shenoy V, *et al.* Pharmacological agents in dentistry: a review. Br J Pharm Res. 2011;1:66-87.
22. Tarighi P, Khoroushi M. A review on common chemical hemostatic agents in restorative dentistry. Dent Res J. 2014;11:423-428.
23. Jokstad A. Clinical trial of gingival retraction cords. J Prosthet Dent. 1999;81:258-261.
24. Bowles W, Tardy S, Vahadi A. Evaluation of new gingival retraction agents. J Dent Res. 1991;70:1447-1449.
25. Polat NT, Ozdemir AK, Turgut M. Effects of gingival retraction materials on gingival blood flow. Int J Prosthodont. 2007;20:57-62.
26. Mohammadzadeh Akhlaghi NSZ SS, Safari S. Evaluation of upper first premolars root thickness (In vitro). J Endod. 2005;31:228.
27. Beier US, Kranewitter R, Dumfahrt H. Quality of impressions after use of the Magic Foam Cord gingival retraction system--a clinical study of 269 abutment teeth. Int J Prosthodont. 2009;22:143-147.
28. Weir DJ, Williams BH. Clinical effectiveness of mechanical-chemical tissue displacement methods. J Prosthet Dent. 1984;51:326-329.
29. Bader JD, Bonito AJ, Shugars DA. A systematic review of cardiovascular effects of epinephrine on hypertensive dental patients. Oral Surg Oral Med Oral Pathol Oral Radiol Endod. 2002;93:647-653.
30. Csillag M, Nyiri G, Vag J, *et al.* Dose-related effects of epinephrine on human gingival blood flow and crevicular fluid production used as a soaking solution for chemo-mechanical tissue retraction. J Prosthet Dent. 2007;97:6-11.
31. Kellam SA, Smith JR, Scheffel SJ. Epinephrine absorption from commercial gingival retraction cords in clinical patients. J Prosthet Dent. 1992;68:761-765.
32. Madrid C, Courtois B, Vironneau M. Recommendations to use vasoconstrictors in dentistry and oral surgery. Med Bucc Chir Bucc. 2003;9:1-30.
33. Hilley M, Milan S, Giescke Jr A, *et al.* Fatality associated with the combined use of halothane and gingival retraction cord. Anesthesiology. 1984;60:587-588.

34. Kopač I, Cvetko E, Pavlica Z, *et al.* Gingival tissue inflammatory response following treatment with chemical retraction agents in Beagle dogs. Pflügers Archiv. 2001;442:145-146.
35. Wassell R, Barker D, Walls A. Crowns and other extra-coronal restorations: impression materials and technique. Br Dent J. 2002;192:679-690.
36. Csempesz F, Vág J, Fazekas Á. In vitro kinetic study of absorbency of retraction cords. J Prosthet Dent. 2003;89:45-49.
37. Conrad HJ, Holtan JR. Internalized discoloration of dentin under porcelain crowns: a clinical report. J Prosthet Dent. 2009;101:153-157.
38. Land MF, Rosenstiel SF, Sandrik JL. Disturbance of the dentinal smear layer by acidic hemostatic agents. J Prosthet Dent. 1994;72:4-7.
39. Farzin M, Safari S, Vojdani M. Bond strength and deflection of two denture base resin material bonded to a hard Relining material. J Isfahan Dent Uni. 2010;6:195-202.
40. Thomas MS, Joseph RM, Parolia A. Nonsurgical gingival displacement in restorative dentistry. Compend Contin Educ Dent. 2011;32:26-34.
41. Sarmento H, Leite F, Dantas R, *et al.* A double-blind randomised clinical trial of two techniques for gingival displacement. J Oral Rehabil. 2014;41:306-313.
42. Nowakowska D, Saczko J, Kulbacka J, *et al.* Dynamic oxidoreductive potential of astringent retraction agents. Folia Biol (Praha). 2010;56:263-268.
43. Gupta G, Sunil Kumar M, Rao H, *et al.* Astringents in dentistry: a review. Asian J Pharm Health Sci. 2012;2:428-432.
44. Fazekas A, Csempesz F, Csabai Z, *et al.* Effects of pre-soaked retraction cords on the microcirculation of the human gingival margin. Oper Dent. 2002;27:343-348.
45. Yang JC, Tsai CM, Chen MS, *et al.* Clinical study of a newly developed injection-type gingival retraction material. Chin Dent J. 2005;24:147-151.
46. Prasanna G, Reddy K, Kumar R, *et al.* Evaluation of Efficacy of Different Gingival Displacement Materials on Gingival Sulcus Width. J Contem Dent Pract. 2013;14:217-221.
47. Ferrari M, Nathanson D. Tissue management and retraction technique combined with all-ceramic crowns: case reports. Pract Periodontics Aesthet Dent. 1995;7:87-94.
48. Ferrari M, Cagidiaco MC, Ercoli C. Tissue management with a new gingival retraction material: a preliminary clinical report. J Prosthet Dent. 1996;75:242-247.
49. Lesage P. Expasyl: protocol for use with fixed prosthodontics. Clinic. 2002;23:97-103.
50. Shannon A. Expanded clinical uses of a novel tissue-retraction material. Compend Contin Educ Dent. 2002;23:3-6.
51. Brady WF. Periodontal and restorative considerations in rotary gingival curettage. J Am Dent Assoc. 1982;105:231-236.
52. Shillingburg HT, Sather DA, Wilson E, *et al.* Fundamentals of fixed prosthodontics: Quintessence Pub.2012.
53. De Vitre R, Galburt RB, Maness WJ. Biometric comparison of bur and electrosurgical retraction methods. J Prosthet Dent. 1985;53:179-182.
54. Parker S. The use of lasers in fixed prosthodontics. Dent Clin North Am. 2004;48:971-998.
55. Chartrand A. Integrating laser dentistry into aesthetic dentistry. Oral Health. 2005;13-18.
56. Jacboson B, Berger J, Kravitz R, *et al.* Laser pediatric crowns performed without anesthesia: a contemporary technique. J Clin Pediatr Dent. 2003;2:11-12.
57. Misch CE. Dental implant prosthetics. 2nd Edition: Elsevier Health Sciences: 2014.
58. Tetè S, Mastrangelo F, Bianchi A, *et al.* Collagen fiber orientation around machined titanium and zirconia dental implant necks: an animal study. Int J Oral Maxillofac Implants. 2009;24:52-58.
59. Linkevicius T, Apse P, Grybauskas S, *et al.* The influence of soft tissue thickness on crestal bone changes around implants: a 1-year prospective controlled clinical trial. Int J Oral Maxillofac Implants. 2009;24:712-719.
60. Subramani K, Jung RE, Molenberg A, *et al.* Biofilm on dental implants: a review of the literature. Int J Oral Maxillofac Implants. 2009;24:616-626.
61. Martin E. Lasers in dental implantology. Dent Clin North Am. 2004;48:999-1015.
62. Chang YS, Bennani V, Tawse-Smith A, *et al.* Effect of a cordless retraction paste material on implant surfaces: an in vitro study. Braz Oral Res. 2011;25:492-499.
63. Deogade SC, Mantri SS, Dube G, *et al.* A New Trend in Recording Subgingival Tissue around an Implant While Making a Direct Abutment Impression. Case Rep Dent. 2014;2014.

Assessing the Effect of Dental Implants Thread Design on Distribution of Stress in Impact Loadings Using Three Dimensional Finite Element Method

Zarei I[a], Khajehpour S[a], Sabouri A[b], Haghnegahdar AZ[c] , Jafari K[d]

[a]Department Of Mechanical Engineering, Collage of Engineering, Shiraz Branch, Islamic Azad University, Shiraz, Iran
[b]Department of Prosthodontics, School of Dentistry, Shiraz University of Medical Sciences, Shiraz, Iran
[c]Department of Oral and Maxillofacial Radiology, School of Dentistry, Shiraz University of Medical Sciences, Shiraz, Iran
[d]Department of Prosthodontics, School of Dentistry, Ardabil University of Medical Sciences, Ardabil, Iran

ARTICLE INFO

Key words:
Dental Implant
Stress
Thread
Finite Element
Cortical Bone

Corresponding Author:
Salar Khajehpour
Department of Mechanical Engineering, Collage of Engineering, Shiraz Branch, Islamic Azad University , Shiraz, Iran.
E-mail: skhajehpour@gmail.com

Abstract

***Statement of Problem*:** Impacts and accidents are considered as the main factors in losing the teeth, so the analysis and design of the implants that they can be more resistant against impacts is very important. One of the important numerical methods having widespread application in various fields of engineering sciences is the finite element method. Among its wide applications, the study of distribution of power in complex structures can be noted.

Objectives: The aim of this research was to assess the geometric effect and the type of implant thread on its performance; we also made an attempt to determine the created stress using finite element method.

Materials and Methods: In this study, the three dimensional model of bone by using Cone Beam Computerized Tomography (CBCT) of the patient has been provided. The implants in this study are designed by Solid Works software. Loading is simulated in explicit dynamic, by struck of a rigid body with the speed of 1 mm/s to implant vertically and horizontally; and the maximum level of induced stress for the cortical and trabecular bone in the ANSYS Workbench software was calculated.

Results: By considering the results of this study, it was identified that, among the designed samples, the maximum imposed stress in the cortical bone layer occurred in the first group (straight threads) and the maximum stress value in the trabecular bone layer and implant occurred in the second group (tapered threads).

Conclusions: Due to the limitations of this study, the implants with more depth thread, because of the increased contact surface of the implant with the bone, caused more stability; also, the implant with smaller thread and shorter pitch length caused more stress to the bone.

Introduction

By entering the engineering science to the medical field, we can see a lot of developments in this field which help the patients and medical science. It is crystal clear that losing teeth has undeniable effects on the patients' aesthetic, and their confidence. The factors such as impact and accident in any age may lead to loss of the human's natural teeth; therefore, to have self-confidence and for cosmetic concerns people decide to plant and replace the artificial tooth.

Based on the conducted researches, the portability success of the implant procedure has been announced between 92 to 97 percent [1]; nevertheless, several factors are involved in the failure of the implant and commonly aging is the most important of them. Also, various factors are effective on the consistency and suitability of the implant, among which being the type of thread and its design [2,3]. As appropriate design can reduce the stress or its distribution can be homogenized, it would be more probable to increase the success of the implant. The failure factors include lack of junction of the implant with the adjacent bone and the excess loads as well as weak health of the mouth and tooth [4].

Considering the biomechanical principles in the implant of the tooth provides the possibility of a better remedy design for patients and dentists. The forces imposed on the implant lead to increase in the stress on it. The type of the load exerted on the implant is effective on the mode distribution of stress. The excess exerted load surrounding the implant causes very small cracks in the bone that leads to loosening and probable breaking of the implant. If as far as possible the forces are exerted vertically to the implant axis, less stress will be imposed on the bone adjacent to the implant [5]. So far, various studies have been conducted on the effects of implant design on distribution of stress and strain surrounding the implant bone. Schrotenboer *et al.* [6] conducted a study on the effect of the platform and tiny teeth on the changes in the level of bone stress by using the finite element.

Ao *et al.* [7] conducted a study on the optimal design of the width and height of the thread, investigating the maximum displacement of the cylindrical implants by using the finite element method. Abuhussein *et al.* [2] also conducted a study on the effect of implant threads assessing thread screw, thread geometry, helix angle, thread lifetime and its width, all of which were effective on the stability of the implant. Various studies have confirmed the advantages of using the thread at the neck of the implant in terms of implant contact and the bone and maintaining the marginal bone area [3]. Several researches have been carried out on treatment through the method of finite element; however, among them, no study has been published on the effect of implant thread type on the distribution of stress on the bone surrounding the implant under the impact of loading yet.

This study aimed to do an accurate review on three different thread design, so that a full recognition would be obtained from the mode of their stress on the jawbone. By using the results of this study, the choice of the implant for patients and dentists is done easier and more accurate.

Materials and Methods

In this study, a three-dimensional model of the bone

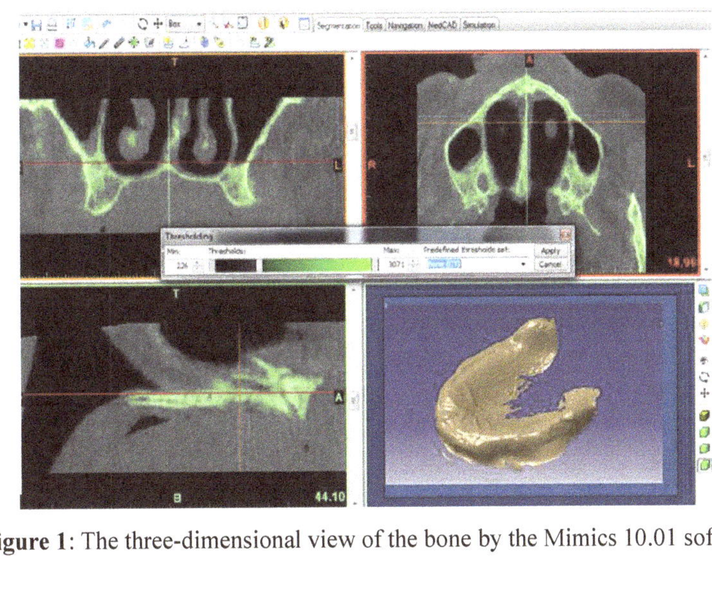

Figure 1: The three-dimensional view of the bone by the Mimics 10.01 software

was designed using CBCT of an old patient by Mimics 10.01 software (Figure 1) . In this design, the bone is designed in the form of dual layer: 1-cortical (outer layer) and 2-trabecular (inner layer). The thickness of the cortical layer was considered 0.75 mm and trabecular 11.74 mm since the cortical bone as a compact shell covers the central part of the trabecular bone.

The articles have suggested several methods for implant modeling [1-5]. The modeling of the implant in some studies is in the form of a simple cylinder [2]. Some have used the obtained data of CT scan of patients' jawbone and transferred them to those from the scan to the software design [8]. The used implants in this study were selected from DENTIS Company (951,Woram-Dong, Dalseo-Gu, Daegu, South Korea). The implants with a length of 10 mm and a diameter of 4.1 mm were used for placing in the jawbone. (Figures 2 and 3)

The analysis of the finite element

In this study, three different types of implants with various threads and one kind of abutment in the explicit dynamic loading depending on time (impact loading) were studied at the angels of 0° (Axial loading) and 90 ° (Bending loading). First group: Straight implant, second group: Tapered implant, third group: Tapered II implant.

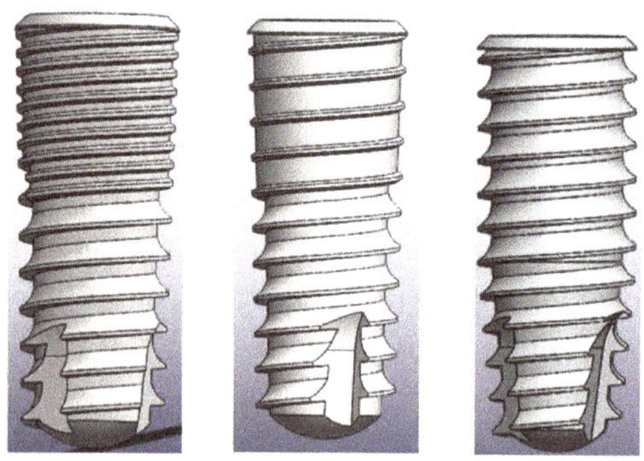

Figure 2: The implants designed in Solid works software

Table 1: The mechanical properties of the materials used in the study

Material	Elastic Moduls (GPa)	Possion Ratio(ν)	Density (g/cm^{-3})
Titanium	110	0.35	4.5
Cortical Bone	1.34	0.30	0.71
Trabecular Bone	0.15	0.30	1.86

The designed models in the Solid Works software were transferred to ANSYS Work bench 14 software to do the finite element analysis. One of the factors causing differences in the results of various analyses is the characteristics of the materials attributed to different components and geometry.

These materials can be introduced in the form of isotropic, anisotropic and orthotropic. The first step for starting the analysis is importing the data related to the mechanical properties of the materials used in the analysis. In this study, the same as many other articles [9-11], the behavior of all materials such as bone and implant in the form of isotropic and linear elastic have been introduced. The properties of materials such as elastic modulus, the Poisson's coefficient and density based on Table 1 were defined for this software Table 1.

After transferring the model to the ANSYS software and attribution of the material properties to its different parts, it was meshed uniformly. Identifying the type and size of the elements in an

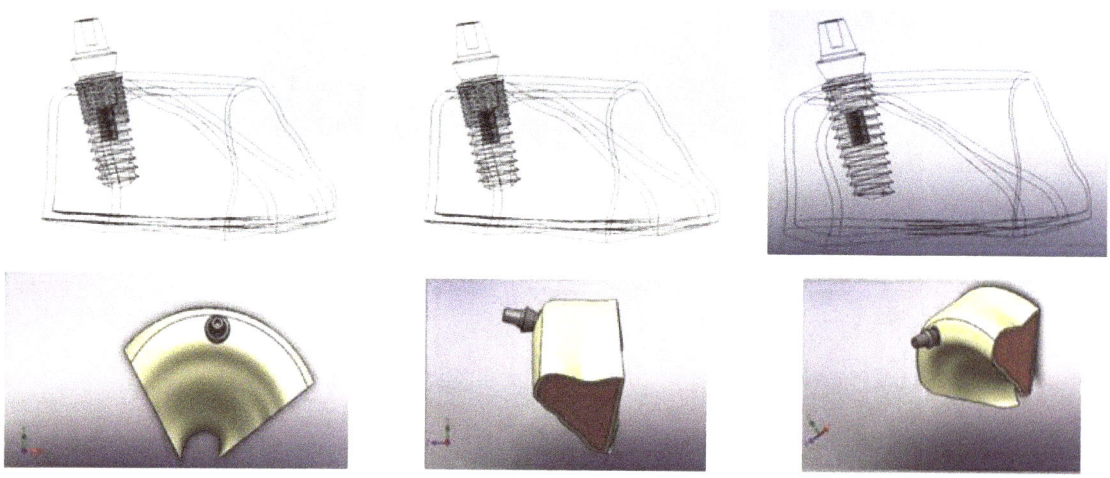

Figure 3: The placement of the implants and abatement in the bone

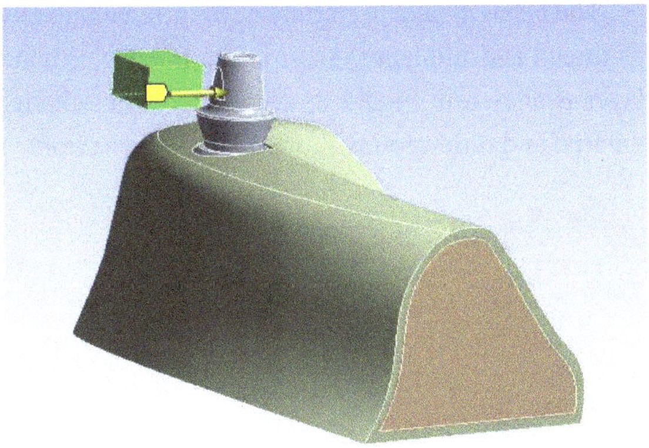

Figure 4: Imposing the bending loading towards the implant

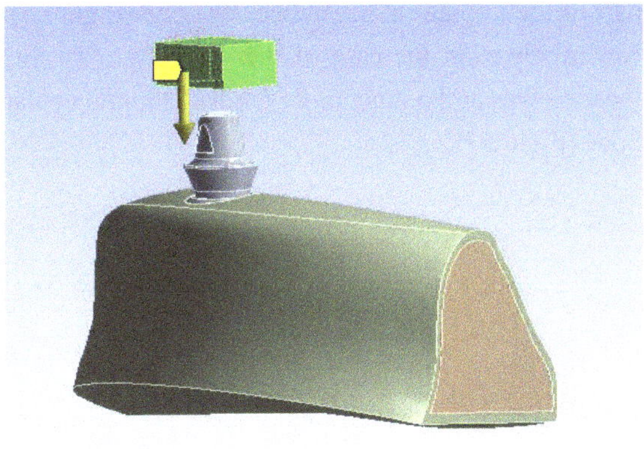

Figure 5: Imposing the axial loading towards the implant

object is the main point of analysis process. Due to the application of tetrahedron three dimensional elements in the objects with complication geometries, in this study the Solid 187 element was used for meshing the different parts.

Solid 187 is a tetrahedral three dimensional element with 10 nodes. Each node in three directions of X, Y, Z can be replaced and because of the existence of 10 nodes, it has a very high ability in matching with figures and compound geometries. This type of element is used for studying the behavior of stress and strain, plastic and hyper-elastic in the complicated geometries and the three dimensional analysis. Noobacky and Sanio used this element for meshing in their study [12,13].

Boundary conditions

The border conditions have a great effect on the distribution of the forces and results. These conditions can be considered as immobile or mobile. The mandible in terms of the border conditions is quite different from the maxilla. In the mandible, the displacement rate is defined in the conditions of being as an abutment because of its mobility and the border conditions for the maxilla have been considered in fixed form.

Loading simulation

The rate and direction of force in different dental models according to the age, gender, type of tooth, etc. are different. In the explicit dynamic analysis to simulate an axial and the bending loading, a rigid body with the speed of 1 mm/s has struck to implant vertically and horizontally (Figures 4 and 5).

Results

The force imposed on the object is called "impact load" that is exerted within short time. The analysis of the impact load is timely and non-linear. In this study, as the aim was to assess the effects of thread type on the stress distribution of the bone and implant.

Axial Loading Simulation

In the analysis of axial load impact, the maximum imposed stress to the different bone layers as well as the implant can be observed in Table 2. In this regard, the minimum value belongs to the third group and its value is 0.8 MPa and the maximum stress occurred in the first group and its value is 2.4 MPa which is two times more than the stress in the third group.

In the axial loading, the maximum stress in trabecular bone occurred in the second group with 8.7 MPa and the minimum amount was observed in the first group with the amount of 4.3 MPa. In the third group the maximum stress in the Trabecular layer was 6.7 MPa (Table2).

According to the stress distribution pattern on the trabecular bone layer among the analyzed models, the location of maximum amount of stress in the first and third groups was the same: at the lowest

Table 2: The maximum amounts of stress imposed on various layers of the bone and implant in the axial loading (MPa)

	Cortical Bone	Trabecular Bone	Implant Titanium
First group: Straight	2.4	4.3	82.1
Second group: Tapered	0.8	8.7	187.4
Third group: Tapered II	0.8	6.7	85.3

part of the implant in the trabecular bone (Figure 6). Nevertheless, in the case of the second group, this location was at the junction of cortical and trabecular bone (Figure 7).

The behavior and performance of different models of thread and implant system in the trabecular bone layer is shown in Figure 8; according to this figure, the first and third groups showed similar behaviors

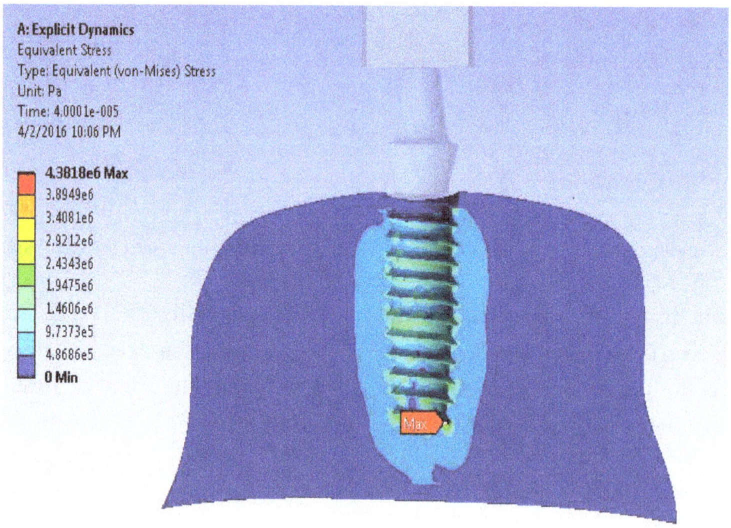

Figure 6: The distribution pattern and place of maximum stress on the trabecular bone layer in the first group

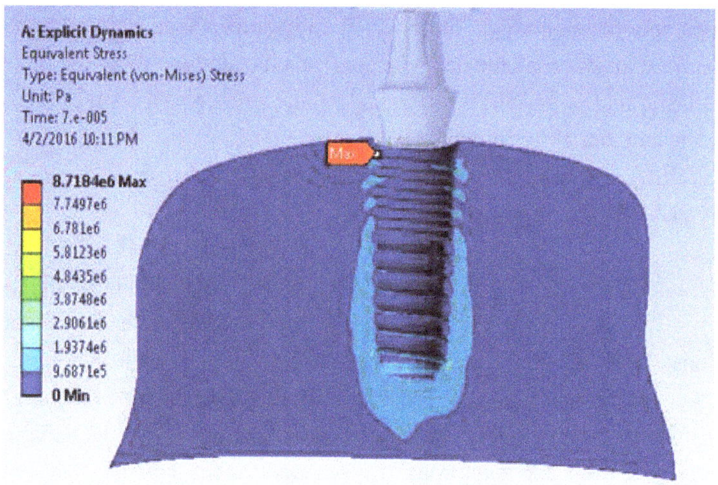

Figure 7: The distribution pattern and place of maximum stress on the trabecular bone in the second group

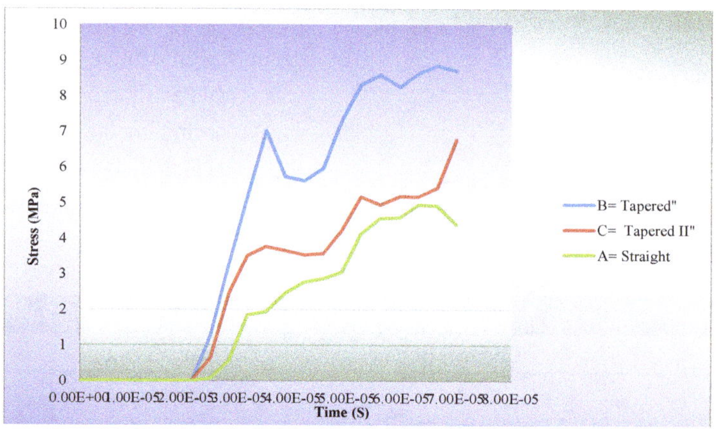

Figure 8: Comparison of behavior in various models of thread regarding the stress distribution on the trabecular bone in the axial loading

Table 3: The maximum stress on different layers of the bone and implant under the bending loading

	Cortical Bone	Trabecular Bone	Implant Titanium
First group: Straight	1.6	5.2	75.9
Second group: Tapered	0.7	7.4	126.9
Third group: Tapered II	1.1	5.1	53.8

Bending Loading Simulation

In the horizontal impact analysis, the maximum amount of stress on different layers of the bone as well as the implant is depicted in Table 3. The bending loading of the first group had maximum stress with the amount of 1.6 MPa; also, minimum stress was imposed on the second group with the amount of 0.7 MPa to the cortical bone.

The third group experienced 1.1 MPa stress on the cortical layer. The stress distribution pattern in this bone layer in all models was the same and its maximum amount was imposed on the first contact area of the implant and bone (Figure 9, Table 3).

In the layer of trabecular bone, no significant difference was observed between the imposed stress in the first and third groups, but the second group exerted the maximum stress with the amount of 7.4 MPa.

Regarding the stress distribution pattern between different models of thread, the first and third groups showed a similar pattern and the location of maximum stress in the bending loading was similar to the axial loading at the bottom part of implant (Figure 6).

The stress distribution behavior in various thread groups in the cortical bone is displayed in Figure 10.

Discussion

The finite element is analyzed in two or three-

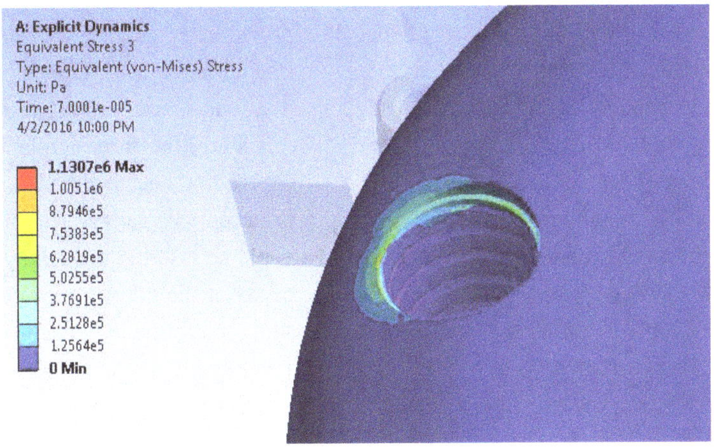

Figure 9: The stress distribution pattern on the cortical bone in the bending loading

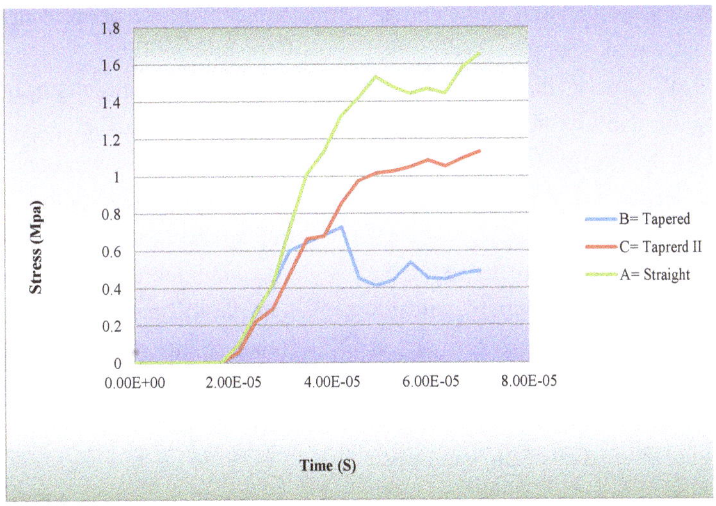

Figure 10: The comparison of stress distribution on the cortical bone in bending loading for various thread design

dimensional form. The choice of two or three-dimensional analysis depends on the complication of the model, the required accuracy rate, application of the results and complication of the structures in the analysis. Based on the results of a study conducted by Meijer, it has been recommended that the two dimensional model should not be used for analysis of the stress on the implant [14]. The difference between modeling in our study and the previous conducted studies is the mode of simulation of software environment with laboratory conditions. In this study, the jaw bone was modeled in an actual form because the figure and geometry of the bone in the mouth and implant system as well as distribution of stress can be effective.

Ozen *et al.* [15] in their study assessed the effect of various materials on the distribution of stress on the implant by using the three dimensional finite element methods. They recommended that the minimum number of elements and nodes for analyzing the stress of the jaw and implant should be 30000 and 200000, respectively. The dimension at which these numbers of elements and nodes are applied should be taken into account. In our study, because of the implication and presence of various layers, in the design of the analyzed model 725047 elements and 1133167 nodes were applied. Change *et al.* [16] in their study assessed the effect of thread deep, figure and length of the cone on the mini implant and found that as the depth of the thread was more, it was more resistance against the exit and replacement.

Schrotenboer *et al.* [6] conducted a study and concluded that the implants with tiny thread in their neck exert more stress on the bone compared to the implant with smooth neck. The result of the mentioned study is consistent with that of the present study. Abuhussein *et al.* [2] found that as the contact area of the implant increased, the stress distribution was more desirable; also, when the ability of the bone for maintaining the stability of the implant and the resistance against the stress was weak, using an implant with the deeper thread can resolve this problem.

These results are consistent with those of the current study. Nokar *et al.* [17] in their study indicated that the cylindrical implant leads to creation of less stress in the contact area of the implant and bone which is in agreement of our current study. Kang *et al.* [18] in their study of "the effect of implant thread size on its adjacent bone atrophy" used two implants. One was with two types of thread (a tiny thread above the implant and a bigger one at the bottom of it) and the other with one type of thread. No significant difference was found between the samples. They found that up to one year after treatment the threads had no any significant effect on the atrophy of the implant's adjacent bone [18]. Their results were in contrast with that of the present study [18]. They studied two implants with similar conditions but different in the thread step in the upper part of the implant clinically within one year after planting the implant in the jaw. One year after planting the implant, they found that during this time, the type of the threads used has not any acceptable effect on the atrophy rate of the implant's adjacent bone [18]. While according to the results of present study there was no significant difference between these two types of implant.

Conclusions

Although the real model of the patient's jaw has been designed in this study and the implants has been modeled with high accuracy, based on engineering principles, choosing the appropriate type of implant is a difficult task. One of the effective parameters that induce stress to the implant, is thread design. In this study the three implant systems were qualified for loading because the level of stress and strain was in acceptable range .Therefore the studied implants could be inserted according to the conditions and the needs of the patient. According to the results of this study the following conclusions are drawn:

1.The implant with smaller threads and the less pitch length leads to an increase of stress on the trabecular bone and implant.

2.Due to increase of its contact area with the bone, the implant with deeper thread, leads to an increase of the implant's stability.

3.The equal pitch length, but different thread depth, had no significant effect on distribution of stress to the implant's adjacent bone.

4.The upper thread of the implant which is near the implant neck, in comparison with the lower threads, plays an important role in the distribution of stress; as a result, this part of the design should be more taken into account.

Acknowledgments

Hereby, the authors appreciate Dr. Jafari for their faithful and sincere cooperation.

References

1. Goodacre JC, Bernal G, Rungcharassaeng K, *et al.* Clinical complications with implants and implant prostheses. J Prosthet Dent. 2003;90:121-132.
2. Abuhussein H, Pagni G, Rebaudi A, *et al.* The effect of thread pattern implant osseointegration. Clin Oral Implants Res. 2010;21:129-136.
3. Ausiello P, Franciosa P, Martorelli M, *et al.* Effects of thread features in osseo-integrated titanium implants using a statistics-based finite element method. Dent Mater. 2012; 28:919-927.
4. Berglundh T, Persson L, Klinge B. A systematic review of the incidence of biological and technical complications in implant dentistry reported in prospective longitudinal studies of at least 5 years. J Clin Periodontol. 2002;29:197-. 212
5. Watanabe F, Hata Y, Komatsu Sh, *et al.* Finite element analysis of the influence of implant inclination, loading position, and load direction on stress distribution. Odontology. 2003;9:31-36.
6. Schrotenboer J, Tsao YP, Kinariwala V, *et al.* Effect of microthreads and platform switching on crestal bone stress levels: a finite element analysis. J Periodontol. 2008;79:2166-2172.
7. Ao J, Li T, Liu Y, *et al.* Optimal design of thread height and width on an immediately loaded cylinder implant: A finite element analysis. Comput Biol Med. 2010;40:681-686.
8. Frisardi G, Chessa G, Barone S, *et al.* Integration of 3D anatomical data obtained by CT imaging and 3D optical scanning for computer aided implant surgery. BMC Med Imaging. 2011;11:5.
9. Hasan I, Bourauel C, Keilig L, *et al.* The influence of implant number and abutment design on the biomechanical behaviour of bone for an implant-supported fixed prosthesis: a finite element study in the upper anterior region. Comput Methods Biomech Biomed Engin. 2011;14:1113-1116.
10. Demenko V, Linetskiy I, Nesvit K, *et al.* Importance of diameter-to-length ratio in selecting dental implants: a methodological finite element study. Comput Methods Biomech Biomed Engin. 2014;17:443-449.
11. Bin D, Keson BCT, Yi L, *et al.* Inverse identification of elastic modulus of dental implant–bone interfacial tissue using neural network and FEA model. Inverse Probl Sci Eng. 2009;17:1073-1083.
12. Sannino G, Pozzi1 A, Schiavetti1 A, *et al.* Stress distribution on a three-unit implant-supported zirconia framework. a 3rd finite element analysis and fatigue test. Oral & implantol. 2012;5:11-20.
13. Okumura N, Stegaroiu R, Kitamura E, *et al.* Influence of maxillary cortical bone thickness, implants design and implant diameter on stress around implants: A three-dimensional finite element analysis. J Prosthodont Res. 2010;54:133-142.
14. Meijer HJ, Starmans FJ, Bosman F, *et al.* A comparison of three finite element models of an edentulous mandible provided two implants. J Oral Rehabil. 1993;20:147-157.
15. Ozen J, Caglar A, Beydemir B, *et al.* Three dimensional finite element stress analysis of different core materials in maxillary implant supported fixed partial dentures. Quintessence Int. 2007;38:355-363.
16. Chang JZ, Chen YJ, Tung YY, *et al.* Effects of thread depth, taper shape, and taper length on the mechanical properties of mini- implant. J Orthod Dentofacial Orthop. 2012;141:279-288.
17. Nokar S, Baghai Naini R. Effects of different designs of implant support fixed partial dentures on peri-implant bone stress distribution during mandibular- flexture. J Dent. 2004;17;36-47.
18. Kang YI, Lee DW, Park KH, *et al.* Effect of thread size on the implant neck area: preliminary results at 1 year of function. Clin Oral Implants Res. 2011;23:1-5.

Combination Effect of Hemostatic and Disinfecting Agents on Micro-leakage of Restorations Bonded with Different Bonding Systems

Farhadpour H[a], Sharafeddin F[b], Akbarian S[c], Azarian B[d]

[a]Department of Dental Materials, School of Dentistry, Shiraz University of Medical Sciences, Shiraz, Iran.
[b]Department of Operative Dentistry and Biomaterials Research Center, School of Dentistry, Shiraz University of Medical Sciences, Shiraz, Iran
[c]Department of Operative Dentistry, School of Dentistry, Shiraz University of Medical Sciences, Shiraz, Iran
[d]Tohid high school, Shiraz, Iran

ARTICLE INFO

Key words:
Chlorhexidine
Hemostatic Agent
Micro-leakage
Self-etching Adhesive
Total-etching Adhesive

Corresponding Author:
Sahar Akbarian
Department of Operative Dentistry, School of Dentistry, Shiraz University of Medical Sciences, Shiraz, Iran.
Email: drakbarian@yahoo.com

Abstract

Statement of Problem: Hemostatic agents may affect the micro-leakage of different adhesive systems. Also, chlorhexidine has shown positive effects on micro-leakage. However, their interaction effect has not been reported yet.

Objectives: To evaluate the effect of contamination with a hemostatic agent on micro-leakage of total- and self-etching adhesive systems and the effect of chlorhexidine application after the removal of the hemostatic agent.

Materials and Methods: Standardized Class V cavity was prepared on each of the sixty caries free premolars at the cemento-enamel junction, with the occlusal margin located in enamel and the gingival margin in dentin. Then, the specimens were randomly divided into 6 groups (n = 10) according to hemostatic agent (H) contamination, chlorhexidine (CHX) application, and the type of adhesive systems (Adper Single Bond and Clearfil SE Bond) used. After filling the cavities with resin composite, the root apices were sealed with utility wax. Furthermore, all the surfaces, except for the restorations and 1mm from the margins, were covered with two layers of nail varnish. The teeth were immersed in a 0.5% basic fuschin dye for 24 hours, rinsed, blot-dried and sectioned longitudinally through the center of the restorations bucco- lingualy. The sections were examined using a stereomicroscope and the extension of dye penetration was analyzed according to a non-parametric scale from 0 to 3. Statistical analysis was performed using Kruskal-Wallis test and Mann-Whitney U-test.

Results: While ASB group showed no micro-leakage in enamel, none of the groups showed complete elimination of micro-leakage from the dentin. Regarding micro-leakage at enamel, and dentin margins, there was no significant difference between groups 1 and 2, 1 and 3, and 2 and 3 ($p > 0.05$). A significantly lower micro-leakage at the enamel and dentin margins was observed in group 3, compared to group 6. No significant difference was observed between groups 4 and 5 in enamel ($p = 0.35$) and dentin ($p = 0.34$). Group 6 showed significantly higher micro-leakage, compared to group 4 and 5 ($p < 0.05$).

Conclusions: Hemostatic agent contamination had no significant effect on micro-leakage of total- and self-etching adhesive systems. Application of chlorhexidine after the removal of hemostatic agent increased micro-leakage in self-etching adhesives but did not affect when total-etching was used.

Introduction

Micro-leakage is the transition of fluids, bacteria, ions or molecules between a cavity wall and the restorative material [1]. In composite restorations, micro-leakage can be caused by polymerization shrinkage, the differences in the coefficient of thermal expansion between tooth structure and the material, and occlusal loads [2]. Contamination in different stages of bonding procedure may also cause micro-leakage [3-5]. Clinically, it can lead to staining around the margins of restorations, margin deterioration, poor aesthetics, post-operative sensitivity, secondary caries, restoration failure, pulpal pathology, and unfavorable effects on clinical performance of composite restorations [6-8]. In most of the current literature on adhesive techniques and materials, the focus is on the elimination of leakage because of its importance for the long-term success of restorations [1].

In order to achieve a durable bond, moisture control is essential. However, isolation against saliva and blood contamination is sometimes difficult, especially at and below the gingival margin [9]. Saliva and blood contamination can reduce the dentin bond strength of total- and self-etching adhesive systems [10-12]. Clinicians may rely on hemostatic agents to avoid blood contamination, particularly near or at the gingival margin where blood contamination is more probable [13]. Hemostatic agents are substances that can be used on hemorrhagic gingival tissues before placing restorations [14-15]. Aluminium chloride with a concentration between 5 and 25% is one of the most frequently used hemostatic agents which, with its minimal systemic effects, can precipitate proteins, constrict blood vessels and extract fluid from tissues [14]. Hemostatic agents are highly acidic and are able to remove smear layer and cause some degree of demineralization [15].

Although the effect of hemostatic agents on micro-leakage and bond strength has been evaluated in several studies, they have reached different results [13,15,16]. If viable microorganisms remain after cavity preparation, micro-leakage may cause more problems which can result in secondary caries [6]. According to some bacteriologic and histologic studies, only a small portion of teeth is sterile after cavity preparation [7]. Proliferation of residual bacteria from the smear layer occurs even when there is a good seal from the oral cavity [17]. This problem can be magnified by micro-leakage of composite restoration at margins not ending on enamel [18]. Treating the cavity preparation with chlorhexidine may solve this problem to some extent. Chlorhexidine has a broad spectrum of action, mostly against Gram-positive bacteria, particularly Streptococcus mutans, which seems to be more sensitive [19]. Currently, chlorhexidine is used not only as an anti-microbial agent, but also as a potential adjuvant to establish a better bond to dentin [20]. However, owing to the lack of consensus existing over the effect of chlorhexidine [20,21], further studies are required in this regard .

Generally, bond degradation occurs because of resin elution and collagen fibrils alteration. Exposed collagen fibrils that are exposed in the hybrid bond layer, and are not completely infiltrated by resin are susceptible to degradation by matrix metalloproteinase (MMP) enzymes of the saliva and dentin [20,22].

MMPs that are host cell-derived proteolytic enzymes have a major role in tissue-destructive inflammatory diseases and are capable of degrading most of the extracellular matrix components, including different types of collagen [23,24]. Chlorhexidine can be used to prevent or minimize the auto-degradation of collagen matrices in incompletely resin-infiltrated dentin [25,26].

Considering the contrasting effects of hemostatic agents on micro-leakage, and the positive effects of chlorhexidine mentioned above, this study aimed to evaluate the effect of hemostatic agent contamination on micro-leakage of total- and self-etching adhesive systems and the effect of chlorhexidine application after the removal of the hemostatic agent.

The null hypothesis was that hemostatic agent contamination would not affect the micro-leakage of total- and self-etching adhesive systems and the application of chlorhexidine after the removal of hemostatic agent would not affect micro-leakage.

Materials and Methods

Sixty extracted non-carious human premolar teeth collected and stored at 4°C were used within one month of extraction. Standardized Class V cavities (2 mm depth, 2 mm mesiodistal, 3 mm occlusogingival) were prepared at the cemento-enamel junction, with the occlusal margin located in enamel and the gingival margin in dentin. In the occlusal cavo surface margin, a bevel was made. Cavities were prepared using a #556 diamond fissure bur in a high-speed handpiece with water coolant. Then, they were randomly divided into 6 groups (n = 10) according to the following factors: Hemostatic agent contamination, chlorhexidine application, and the adhesive systems used. Group 1- Adper Single Bond system (ASB) (3M,ESPE,USA) was applied as recommended by the manufacturer (Table 1). Group 2- One drop of hemostatic agent solution (Hemostop,Dentsply. Argentina) was applied on the dentin surface for 2 minutes and rinsed for 30s and air-dried .Then, the cavity surface was etched with 37% phosphoric acid gel for 15s. After rinsing and air-drying, ASB was applied (H + ASB). Group 3- One drop of the hemostatic agent solution was applied into the cavity for 2 minutes, rinsed for 30s and air-dried. After that, CHX 0.2% solution was applied with a microbrush.The next steps were similar to group 1 (H+CHX+ASB). Group 4- Clearfil SE Bond system (CSB) (Kuraray,Japan) was applied as recommended by the manufacturer (Table 1). Group 5- One drop of hemostatic agent solution was applied into the cavity for 2 minutes and rinsed for 30s and air-dried. Then, CSB was applied (H+CSB).Group 6- One drop of hemostatic agent solution was applied into the cavity for 2 minutes and rinsed for 30s and air-dried. After that, CHX 0.2% solution was applied with a microbrush. Then, CSB was applied (H+CHX+CSB).

After the adhesive application and light curing for 20s with an LED light curing system (Demetron,Kerr)(1200 mW/cm2), the cavities were bulk filled with one increment of resin composite (Filtek Z250, 3M, ESPE, St Paul, MN, USA). Excess composite was removed with an explorer and then light cured with an LED for 20s. All procedures were performed by one operator at room temperature and during procedures, the cavities were kept moist. After the restoration, the samples were stored for 24 hours in distilled water.

Afterwards, the root apices were sealed with utility wax, and all the surfaces, except for the restorations and 1mm from the margins, were covered with two layers of nail varnish. The teeth were immersed in a 0.5% basic fuschin dye for 24 hours. Then, they were rinsed, blot-dried and sectioned longitudinally through the center of the restorations from the buccal to lingual surface with a water-cooled diamond saw (Leitz 1600, Wetzlar, Germany).

The sections were examined for dye penetration by two independent researchers using a stereomicroscope (Carl ZiessInc, Oberkochen, Germany) at 20× magnification. The extent of the dye penetration was analyzed according to a non-parametric scale from 0 to 3 (0 = no dye penetration, 1 = dye penetration less than 1/2 of the cavity depth, 2 = dye penetration more than 1/2 of the cavity depth, 3 = dye penetration spreading along the axial wall).

Statistical analysis was performed using Kruskal-Wallis H test and Mann-Whitney U-test. Significance level for all statistical tests was predetermined at $p < 0.05$.

Table 1: Adhesive Systems, Composition, and Application Mode

Adhesive Systems	Composition	Application mode
Adper Single Bond (3M, ESPE, St Paul, MN, USA)	Scotchbond etchant:37% phosphoric acid Adhesive:Bis-GMA, HEMA, dimethacrylates, polyalkenoic acid copolymer, initiators, water, and ethanol	1.Apply acid etch for 15s 2.Rinse for 15s. 3.Blot dry for 30s. 4.Apply one coat of adhesive for 10s. 5.Airdry for 10s at 20cm. 6.Light cure.
Clearfil SE Bond (Kuraray, Okayama, Japan)	Primer:MDP,HEMA,dimethacrylate Monomer,water,catalyst Bond:MDP,HEMA, dimethacrylate Monomer,microfiller,catalyst	1.Apply primer and leave for 20s. 2.Drythorouly with mild air flow. 3.Apply bond. 4.Gentle air flow. 5.Light cure.

Table 2: Micro-leakage scores of enamel and dentin

Group	Material	Enamelscores				Mean	Mediam	Dentinscores				Mean	Mediam
		0	1	2	3			0	1	2	3		
1	ASB	12	0	0	0	0	0	5	6	1	0	0.6	1
2	H+ASB	10	2	0	0	0.16	0	3	7	2	0	0.91	1
3	H+CHX+ASB	10	1	1	0	0.25	0	8	4	0	0	0.33	0
4	CSB	8	4	0	0	0.33	0	7	5	0	0	0.41	0
5	H+CSB	6	5	1	0	0.58	0.5	5	6	1	0	0.66	1
6	H+CHX+CSB	0	9	1	2	1.41	1	0	8	3	1	1.41	1

ASB=Adper Single Bond, CSB=Clearfil SE Bond, CHX= Chlorhexidine, H= Hemostatic

Results

Dye penetration scores for the enamel and dentinal margins are presented in Table 2. Whereas ASB group showed no micro-leakage in enamel, none of the groups showed complete elimination of micro-leakage in dentin. Pairwise multiple comparisons of the six groups were performed using the Mann-Whitney test between treatment groups for both enamel and dentinal margins.

There was no significant difference between groups 1 and 2 neither in enamel (p = 0.51) nor in dentin (p=0.41). Moreover, there was no significant difference between groups 1 and 3 concerning enamel (p = 0.51), and dentin (p = 0.26). Also, no significant difference was seen between groups 2 and 3 regarding enamel (p = 0.97) and dentin (p = 0.52) margins. However, significantly lower micro-leakage at enamel and dentin margins was observed in group 3, compared to group 6 ($p < 0.05$).

No significant difference was observed between groups 4 and 5 in enamel (p = 0.35) and dentin (p = 0.34) margins. Group 6 showed significantly higher micro-leakage, compared to group 4. ($p < 0.05$) and group 5 ($p < 0.05$).

Discussion

In the first part of this study, we evaluated the effect of hemostatic agent contamination on the micro-leakage of total- and self-etching adhesive systems to dentin. As the findings of the study failed to reject the first part of the null hypothesis, it is concluded that hemostatic agent contamination had no significant effect on the micro-leakage of total- and self-etching adhesive systems. These findings are in line with a previous study performed by Arslan *et al*. that reported no significant changes in micro-leakage scores after the application of the hemostatic agent, with self-etching adhesives [13]. In another study, the researchers used Viscostat as a hemostatic agent and contrary to our findings; they reported significant increase in micro-leakage [3]. The difference in the results of that study and the present study may be attributed to differences in the hemostatic agents used.

The increased micro-leakage might be because of the fact that Viscostat, contrary to Hemostop, is a viscous gel composed of ferric sulphate and the viscosity makes its removal from the dentin surface harder, and may lead to coagulation of proteins present in the dentinal fluid. The coagulated proteins and residues of ferric sulfate may result in the inhibition of the infiltration of the bonding agent into the etched enamel surfaces and dentinal tubules.

Evaluation of the effect of chlorhexidine application after the removal of hemostatic agent revealed that the use of chlorhexidine after astringent removal did not have any significant effects on micro-leakage when ASB was used as adhesive system and the second part of the null hypothesis was accepted for ASB.

But regarding CSB, chlorhexidine application increased micro-leakage and the null hypothesis was rejected in this regard.

For deciding the step in which chlorhexidine is applied, in some studies, chlorhexidine has been used after etching [26,27]. The rationale for the application of chlorhexidine in this step is the ability of chlorhexidine to inhibit enzyme activities directly; inhibiting the inherent collagenolytic activity of mineralized dentin would reinforce the bond of resin composite to dentin. In some other investigations, chlorhexidine has been used before etching with the purpose of the disinfection and cleansing of the dentin surface [21,28]. Also, according to some other investigators, there is no significant difference between the application of chlorhexidine before or after etching of dentin [29,30]. In this study, chlorhexidine was used after removing the hemostatic agent and before etching in order to disinfect the dentin surface and remove the microorganisms and thus to reduce the probability of recurrent caries and restoration failure as well as eliminating the remnants of hemostatic agent that could interfere with the bond of composite to dentin.

In a study by Sung *et al.*, the researchers concluded that application of chlorhexidine had no significant effect on micro-leakage of total-etching system [31]. Siso *et al.* reported that chlorhexidine solution had no effect on micro-leakage of composite restorations [32].

Although a number of studies obtained different results after chlorhexidine use [31-33], some other studies reported findings similar to ours. For instance, Tulunoglu *et al.* concluded that chlorhexidine solution had an adverse effect on self-etching adhesive systems and produced higher micro-leakage [33]. Singla *et al.* also reported higher micro-leakage when using chlorhexidine with self-etching adhesives [34].

Further in vitro and in vivo studies are recommended to improve the understanding of the interaction effect of different hemostatic agents and chlorhexidine with bonding systems which have different acidities.

Conclusions

Considering the limitations of this in vitro study, we found that hemostatic agent contamination had no significant effect on micro-leakage of total- and self-etching adhesive systems. Application of chlorhexidine after the removal of hemostatic agent could increase micro-leakage in self-etching adhesives but did not affect the micro-leakage when using total-etching adhesive systems.

Acknowledgements

The authors thank the Vice-Chancellory of Shiraz University of Medical Science and Biomaterial Research Center of Shiraz University of Medical Sciences for supporting this research (Grant# 5455). The authors also thank Dr. M. Vossoughi for the statistical analysis and Dr. Ehya Amalsaleh for improving the use of English in the manuscript.

Conflict of Interest: None declared.

References

1. Kidd EA. Microleakage: a review. J Dent. 1976; 4:199-206.
2. Ben-Amar A. Microleakage of composite resin restorations. A status report. Am J Dent. 1989;2:175-180.
3. Kumar P, Shenoy A, Joshi S. The effect of various surface contaminants on the microleakage of two different generation bonding agents: A stereomicroscopic study. J Conserv Dent. 2012;15:265-269.
4. Sharafeddin F, Koohpeima F, Palizian B. Evaluation of Microleakage in Class V Cavities Filled with Methacrylate-based versus Silorane-based Composites. J Dent Biomater. 2015;2: 67-72.
5. Sharafeddin F, Darvishi F, Malekzadeh P. The Effect of Incorporation of Polyethylene and Glass Fiber on the Microleakage of Silorane-based and Methacrylate-based Composites in Class II Restorations: An in Vitro Study. J Dent Biomater. 2015;2:39-46.
6. Moreira Jr G, Sobrinho AP, Nicoli JR, *et al.* Evaluation of microbial infiltration in restored cavities-An alternative method. J Endod. 1999; 25:605-608.
7. Kihn P, Spanganberg P, von Fraunhofer J. The role of cavity preparation and conditioning in the leakage of restorations. J Adhes Dent. 2004;6:287-291.
8. Eick JD, Welch FH. Polymerization shrinkage of posterior composite resins and its possible influence on postoperative sensitivity. Quintessence Int. 1986;17:103-111.
9. Yoo H, Pereira P. Effect of blood contamination with 1-step self-etching adhesives on micro-

tensile bond strength to dentin. Oper Dent. 2006;31:660-665.

10. de Carvalho Mendonça EC, Vieira SN, Kawaguchi FA, *et al.* Influence of blood contamination on bond strength of a self-etching system. Eur J Dent. 2010;4:280-286.
11. Chang S, Cho B, Lim R, *et al.* Effects of blood contamination on microtensile bond strength to dentin of three self-etch adhesives. Oper Dent. 2010;35:330-336.
12. Neelagiri K, Kundabala M, Shashi RA, *et al.* Effects of saliva contamination and decontamination procedures on shear bond strength of self-etch dentine bonding systems: An in vitro study. J Conserv Dent. 2010;13:71-75.
13. Arslan S, Ertaş H, Zorba YO. Effect of a plant-based hemostatic agent on microleakage of self-etching adhesives. Med Oral Patol Oral Cir Bucal. 2013;18:124-129.
14. Gupta G, Kumar S, Rao H, *et al.* Astringents in dentistry: a review. Asian J Pharm Hea Sci. 2012;2:428-432.
15. Harnirattisai C, Kuphasuk W, Senawongse P, *et al.* Bond strengths of resin cements to astringent-contaminated dentin. Oper Dent. 2009;34:415-422.
16. Sharafeddin F, Farhadpour H. Evaluation of Shear Bond Strength of Total- and Self-etching Adhesive Systems after Application of Chlorhexidine to Dentin Contaminated with a Hemostatic Agent. J Dent (Shiraz). 2015;16: 175–181.
17. Brannstrom M. The cause of postrestorative sensitivity and its prevention. J Endod. 1986; 12:475-481
18. Boston D, Graver H. Histological study of an acid red caries-disclosing dye. Oper Dent. 1989;14:186-192
19. Fardal O, Turnbull R. A review of the literature on use of chlorhexidine in dentistry. J Am Dent Assoc. 1986;112:863-869.
20. Herênio SS, de Carvalho NMP, Lima DM. Influence of chlorhexidine digluconate on bond strength durability of a self-etching adhesive system. Rev Sulbras Odontol. 2011; 8:417-424.
21. Ercan E, Erdemir A, Zorba YO, *et al.* Effect of different cavity disinfectants on shear bond strength of composite resin to dentin. J Adhes Dent. 2009; 11: 343-346.
22. Brackett WW, Tay FR, Brackett MG, *et al.* The effect of chlorhexidine on dentin hybrid layers in vivo. Oper Dent. 2007; 32:107-111.
23. Moon PC, Weaver J, Brooks CN. Review of matrix metalloproteinases' effect on the hybrid dentin bond layer stability and chlorhexidine clinical use to prevent bond failure. Open Dent J. 2010;4:147-152.
24. Gendron R, Grenier D, Sorsa T, *et al.* Inhibition of the activities of matrix metalloproteinases 2, 8, and 9 bychlorhexidine. Clin Diagn Lab Immunol. 1999;6:437-439.
25. Hebling J, Pashley DH, Tjäderhane L, *et al.* Chlorhexidine arrests subclinical degradation of dentin hybrid layers in vivo. J Dent Res. 2005; 84: 741-746.
26. Komori PC, Pashley DH, Tjäderhane L, *et al.* Effect of 2% chlorhexidine digluconate on the bond strength to normal versus caries-affected dentin. Oper Dent. 2009;34:157-165.
27. Loguercio AD, Stanislawczuk R, Polli LG, *et al.* Influence of chlorhexidine diglu-conate concentration and application time on resin-dentin bond strength durability. Eur J Oral Sci. 2009;117:587-596.
28. Breschi L, Cammelli F, Visintini E, *et al.* Influence of chlorhexidine concentration on the durability of etch-and-rinse dentin bonds: a 12-month in vitro study. J Adhes Dent. 2009;11: 191-198.
29. de Castro FL, de Andrade MF, Duarte Júnior SL, *et al.* Effect of 2% chlorhexidine on microtensile bond strength of composite to dentin. J Adhes Dent. 2003;5:129-138.
30. Campos EA, Correr GM, Leonardi DP, *et al.* Influence of chlorhexidine concentration on microtensile bond strength of contemporary adhesivesystems. Braz Oral Res. 2009;23:340-345.
31. Sung EC, Chan SM, Tai ET, *et al.* Effects of Various irrigation solutions on microleakage of Class V composite restoration. J Prosthet Dent. 2004;91:265-267
32. Siso HS, Kustarci A, Göktolga EG. Micro-leakage in resin composite restorations after antimicrobial pretreatments: effect of KTPlaser, chlorhexidine gluconate and Clearfil

Protect Bond. Oper Dent. 2009;34:321-327
33. Tulunoglu O , Ayhan H , Olmez A , *et al.* The effect of cavity disinfectants on microleakage in dentin bonding systems. J Clin Pediatr Dent. 1998;22:299-305
34. Singla M, Aggarwal V, Kumar N. Effect of chlorhexidine cavity disinfection on microleakage in cavities restored with composite using a self-etching single bottle adhesive. J Conserv Dent. 2011;14:374-377.

18

Chemical Stability of Bioglass in Simulated Oral Environment

Moazzami SM[a], Sadid Zadeh R[b], Kianoush K[c], Sarmad M[d], Barani Karbaski F[e], Amiri Daluyi R[a], Kazemi RB[f]

[a]Dental Research Center and Department of Operative and Esthetic Dentistry, Mashhad Dental School, Mashhad University of Medical Sciences, Mashhad, Iran
[b]Department of Restorative Dentistry, School of Dental Medicine, Buffalo, NY
[c]Biomedical Engineering Student, Biomechanics Research Assistant, Adelaide, SA, Australia
[d]Faculty of Mathematical Sciences, Ferdowsi University of Mashhad, Mashhad, Iran
[e]Dental Research Center and Department of Pediatric Dentistry,Mashhad Dental School, Mashhad University of Medical Sciences, Mashhad, Iran
[f]Operative Dentistry D200, Department of Craniofacial Sciences, UCONN Health, School of Dental Medicine, Farmington CT, USA

ARTICLE INFO

Key words:
Bioglass
Resin Composite
Dental Porcelain
Chemical Stability

Corresponding Author:
Saied Mostafa Moazzami
Dental Research Center and Department of Operative and Esthetic Dentistry, Mashhad Dental School, Mashhad University of Medical Sciences (MUMS), Mashhad, Iran.
Email: MoazzamiM@mums.ac.ir

Abstract

***Statement of Problem*:** Bioglasses are a series of biocompatible dental materials, which are considered as light conducting inserts in resin composite restorations. Consequently, their chemical stability is more essential when they are used in conjunction with resin composite.

Objectives: The aim of this study was to evaluate and compare the chemical stability of Bioglass with dental porcelain and resin composite by determining the amount of released K^+, Na^+, Ca^{2+} ions and silicone elements from these materials as a result of exposure to tested solutions with different pH levels including: Sodium Bicarbonate [SB, (pH=9.2)], Sodium Buffer Lactate [SBL, (pH=2.4)], Acetic Acid [AA, (pH=2.4)], and Distilled Water [DW, (pH=6.2)].

***Materials and Methods*:** In this experimental study, forty 2.0 × 4.0 cylindrical rods for each tested material group (Dental porcelain, Resin composite and Bioglass) were prepared. They were divided into four subgroups of 10 rods each, which immersed in one of the four testing solutions in a designated container. The containers were stored at 50°C and 100% humidity for one week. The released ions were measured by using a spectrophotometer ($\mu g/cm^2/ml$). The data were statistically analyzed by nonparametric Kruskal-Wallis H test.

***Results*:** It was observed that the tested materials released ions at different levels of concentration. The significant amounts of Sodium, Calcium, and Silicon ions release were measured in Bioglass subgroups in all the tested solutions ($p < 0.001$). Potassium ion release from dental porcelain was the largest in all solutions except for AA in which Bioglass had the greatest potassium ion release ($p < 0.001$).

Conclusions: A greater structural instability was observed for Biogalss group than dental porcelain and resin composite in testing solutions with different pH levels.

Introduction

Ceramics are categorized into crystalline, non-crystalline (vitreous) and compound forms based on their chemical structures. Glass is an example of non-crystalline ceramics [1,2]. Degradation of dental ceramics is generally due to mechanical forces or chemical attacks within the oral environment. Dental ceramics chemical durability has also been shown to be great except when in contact with acidic fluoride, ammonium bifluoride and hydrofluoric acid which have professional use [3].

Bioglasses are a type of non-crystalline ceramics which are series of bioactive/biocompatible glasses, composed of SiO_2, Na_2O, CaO and P_2O_5 in different proportions from low ratio of silica in one product to high sodium/calcium or calcium/phosphorus ratios in other products [1,2].

With the advent of bioactive glass in 1969 by Hench *et al.*, one of the first completely synthetic materials that seamlessly bonds to the bone and is able to integrate with host tissues, as a new rehabilitating procedure was introduced to the field of medicine [4]. Bioglasses were used to reconstruct tissue deficiencies such as mid-ear bony defects [5]. Later, its application was extended to dentistry in procedures such as ridge augmentation and reconstruction of the alveolar bone defects [4,6-9].

Bioglasses are a series of promising materials used in oral cavity which are used as restorative material as well. Therefore, the concept of using Bioglasses in a restorative material to conduct light in light cured resin composite restorations as a glass insert addressed as "Light Conducting Bioglass Insert" (LCBI) was firstly introduced in 1996 [10]. It was observed that hardness of these restorations, especially in the deepest areas, was significantly improved by LCBI. These findings also confirmed the reduction of micro-leakage, discussed by better polymerization, along the gingival margins of the posterior resin composite restorations [11]. Because some parts of the LCBI might be exposed to the oral environment, the chemical and physical stability of LCBI must to be also at an acceptable level.

High resistance to chemical attack is one of the critical and desirable properties of restorative materials. Dental ceramics have to provide an acceptable tolerance against different solutions with different pH levels in the oral cavity. Generally, there are two accepted mechanisms for glass degradation in aqueous solutions: selective alkaline ion release and glass lattice solubility [3].

The rate of degradation of dental material when used as a restoration is an important issue. As to bioglass as a LCBI, it must be acceptable and at least in the same rate of other restorative materials such as resin composite and dental porcelain. Degradation is generally due to mechanical forces or chemical attacks within the oral environment [3].

The most commonly employed test set-up for this purpose is wear analysis and ion release analysis. Because of the lack of an internationally acceptable method, different methods have been used for assessing the chemical stability of dental materials which can be categorized in two distinct classes: clinical and laboratory test methods. The clinical testing is complex and time consuming (up to six years). Laboratory methods can simply simulate the oral condition and give some reasonable results to compare different dental materials. *In-vitro* chemical tests were of utmost importance in evaluation and comparison of the chemical behavior of such newly introduced material to determine its compatibility with the oral cavity environment and other restorative materials. These methods include visual examination, weight changes observation, dye penetration assessment, physical and mechanical measurements, instrumental methods, and chemical analysis of the reactant [12-14]. Atomic absorption spectrophotometer or an atomic emission spectrometer (flame photometer) is a simple and an appropriate method.

The aim of this study was to evaluate the chemical stability of newly introduced LCBI in comparison with resin composite and dental porcelain in four different solutions with different pH levels: Sodium Bicarbonate [(SB), (pH = 9.2)], Sodium Buffer Lactate [(SBL), (pH = 2.4)], Acetic Acid [(AA), (pH = 2.4)], and Distilled Water [(DW), (pH = 6.2)] using Atomic absorption spectrophotometer. The null hypothesis was that the three materials show similar chemical stability in the simulated oral environment.

Materials and Methods

Specimen preparation

One hundred twenty 2.0 × 4.0 mm rods were prepared

using three tested material groups (n = 40) as follows: a- Dental Porcelain group (DP): Forty specimens were fabricated of Vita porcelain (217 VMK 68N B3+4, Germany) by packing the porcelain powder in prefabricated copper cylinders with an inner diameter of 3.0 mm and height of 12.0 mm in order to make 2.0 × 4.0 mm rods. The cylinders were placed in a dental porcelain furnace (VITA- Vacumat 200, Vita Zahnfabrik H. Rauter GmbH & Co. KG 79704 Bad Sackingen, Germany) and fired in compliance with the manufacturers' recommendations at 920°C in10 minutes. The details of the procedure have already been described [10]. b- Resin Composite group (RC): Forty specimens were fabricated of resin composite (Filtek ™ Z250, USA) by bulk placing the material in transparent plastic cylinders with internal diameter of 3.0 mm and height of 9.0 mm in order to make 2.0 × 4.0 mm rods. The curing step was then performed using a visible light curing unit (Coltolux50), for 80 seconds in a scan mode from one side/end to the other from both sides. c- Bioglass Insert group (BI): Forty specimens were fabricated by cutting off the bioglasss block (Pare-e-Tavoos, Mashhad, Iran) into cylinders of 3.0 mm diameter and 10.0 mm length in order to make 2.0 × 4.0 mm rods using diamond disks (D&Z, Darmstadt, Germany).

Preparation of the rod specimens of the same dimensions: The cylindrical specimens of all groups were cut, ground and shaped into rods with a diameter of 2.0 mm. To fabricate the specimens precisely, we held them in a fixed position handpiece. While the specimens were put in rotating mood, an adjustable high-speed air motor was run to grind the specimens to the desired dimension [10]. Subsequently, the samples were cut short to a length of 4.0 mm using diamond bur (# 450213-BD1, Kerr Corporation 1717 West Collins, Orange, CA, USA) (Figure 1).

Ion release test

Forty prepared rods of one of the three groups were randomly divided into four subgroups of 10 rods each and transferred into a 20 ml laboratory plastic container. Fifteen milliliters of each testing solutions AA, SBL, DW and SB were added to each subgroup of testing materials, each consisting of 10 samples. The containers were subsequently sealed tightly to prevent evaporation. In order to maintain 100% humidity at 50°C, we put the containers into an incubator, especially designed for this study, for a period of seven days (Figure 2). The containers were automatically shaken with a platform shaker (F37041-0000 Spindrive Orbital Shaker Platform, Bel-Art – SP Scienceware. USA) for 10 minutes to accelerate the diffusion process every 12 hours, homogenize the

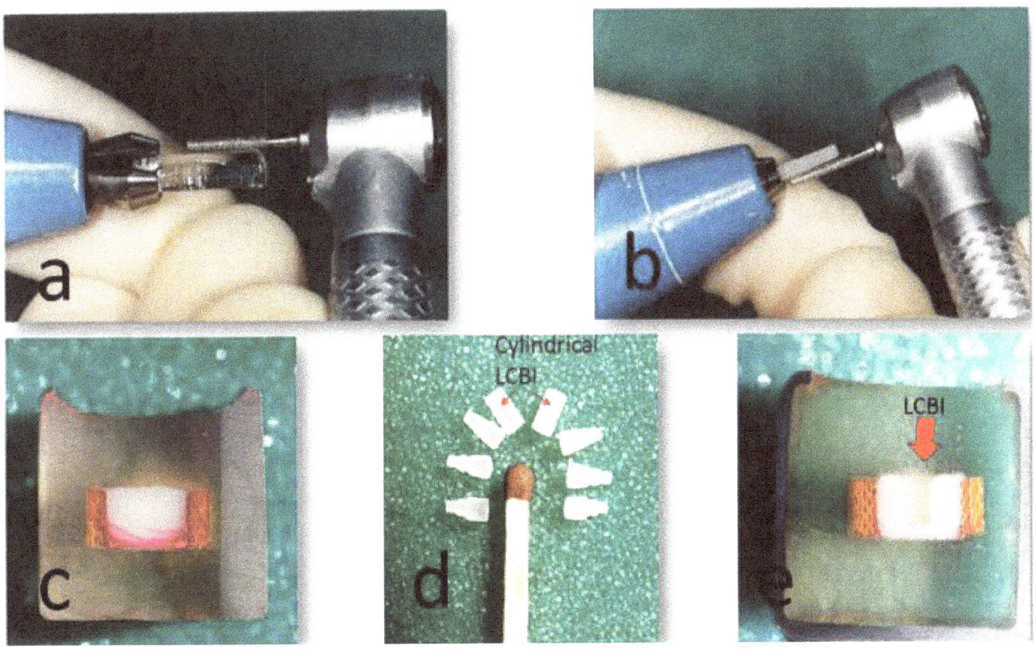

Figure 1: All cylindrical Bioglass rods were cut and shaped into a diameter of exactly 2.0 mm by using a combination of a low-speed hand-piece to hold the specimen and a high-speed air motor to grind the samples while they were run in the opposite directions as Moazzami *et al*. described (a and b of reference "10"). Subsequently, they were cut into a length of 4.0 mm using a diamond disk (Figure 1d). The same procedure was done for preparing the porcelain and composite rods. Figures 1c and 1e are related to the study with reference "10", showing the use of LCBI for increasing the bottom hardness of composite. Courtesy of Moazzami *et al*.

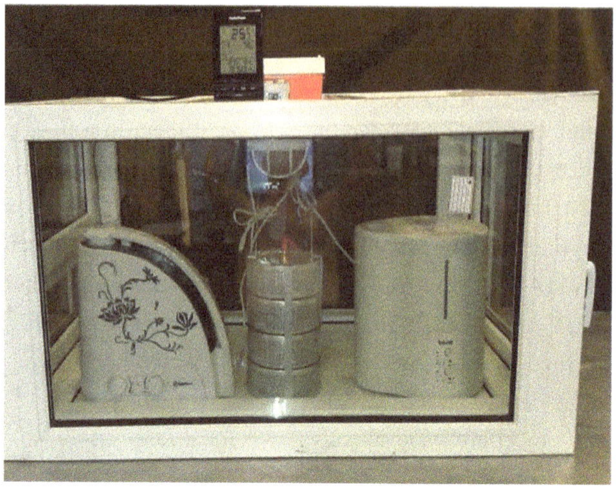

Figure 2: Humidity and temperature simulator for oral cavity which were especially designed for this study by Moazzami *et al.*

solution and help renew the material-solution contact.

After seven days, the specimens were removed from the containers to allow the solutions to be analyzed by the atomic absorption spectrophotometer (AA-680 atomic absorption/flame emission spectrophotometer, Shimadzu/Japan). Prior to testing, the solutions were prepared by diluting in accordance with the original element concentration, as shown in Table1. The sodium concentration in SB and SBL solutions could not be accurate because of the previous presence of this element in the solution. Silicon concentration was below the measurable amount in the resin composite and dental porcelain subgroup solutions; thus, its value was considered zero (Table 1).

The data distribution was not normal and the sample size was not large enough; therefore, they were statistically analyzed by non-parametric Kruskal-Wallis H test.

Results

Kruskal-Wallis H tests showed that ions released from all the testing materials in different solutions were significantly different (Table 1 and Figures 3-6) and ions released in all solutions (except Potassium ion in DW ($p = 0.095$) from different testing materials were significantly different as well ($p = 0.001$).

Maximum potassium ion release form Bioglass, resin composite and dental porcelain was in SBL,

Table 1: The average of different ion release in different solutions by various materials after one week at 50°C (µg/cm2/ml).

Materials	Solutions	K^+	Na^+	Ca^{2+}	Si^{4+}
Bioglass	AA	133.12	4584.40	5996.18	2664.81
	SBL	149.46	------------	5268.63	1879.38
	DW	22.04	369.08	260.10	1678.42
	SB	134.27	------------	43.88	216.53
***p*-value**		<0.001	<0.001	<0.001	<0.001
Resin Composite	AA	43.90	82.72	187.89	0.00
	SBL	90.06	------------	92.72	0.00
	DW	19.24	176.69	107.36	0.00
	SB	123.87	------------	41.14	0.00
***p*-value**		<0.001	<0.001	<0.001	------------
Dental Porcelain	AA	112.66	109.30	196.15	0.00
	SBL	268.38	------------	117.24	0.00
	DW	24.17	135.92	99.41	0.00
	SB	145.80	------------	76.45	0.00
***p*-value**		<0.001	0.003	<0.001	------------

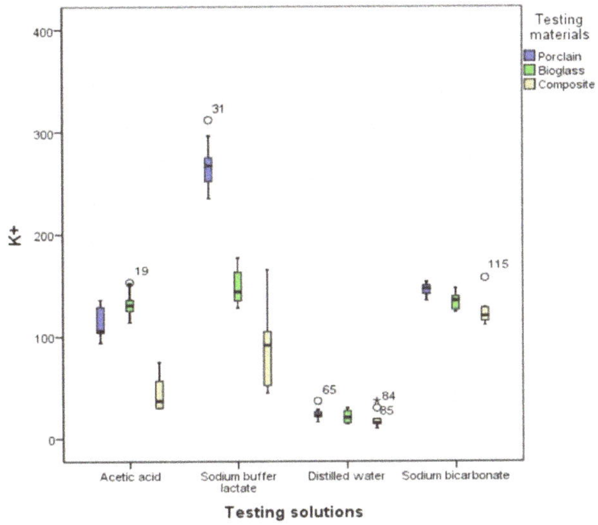

Figure 3: Potassium ion release of porcelain, Composite and Bioglass in different testing solutions (μg/cm²/ml). The numbers (the small circles and star) shows the observation (sample) which is far from the others (suspected as an outlier).

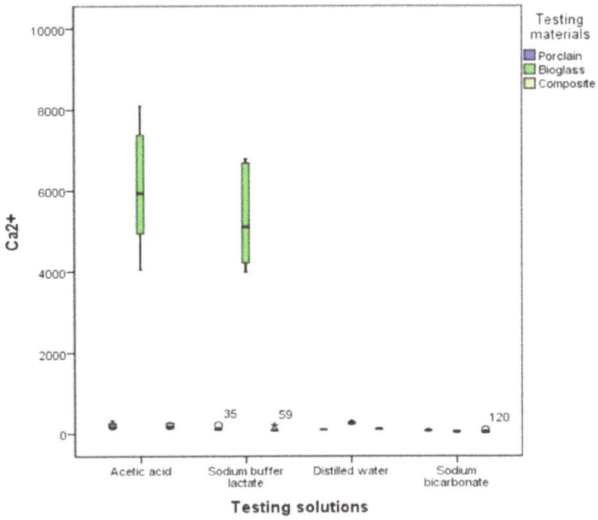

Figure 5: Calcium ion release of porcelain, composite and Bioglass in different testing solutions (μg/cm²/ml). The numbers (the small circles and star) shows the observation (sample) which is far from the others (suspected as an outlier).

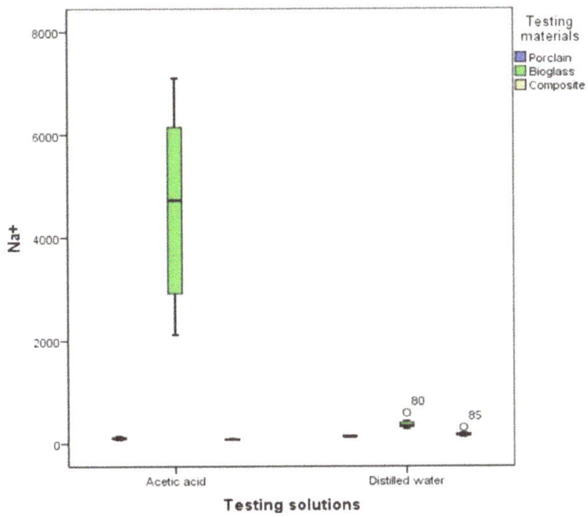

Figure 4: Sodium ion release of porcelain, composite and Bioglass in different testing solutions (μg/cm²/ml). SB and SBL were not tested because of their sodium content. The numbers (and the circles) shows the observation (sample) which is far from the others (suspected as an outlier).

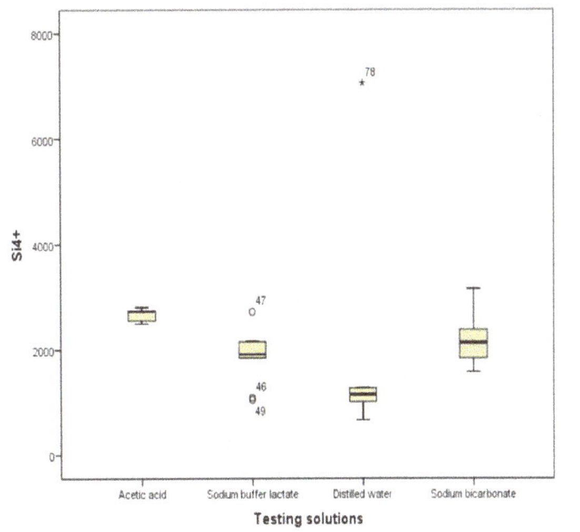

Figure 6: Silicon ion release of Bioglass in different testing solutions (μg/cm²/ml). Silicon ion release of porcelain and composite were not at measurable levels. The numbers (and the small circles) shows the observation (sample) which is far from the others (suspected as an outlier).

SB and SBL with 149, 123 and 268; their minimum release was in DW with 22, 19 and 24 (μg/cm²/ml), respectively (Table 1and Figure 3).

Maximum sodium ion release from Bioglass, resin composite and dental porcelain was found in AA, DW and DW subgroups in the order of 4584, 176,135 (μg/cm²/ml) where the minimum release was measured in DW, AA and AA subgroups in the same order of 369, 82 and 109 (μg/cm²/ml), respectively (Table 1 and Figure 4). The least values were found in resin composite and dental porcelain in AA subgroups, which were significantly different from the one in Bioglass in the same subgroup ($p < 0.001$). Due to sodium component in the formulation of SBL and SB solutions, sodium ion release in these two subgroups was not tested (Table 1 and Figure 4).

Maximum calcium ion release from Bioglass, resin composite and porcelain was found in AA subgroups in the order of 5996, 187 and 196 (μg/cm²/ml), where the minimum release was measured in the SB subgroup with the same order of 43, 41 and 76 (μg/cm²/ml), respectively (Table 1 and Figure

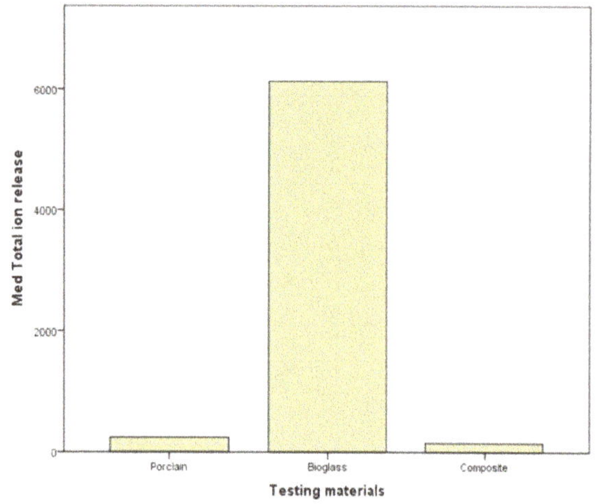

Figure 7: Total ion release from different materials regardless of solutions (μg/cm2/ml).

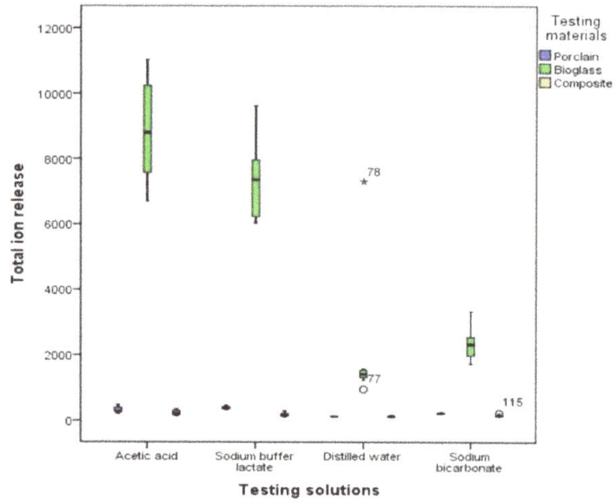

Figure 8: Total ion release from Porcelain, Composite and Bioglass in different testing solutions (μg/cm2/ml). The numbers (and the small circles) shows the observation (sample) which is far from the others (suspected as an outlier).

5). Maximum calcium release from Bioglass was significantly higher in AA and SBL than DW and SB subgroups ($p < 0.001$), (Table 1 and Figure 5).

Maximum silicon ion release was measured for Bioglass in all subgroups in order of AA; 2664, SBL; 1879, SB; 216 and DW; 1678 (μg/cm^2/ml), respectively (Tables1 and Figure 6). As to silicon ion release, Bioglass showed the maximum release in all solutions. Silicon ion release was hardly measurable for resin composite and dental porcelain; therefore, it was considered zero (Table 1 and Figure 6).

In Bioglass in comparison with resin composite and dental porcelain groups, regardless of the subgroup solutions used, the total ion release was significantly different ($p < 0.001$) (Table 1 and Figure 7). Furthermore, the total ion release in different solutions by different materials is shown Figure 8.

Discussion

Deterioration of dental materials is a complex process depending not only on the materials' compositions and structures, but also on many other factors related to the oral environment, such as surface exposure to different oral conditions (e.g. acidity of the saliva, its composition, etc.).

In the present research study, a variety of solutions with different pH levels were used to investigate the chemical behaviour of the testing materials in simulated oral cavity conditions, replicating the regular occurrence of pH level fluctuations resulting from different foods and beverages. The acidity of the environment (low pH) leads to a shift in the electrochemical equilibrium potential towards further ion release [15].

In the present study, the selected testing dental materials belonged to different classes of dental material chemical structures. Considering the limitation of this study, a series of procedures were carried out to investigate the Bioglass chemical durability and stability in comparison with dental porcelain and resin composite.

As anticipated, Bioglass showed the "lowest chemical stability" because of the "highest ion release". This can be explained by its chemical property of the non-crystalline three-dimensional structure [1]. However, for porcelain which exhibited the "highest chemical stability" because of the "lowest ion release", it could be explained by its chemical property of the structural integrity and crystalline three-dimensional atomic arrangement.

The main components of ceramics are silicon, aluminum, and potassium [15,16]. Bioglass, resin composite and dental porcelain all contain ceramic particles. The solubility of these components is high in acidic solutions [16,17]. The highest sodium, calcium and silicon ion were also released from Bioglass in all the tested solutions ($p < 0.001$) that may contribute to more instability of this type of dental material.

The potassium releases from bioglass, in comparison with resin composite and porcelain, is not the same as other ion releases. Porcelain ranked first for potassium release in SBL and SB solutions. Bioglass, ranked second with not a very significant difference in all solutions except for AA, which in Bioglass ranked first. Lower Bioglass potassium release among other alkaline elements (Ca, Na) could be explained well by its lower containing percentage of K_2O rather than Na_2O and CaO [3].

It was anticipated that silicon ion release from Bioglass would be higher in pH levels above 9, but in this study, it was observed that the highest silicon release was obtained in AA (pH = 2.4) and next in SB (pH = 9.2); this is probably due to different contents and molecular arrangements [3]. The same study also revealed that the calcium ion release, as it had been anticipated, decreased as pH increased [3]. These findings were confirmed by the results of our study.

However, our results of potassium ion release were in contrast with their findings [3,16]. Considering all the ions released from Bioglass (except for potassium) in all solutions, the chemical durability of Bioglass in different solutions may be concluded as follows: AA < SL< SB < DW. It means that stronger acidic environments impose greater deterioration of Bioglass material. The potassium release rate from all materials was observed as "SB > SBL> AA > DW", except in the porcelain group which was "SBL> SB > AA > DW"; these results are in contrast with Anusavise's findings [3].

Further studies are required to enhance Bioglass chemical stability and bonding capacity along with its light conductivity behaviour. It is also of importance to investigate the physico-mechanical properties of Bioglass in relationship with other dental materials, especially resin composite, in favor of improving its unique dental application.

Conclusions

Based on the limitation of this study, greater structural instability and less durability in simulated oral cavity conditions were observed for Bioglass compared to resin composite and dental porcelain in testing solutions with different pH levels. In the control solution (DW), durability of the testing materials, including Bioglass, was not compromised. Efforts are needed to improve the chemical resistance of Bioglass in more acidic environments to make it a stable material for in-mouth usage.

Acknowledgements

This study was supported by the Research Council of Mashhad University of Medical Sciences and Mashhad Dental Research Center, Mashhad, Iran. Authors wish to thank to Pare-Tavous Research Institute for their laboratory supports.

Conflict of Interest: None declared.

References

1. Ma L. Dissolution behavior of phosphate glasses. 2014.Doctoral Dissertations. Paper 2349.
2. McLean JW. The science and art of dental ceramics. Oper Dent. 1991;16:149-156.
3. Anusavice KJ. Degradability of dental ceramics. Adv Dent Res. 1992;6:82-89.
4. Baino F, Novajra G, Vitale-Brovarone C. Bioceramics and Scaffolds: A Winning Combination for Tissue Engineering. Front Bioeng Biotechnol. 2015;3:202.
5. Merwin GE. Bioglass middle ear prosthesis: preliminary report. Ann Otol Rhinol Laryngol. 1986;95:78-82.
6. Fathi M, Mortazavi V, Doostmohammadi A. Bioactive Glass Nanopowder for theTreatment of Oral Bone Defects. J Dent Med Tehran Univ Med Sci. 2007;4:115-122.
7. Hench LL. Chronology of bioactive glass development and clinical applications. 2013;3: 67-73.
8. Schepers EJ, Ducheyne P. Bioactive glass particles of narrow size range for the treatment of oral bone defects: a 1-24 month experiment with several materials and particle sizes and size ranges. J Oral Rehabil. 1997;24:171-181.
9. Zamet JS, Darbar UR, Griffiths GS, *et al.* Particulate bioglass as a grafting material in the treatment of periodontal intrabony defects. J Clin Periodontol. 1997;24:410-418.
10. Bagheri J, Moazzami S. Effect of light conducting intrawedge on hardness increase of the depth of the posterior composite resin restorations. J Mashhad Dent Sch. 1996;20:27-37.
11. Moazzami SM, Alaghehmand H. Effect of Light Conducting Cylindrical Inserts on Gingival Microleakage. J Dent Tehran Univ Med Sci. 2007;4:32-36.
12. Lay L. Corrosion resistance of technical ceramics. 1st Edition. 1991.
13. Bonsor SJ. Bonded amalgams and their use in clinical practice. Dent Update. 2011;38:222-224,

226-228, 230.

14. Wu C, Chang J. Degradation, bioactivity, and cytocompatibility of diopside, akermanite, and bredigite ceramics. J Biomed Mater Res B Appl Biomater. Journal of biomedical materials research Part B, Applied biomaterials. 2007;83:153-160.
15. Kukiattrakoon B, Hengtrakool C, Kedjarune-Leggat U. The effect of acidic agents on surface ion leaching and surface characteristics of dental porcelains. J Prosthet Dent. 2010;103:148-162.
16. Kukiattrakoon B, Hengtrakool C, Kedjarune-Leggat U. Chemical durability and microhardness of dental ceramics immersed in acidic agents. Acta Odontol Scand. 2010;68:1-10.
17. Kukiattrakoon B, Hengtrakool C, Kedjarune-Leggat U. Degradability of fluorapatite-leucite ceramics in naturally acidic agents. Den Mater J. 2010;29:502-511.

19

Effect of Different Irrigation Solutions on the Colour Stability of Three Calcium Silicate-Based Materials

Sobhnamayan F[a], Adl A[b], Ghanbaran S[a*]

[a]Department of Endodontics, School of Dentistry, Shiraz University of Medical Sciences, Shiraz, Iran
[b]Department of Endodontics and Biomaterials Research Center, School of Dentistry, Shiraz University of Medical Sciences, Shiraz, Iran

ARTICLE INFO

Key words:
Biodentine
Calcium Enriched Mixture
Discoloration
Mineral Trioxide Aggregate
Spectrophotometric Analysis

Corresponding Author:
Sahar Ghanbaran
Department of Endodontics, School of Dentistry, Shiraz University of Medical Sciences, Shiraz, Iran
Email: ghanbaran@sums.ac.ir

Abstract

***Statement of Problem*:** Previous studies have shown discoloration of mineral trioxide aggregate (MTA) in contact with root canal irrigation solutions. However, there are limited data on colour stability of other calcium silicate–based materials (CSMs).

Objectives: This in vitro study aimed to evaluate the colour stability of three CSMs in contact with different irrigation solutions.

***Materials and Methods*:** Three CSMs including White MTA (wMTA) Angelus, calcium enriched mixture (CEM), and Biodentine were assessed in this study. Forty five samples of each material were mixed according to the manufactures' instructions and then placed in silicone tubes. After 24 hours, the materials were removed from the moulds and 9 samples of each material left dry or immersed in normal saline, 5% sodium hypochlorite (NaOCL), 2% chlorhexidinegluconate (CHX), or 17%EDTA for 24 hours. Colour changes were measured with a spectrophotometer. Data were evaluated with 2-way analysis of variance, one way analysis of variance and Tukey post hoc tests.

***Results*:** The highest discoloration of all materials was observed after contact with CHX. In the MTA Angelus and CEM cement groups, significant differences were observed between CHX and NaOCl and also between these two irrigants with the other three irrigants ($p < 0.05$).

In the Biodentine group, CHX created statistically significant discoloration compared to other irrigants ($p < 0.05$). Only wMTA Angelus showed a significantly higher discoloration in contact with EDTA compared to normal saline and dry condition ($p < 0.05$).

wMTA Angelus showed a significantly higher colour change compared with CEM cement and Biodentine after contact with NaOCl, CHX, and EDTA ($p < 0.05$).

***Conclusions*:** The contact of wMTA, CEM cement, and Biodentine with CHX should be avoided because this leads to severe discoloration. Contact with sodium hypochlorite also leads to discoloration of wMTA and CEM cements. Among of the three tested materials, wMTA showed the highest discoloration after contact with NaOCl, CHX, and EDTA.

Introduction

Nowadays, aesthetics is an important concern to both patient and dentist. Tooth discoloration after endodontic treatment is a common problem that damages the quality of treatment, resulting in dissatisfaction in 31.6%-57% of the patients [1,2].

Many materials used in endodontics may cause tooth discoloration [1]. Therefore, colour stability of endodontic materials is considered as an important factor for clinical success [3]. A progressive discoloration is proposed to be the result of penetration of materials into dentinal tubules [4].

Endodontic procedures such as direct pulp capping, Cvek pulpotomy, perforation repair, and regenerative endodontics lead to the placement of some biomaterials in the coronal part of the tooth, which may cause discoloration [5,6].

Mineral trioxide aggregate (MTA) was first introduced in a grey form (gMTA). After reports of tooth discoloration caused by gray MTA [5,7], wMTA (wMTA) with a reduction ofAl_2O_3, MgO, and FeO was developed with an off-white colourto overcome this shortcoming [8]. However, several studies reported tooth discoloration induced even bywMTA[1,3,8-12].

In recent years, other new calcium silicate-based materials (CSMs) such as Biodentine (Septodent, Saint Maura des Fosses, France) and Calcium-Enriched Mixture (CEM)(BioniqueDent, Tehran, Iran)have been introduced to overcome the shortcoming of MTA [13-16].

CEM cement is a biomaterial [17] with different chemical composition but similar clinical applications to those of MTA [18-22]. According to the result of a recent study, CEM cement did not induce tooth discoloration after six months. Therefore, it can be used in the vital pulp therapy of aesthetically sensitive teeth [23]. Biodentine is a dentin restorative material which has indications similar to MTA in addition to the advantage of a shorter setting time(13). High colour stability of Biodentine has been reported in previous studies [11,24,25].

A recent study showed that endodontic irrigation solutions; sodium hypochlorite (NaOCl) and chlorohexidine (CHX) caused clinically perceptible colour changes in Pro Root wMTA(DENTSPLY, Tulsa Dental), wMTA Angelus, Bioaggregate, and Biodentine. However, Pro Root MTAshowed morecolour change which was attributed to the higher amounts of bismuth oxide in its composition [24].

To the best of our knowledge, there is no published study on the colour stability of CEM cement in contact with different irrigation solutions. In addition, the effect of ethylene diamine tetra acetic acid (EDTA) on the colour stability of CSMs has not been yet investigated. Therefore, the aim of this in vitro study was to evaluate colour stability of three CSMs (MTA Angelus (Angelus Solucoes Odontologicas, Londrina, Brazil), Biodentine (Septodent, Saint Maura des Fosses, France), and CEM (BioniqueDent, Tehran, Iran) in contact with different irrigation solutions (EDTA, NaOCl, CHX, Normal Saline).

Materials and Methods

Sample Preparation

Forty five specimens of each material to be tested (MTA, Biodentine, CEM cement were mixed according to the manufactures' instructions and then placed in 15 mm diameter and 2mm high silicone tubes. The specimens were stored at 37°C and 100% humidity during the setting to reach their optimal mechanical properties [25]. After 24 hours, the materials were removed from the moulds and 9 samples from each group were left dry (as control) or immersed in the following 4 irrigation solutions for 24 hours:

Normal saline(Darou pakhsh, Tehran, Iran), 5% NaOCl (Cerkamed, Pawłowski, Poland), 0.2% CHX (Cerkamed, Pawłowski, Poland), EDTA (Cerkamed, Pawłowski, Poland).

Spectrophotometric Analysis

Measurement of colour was performed and repeated 3 times with a spectrophotometer (VITA Easy shade Advance 4.0 Germany) under constant laboratory light by the same operator. The device was calibrated before each measurement. The Commission Internationale de l'eclairage (CIE) system was used to calculate the differences in colour. The colour differences (ΔE) of the samples were calculated using the following formula:

$$\Delta E = [(\Delta a)^2 + (\Delta b)^2 + (\Delta L)^2]^{1/2}$$

where $\Delta L^* = (L^*_1 - L^*_0)$, $\Delta a^* = (a^*_1 - a^*_0)$, and $\Delta b^* = (b^*_1 - b^*_0)$.

ΔL shows the change in luminosity, Δa is the change in the red-green parameter, and Δb shows the change in the yellow-blue parameter. Images of the samples were taken before and after immersion,

Table 1: Mean value and standard deviation (± SD) of colour changes (ΔE) in different groups

	Normal saline	Naocl	CHX	EDTA	Dry
CEM	5.4 ± 0.78^{Ad}	9.1 ± 0.40^{Bb}	14.6 ± 0.88^{Ba}	6.0 ± 0.52^{Bc}	4.9 ± 1.10^{Ad}
MTA	5.1 ± 1.02^{Ad}	15.2 ± 1.11^{Ab}	18.4 ± 1.1^{7Aa}	10.9 ± 0.61^{Ac}	4.4 ± 0.48^{Ad}
Biodentin	5.2 ± 0.93^{Ab}	4.5 ± 0.98^{Cb}	14.6 ± 1.31^{Ba}	5.3 ± 0.64^{Ab}	4.9 ± 0.87^{Ab}

Upper case letter shows a significant deference in a column and lower case letter shows a significant difference in a row

using a digital camera (Cybershot DSC-W220; Sony, Tokyo, Japan).

Statistical Analysis

The data were analyzed with two-way ANOVA using SPSS software (PASW Statistics 20; SPSS Inc, Chicago, IL). There was an interaction effect between the material and irrigation soloution. ($p \leq 0.05$). Therefore, one-way ANOVA and Tukey post hoc tests were used to perform multiple comparison tests. The level of statistical significance was set at $p < 0.05$.

Results

Table 1 shows the mean value and standard deviation of colour changes in different groups. The mean values for changes in the colour of materials are shown in Figure 1. All materials showed the highest discoloration after contact with CHX.

In the MTA Angelus and CEM cement groups, significant differences were observed between CHX and NaOCl and also between these two irrigants with the other three irrigants ($p < 0.05$).

In the Biodentine group, CHX showed statistically significant differences with the other irrigants ($p < 0.05$). Only wMTA Angelus showed a significantly higher discoloration in contact with EDTA compared to normal saline and dry condition ($p < 0.05$)

There were no significant differences in the ΔE values of three materials in the presence of normal saline and in the dry condition ($p = 0.715$, $p = 0.298$, respectively).

White MTA Angelus showed a significantly higher ΔE value compared with CEM cement and Biodentine after contact with NaOCl, CHX, and EDTA ($p < 0.05$).

Discussion

Tooth discoloration has been reported with the use of a number of endodontic materials; therefore, material selection should not rely solely on biological and functional criteria but also aesthetic considerations should be taken into account [26]. Colour changes in different types of dental materials has been measured using spectrophotometer [27-29]. In the current study, a spectrophotometer was used to evaluate the colour change of three dental cements after contact

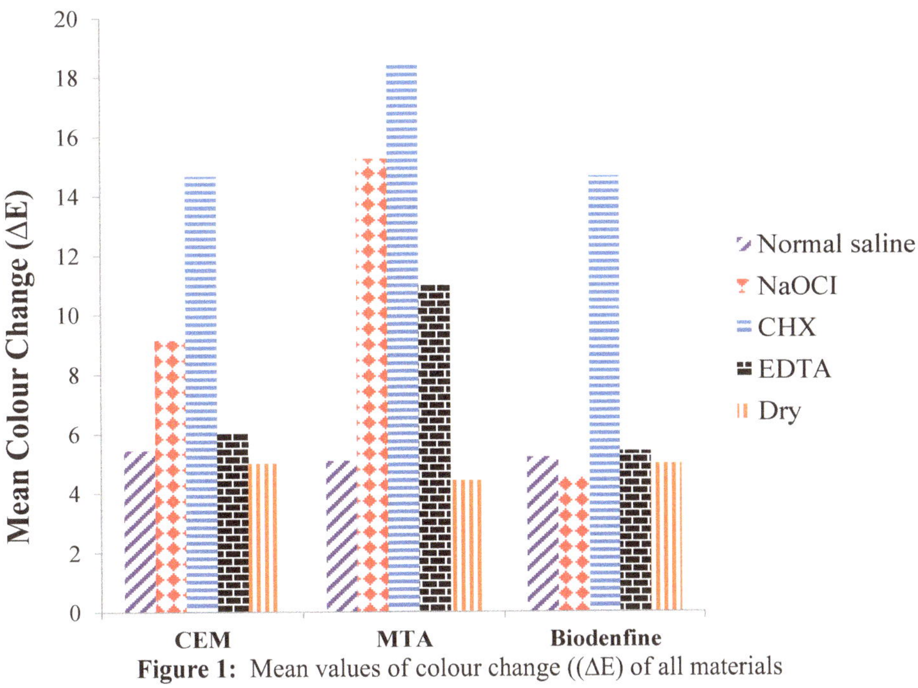

Figure 1: Mean values of colour change ((ΔE) of all materials

with different irrigation solution. Spectrophotometric analysis was applied because of its sensitivity to small changes in colour, repeatability, and objectivity [30].

This study showed that MTA Angelus, CEM cement, and Biodentinerevealed the most severe discoloration in contact with CHX. MTA Angelus and CEM cement also showed severe discoloration in contact with NaOCl, while Biodentine was not affected by NaOCl. This finding is in the same line with those of Keskinet a. who reported that Biodentine exhibited more discoloration when immersed in CHX compared with NaOCl [24].

Chlorhexidine has been shown to cause extrinsic discoloration of silicate filling materials [31] and dental tissues at varying concentrations by affecting dental pellicle or plaque [32]. However, the exact mechanism of discoloration of dental cements in the presence of CHX is not well defined [24]. The current study has also shown that wMTA and CEM cement exhibited higher discoloration in contact with NaOCl when compared with dry condition, normal saline, and EDTA.

Previously, it had been shown that immersion of wMTA in sodium hypochlorite resulted in the formation of a dark brown discoloration. It has been speculated that the discoloration was attributed to the reaction of sodium hypochlorite with bismuth oxide which is a part of MTA [26].

In contrast to MTA, CEM cement has no bismuth oxide in its content [11]; therefore, the reason of its discoloration in contact with NaOCl is not yet understood.

The current study also evaluated the effect of EDTA on the colour stability of wMTA, CEM cement, and Biodentine. EDTA is normally used for removal of the mineralized portion of smear layer. Recently, EDTA was introduced to regenerative endodontic procedures as the only irrigant in the second visit based on its ability in releasing growth factors from the dentin and also inducing cell attachment and differentiation [33,34].

According to the results, CEM cement and Biodentine exhibited colour stability in contact with EDTA while wMTA Angelus showed higher discoloration compared to normal saline and dry condition. It should be noted that 2 samples of Biodentine were eroded in contact with EDTA and deleted from the study. Therefore, the effect of EDTA on the microstructure of Biodentine should be investigated.

In the dry condition and in the presence of normal saline, no differences were found between three cements; however, in contact with NaOCl and CHX, wMTA Angelus showed significantly more discoloration than the other materials. This is somehow in contrast to a previous study reporting no statistically significant difference between discoloration of wMTA Angelus and Biodentine in contact with NaOCl and CHX[24] .

It is well defined that contact of bismuth oxide–containing products with NaOCl and CHX leads to material discoloration [24].Therefore, the higher discoloration of wMTA Angelus which was found in this study may be attributed to the fact that neither CEM cement [11] nor Biodentine [35] contains bismuth oxide as radiopacifire [35].

Conclusions

Under the limitation of this study, contact of wMTA, CEM cement, and Biodentine with CHX should be avoided because this leads to severe discoloration. Contact with sodium hypochlorite also leads to discoloration of wMTA and CEM cements. White MTA showed significantly higher discoloration compared with other materials after contact with NaOCl, CHX, and EDTA.

Conflict of Interest: None declared.

References

1. Lenherr P, Allgayer N, Weiger R, *et al*. Tooth discoloration induced by endodontic materials: a laboratory study. Int Endod J. 2012;45:942-949.
2. Thomson AD, Athanassiadis B, Kahler B, *et al*. Tooth discolouration: staining effects of various sealers and medicaments. Aust Endod J. 2012;38:2-9.
3. Eghbal MJ, Torabzadeh H, Bagheban AA, *et al*. Color stability of mineral trioxide aggregate and calcium enriched mixture cement. J Invest Clin Dent. 2016;7:341-346.
4. Van der Burgt T, Mullaney T, Plasschaert A. Tooth discoloration induced by endodontic sealers. Oral Surg Oral Med Oral Pathol. 1986;61:84-89.
5. Karabucak B, Li D, Lim J, *et al*. Vital pulp therapy with mineral trioxide aggregate. Dent Traumatol. 2005;21:240-243.
6. Belobrov I, Parashos P. Treatment of tooth discoloration after the use of white mineral trioxide aggregate. J Endod. 2011;37:1017-1020.

7. Bortoluzzi EA, Araújo GS, Guerreiro Tanomaru JM, *et al*. Marginal gingiva discoloration by gray MTA: a case report. J Endod. 2007;33:325-327.
8. Akbari M, Rouhani A, Samiee S, *et al*. Effect of dentin bonding agent on the prevention of tooth discoloration produced by mineral trioxide aggregate. Int J Dent. 2011;2012.
9. Moore A, Howley MF, O'Connell AC. Treatment of open apex teeth using two types of white mineral trioxide aggregate after initial dressing with calcium hydroxide in children. Dent Traumatol. 2011;27:166-173.
10. Felman D, Parashos P. Coronal tooth discoloration and white mineral trioxide aggregate. J Endod. 2013;39:484-487.
11. Kohli MR, Yamaguchi M, Setzer FC, *et al*. Spectrophotometric analysis of coronal tooth discoloration induced by various bioceramic cements and other endodontic materials. J Endod. 2015;41:1862-1866.
12. Ioannidis K, Mistakidis I, Beltes P, *et al*. Spectrophotometric analysis of coronal discolouration induced by grey and white MTA. Int Endod J. 2013;46:137-144.
13. Laurent P, Camps J, De Méo M, *et al*. Induction of specific cell responses to a Ca 3 SiO 5-based posterior restorative material. Dent Mater. 2008;24:1486-494.
14. Koubi G, Colon P, Franquin JC, *et al*. Clinical evaluation of the performance and safety of a new dentine substitute, Biodentine, in the restoration of posterior teeth-a prospective study. Clinl Oral Investig. 2013;17:243-249.
15. Pradelle-Plasse N, Tran X, Colon P, *et al*. Biocompatibility or cytotoxic effects of dental composites. 2009.
16. Shokouhinejad N, Nekoofar MH, Pirmoazen S, *et al*. Evaluation and Comparison of Occurrence of Tooth Discoloration after the Application of Various Calcium Silicate–based Cements: An Ex Vivo Study. J Endod. 2016;42:140-144.
17. Asgary S, Shahabi S, Jafarzadeh T, *et al*. The properties of a new endodontic material. J Endod. 2008;34:990-993.
18. Asgary S, Eghbal MJ, Parirokh M. Sealing ability of a novel endodontic cement as a root-end filling material. J Biomed Mater Res A. 2008;87:706-709.
19. Malekafzali B, Shekarchi F, Asgary S. Treatment outcomes of pulpotomy in primary molars using two endodontic biomaterials. A 2-year randomised clinical trial. Eur J Paediatr Dent. 2011;12:189-193.
20. Asgary S, Eghbal MJ, Ghoddusi J. Two-year results of vital pulp therapy in permanent molars with irreversible pulpitis: an ongoing multicenter randomized clinical trial. Clin Oral Investig. 2014;18:635-641.
21. Haghgoo R, Arfa S, Asgary S. Microleakage of CEM cement and ProRoot MTA as furcal perforation repair materials in primary teeth. Iran Endod J. 2013;8:187-190.
22. Guler AU, Kurt S, Kulunk T. Effects of various finishing procedures on the staining of provisional restorative materials. J Prosthet Dent. 2005;93:453-458.
23. Rouhani A, Akbari M, Farhadi-faz A. Comparison of tooth discoloration induced by calcium-enriched mixture and mineral trioxide aggregate. Iran Endod J. 2016;11:175-178.
24. Keskin C, Demiryurek EO, Ozyurek T. Color Stabilities of Calcium Silicate–based Materials in Contact with Different Irrigation Solutions. J Endod. 2015;41:409-411.
25. Vallés M, Mercadé M, Duran-Sindreu F, *et al*. Influence of light and oxygen on the color stability of five calcium silicate–based materials. J Endod. 2013;39:525-528.
26. Camilleri J. Color stability of white mineral trioxide aggregate in contact with hypochlorite solution. J Endod. 2014;40:436-440.
27. Deljoo Z, Sadeghi M, Azar MR, *et al*. The Effect of Different Polishing Methods and Storage Media on Discoloration of Resin Composites. J Dent Biomater. 2016;3;226-232.
28. Khaledi AAA, Safari A, Adibi A, *et al*. The Effect of Chlorhexidine Mouth Rinse on the Colour Stability of Porcelain with Three Different Surface Treatments: An in Vitro Study. J Dent Biomater. 2014;1:3-8.
29. Mousavi S, Narimani S, Hekmatfar S, *et al*. Colour Stability of Various Types of Acrylic Teeth Exposed to Coffee, Tea and Cola. J Dent Biomater. 2016;3:335-340.
30. Khokhar Z, Razzoog M, Yaman P. Color stability of restorative resins. Quintessence Int. 1991;22;733-777.
31. Heyden G. Relation between locally high concentration of chlorhexidine and staining as seen in the clinic. J Periodontal Res Suppl. 1973;12:76-80.
32. Bagis B, Baltacioglu E, Oezcan M, *et al*.

Evaluation of chlorhexidine gluconate mouthrinse-induced staining using a digital colorimeter: An in vivo study. Quintessence Int. 2011;42:213-223.

33. Martin DE, De Almeida JF, Henry MA, *et al.* Concentration-dependent effect of sodium hypochlorite on stem cells of apical papilla survival and differentiation. J Endod. 2014;40:51-55.

34. Zhao S, Sloan A, Murray P, *et al.* Ultrastructural localisation of TGF-β exposure in dentine by chemical treatment. Histochem J. 2000;32:489-494.

35. Camilleri J, Kralj P, Veber M, *et al.* Characterization and analyses of acid-extractable and leached trace elements in dental cements. Int Endod J. 2012;45:737-743.

20

Fractography and Mechanical Properties of Urethane Dimethacrylate Dental Composites Reinforced with Glass Nanoparticles

Monfared M*, Bahrololoom ME

Department of Materials Science and Engineering, School of Engineering, Shiraz University, Shiraz, Iran

ARTICLE INFO

Key words:
Dental Composite
Glass Nanoparticles
Mechanical Properties
Fractography
Biomaterials

Corresponding Author:
Marzieh Monfared
Department of Materials Science and Engineering, School of Engineering, Shiraz University, Shiraz, Iran
Email: mamonfared@gmail.com

Abstract

***Statement of Problem*:** Dental resin composites are becoming prevalent in restorative dentistry and have almost replaced amalgam nowadays. Consequently, their mechanical properties and durability are critical.

***Objectives*:** The aim of this study was to produce Pyrex glass nano-particles by wet milling process and use them as reinforcement in dental resins for anterior restorations and then examination of fractographic properties of these composites.

***Materials and Methods*:** The glass nano-particles were achieved via wet milling. The surface of the particles was modified with 3-(Trimethoxysilyl) propyl methacrylate (γ-MPTMS) silane in order to improve their surface. Fourier transform infra-red (FTIR) analysis showed that the silane groups provided double bonds to the surface of the particles and prevented agglomeration. Then, the composite resins were made with different weight percentages of Pyrex glass. The mechanical properties of samples flexural test were evaluated. The required energy for fracture of the specimens was achieved via this test. The fracture surfaces of the samples were analyzed using a scanning electron microscope (SEM) in order to explain the mechanisms of fracture.

Results: The results and analysis showed that increasing the glass nano-particles mass fraction had a great effect on mechanical properties of the composites due to the mechanisms of crack propagation and crack deflection as well as preventing void formation. The effective energy dissipation mechanisms such as crack pinning and deflection, was observed in SEM micrographs.

Conclusions: Void formation in the low filler content composite is one of the mechanisms to decrease the energy required for fracture of these composites and eventually weaken them.

Introduction

Dental resin composites consisting of a polymerizable resin matrix and appropriate filler are becoming prevalent in modern dentistry [1]. To-date, dental resin composites have almost replaced dental amalgam as filling materials in small-sized operations due to the fact that an amalgam filling has disadvantages such as toxicity, difficulty in fixing and lack of bioactivity [2]. Since the invention of resin composites in the 1960s by Bowen [3], there has been great progress both in research and application of these materials. However, using these materials in heavy-load (such as, posterior areas) and large area restorations has been limited because of several disadvantages like high polymerization shrinkage, low wear resistance and secondary caries. Studies on modifications in resins and inorganic fillers have been increased significantly to improve the mechanical properties due to the function of resin composites [2].

Resin composites typically consist of a dispersed phase composed of glass filler particles such as zirconia/silica based that are distributed to reinforce a polymerizable resin matrix, and silane coupling agents. The organic compounds are glycidyl methacrylate (BIS-GMA), urethane dimethacrylate (UDMA), and triethylene glycol dimethacrylate (TEGDMA), which are cured during application. Due to the good aesthetic properties and strength of these composites, they are the most commonly used materials to restore hard tissues like dentin and enamel [4].

In addition, since particles in nano scale improve the strength and wear resistance, they are attractive as filler for dental composites [5]. Many different methods are used for the production of inorganic nano-particles [6]. One of the most convenient and promising techniques to produce nano-particles powder is mechanical milling [7]. Planetary milling is an efficient method to produce nano-particles, among the high-energy milling such as oscillating, attrition jetting and vibration milling. The selection of the appropriate milling parameters for specific equipment to produce fine powders, especially dry nanoparticles, is necessary. Drying generally causes agglomeration of fine particles due to high interaction between them [8]. Compounds such as alcohol, ketones, amines, carboxylic acids, and esters are used to prevent particle agglomeration during the production of fine particles [9].

In order to appropriately disperse nano-particles in a polymer matrix and improve compatibility between the nano-fillers and polymer matrix, using several coupling agents including silanes to modify the nano-particle's surface is very common. The proper modification of nano-particle's surface can also make a durable chemical junction between the two phases because of chemical and physical interactions with the inorganic matrix [10].

Although many studies have focused on the strength values of dental composite, little has been done about fractographic analysis. This is really critical, since material strength alone is not sufficient to show the causes of restoration failure or clinical durability [11]. Outside the dental field, fractographic analysis is commonly used to make systematic relations between strength test values and performance of components in brittle materials [12]. A study on commercial glass-ceramics that are usually used in dental field showed that while different batches had identical properties like elastic moduli, microstructures, and fracture toughness, they had highly different failure loads because of the difference in defect type [13]. In order to determine the critical flaw and prediction of component strength in brittle materials, fractographic analysis is essential. Among all brittle materials, resin composites with high filler ratio are quite neglected in fractographic studies [14]. This group of materials is put between polymeric and ceramic materials. Fractographic specialists in both fields discover the issues difficult to distinguish when they are covered by rough microstructures that are so common in failed composite materials [15].

The present study first aimed to modify the glass nano-particles which were produced via wet comminution process and use them as fillers to reinforce dental polymers. We also aimed to observe the fractured surfaces of these new composites after failure under flexural tests and study the mechanisms of their fracture.

Materials and Methods

Production of glass powder

A borosilicate Pyrex glass (Schott Co., Mainz, Germany) with composition of 81 wt% SiO_2, 13 wt% B_2O_3, 4 wt% Na_2O + K_2O and 2 wt% Al_2O_3 was utilized. A planetary mill (Fritsch-GMBH, Idar-Oberstein, Germany) was employed for glass comminution experiments. The grinding bowl volume was 500 ml and the grinding balls were made of tungsten carbide (wolfram carbide: WC). The comminution process was performed with 7.5 weight ratios of balls to glass particles in the 500 ml grinding bowl and WC grinding balls. The glass was milled for 30 hours with 400 rpm speed. Hexane was used as the liquid dispersion medium.

Modification of glass particle size

Having been milled, the glass particles were silanized with γ-MPTMS; then, the particle size and distribution were determined according to the previous work [16]. Fourier transforms infrared spectroscopy (FTIR) of glass particles and SEM photos were recorded before and after silanization.

Production of composites

Producing dental matrices with uniformly dispersed nano-scaled fillers has always been a challenge [17]. Acetone was a medium to explore the optimal procedure for dispersing the silanized glass particles in the resin matrix. Although the silanized particles could be highly separated and uniformly dispersed in acetone, it might not be able to achieve the same high degree of separation and dispersion in UDMA/TEGDMA. Hence, the modified glass particles with different weight fractions (5, 7.5 and 10 wt %) were dispersed in acetone by sonication to achieve uniform dispersion and the solution was added to the resin (70/30 UDMA, TEGDMA in weight percentage). Surrounding the mixture by an ice enclosure inhibits heating of the mixture. Then, acetone was removed by evaporation. This was followed by addition of camphorquinone (CQ) and ethyl 4-(dimethylamino) benzoate (4EDMAB) (in 0.5/0.5 weight ratio). Finally, the composite was placed in an ultrasonic bath to remove air bubbles and better mixing.

Fabrication of samples and flexural test

Composite bars with 2mm × 2mm × 25mm dimensions were fabricated in steel moulds for flexural strength test, according to ISO 4049. Three bar-shaped samples were made in each group. These specimens were light cured with 520 mW/cm^2 intensity (Demetron LC Curing light) for 45 seconds on each side, and then carefully removed from the moulds. In order to simulate the mouth environment, the samples were stored in distilled water at 37°C incubator for 24 hours. The flexural strength was measured via 3-point bending test using a universal testing machine (STM-20 Santam) with a span of 20 mm, at 60 N load cell and a cross-head speed of 0.5 mm/min. Force-displacement curves of all specimens were recorded during the tests and the amounts of work-of-fracture of the samples were calculated by dividing the area under these curves by the specimen's cross-sectional area. Work-of-fracture is the energy required to fracture a specimen [17]. The flexural strength is calculated by:

$F.S. = 3PL/2bh^2$

Where, F.S. is flexural strength, P is force at fracture point, L is span distance (20 mm), b is width of sample and h is the height of the sample.

Morphology

A VEGA//TESCAN Scanning electron microscope (SEM) was employed to examine the morphologies of glass particles and the fractured surfaces of the UDMA/TEGDMA dental resins composites containing various mass fractions of glass particles. Prior to SEM examination, the specimens were sputter-coated with gold to avoid charge accumulation.

Results

FTIR analysis of particles

The FTIR spectra of glass particles before and after milling are given in Figure 1. These spectra show that hexane has no significant effect on glass structures

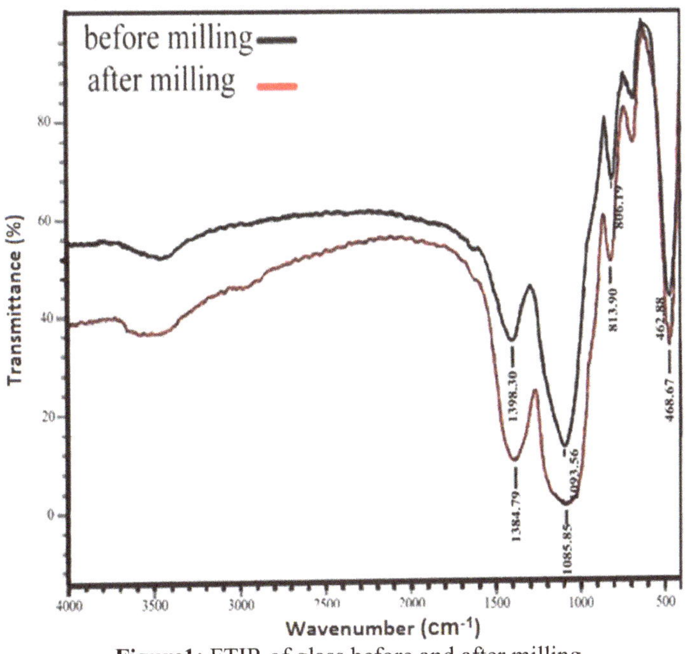

Figure1: FTIR of glass before and after milling

because of the fact that there is no new peak resulting from a new functional group after milling process. Figure 2 shows the FTIR of glass particles after modification with silane.

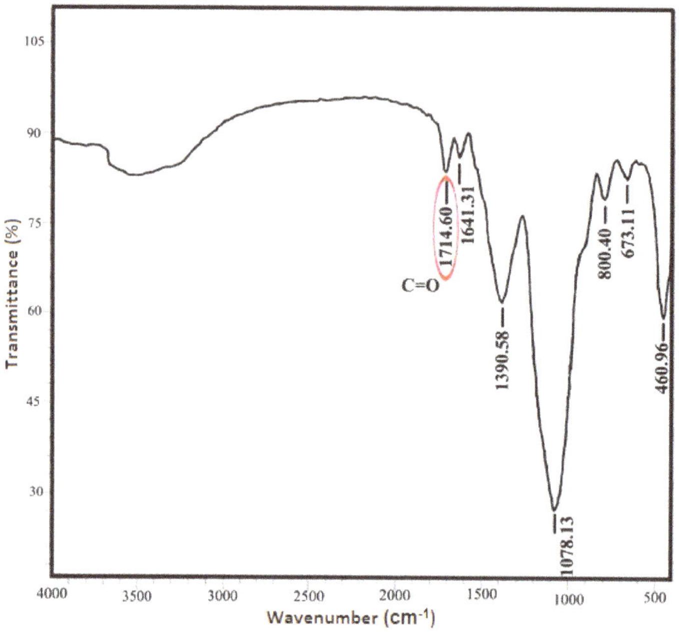

Figure 2: FTIR of silanized glass particles and existance of C = O bond

Morphology of particles

Figures 3A and 3B show the SEM micrographs of the glass particles before and after silanization, respectively.

Flexural strength and work-of-fracture

The flexural strength and flexural modulus of the specimens were calculated using 3-point bending formula; the results have been reported in the previous work [16]. Several curves of force-displacement obtained from the flexural tests of the samples are displayed in Figure 4 as examples. According to these curves, the maximum force and extension at which a composite sample failed were obtained and the values of force and displacement at the failure point and mean value of work-of-fracture for each group are summarized in Table 1.

Fractography

SEM photos of the fractured surfaces emanate from 3-point bending tests are shown in Figure 5. Columnar photos in Figures 5 (a), (b), and (c) show the fractured surfaces of 5, 7.5, and 10 wt% glass filler composites, respectively.

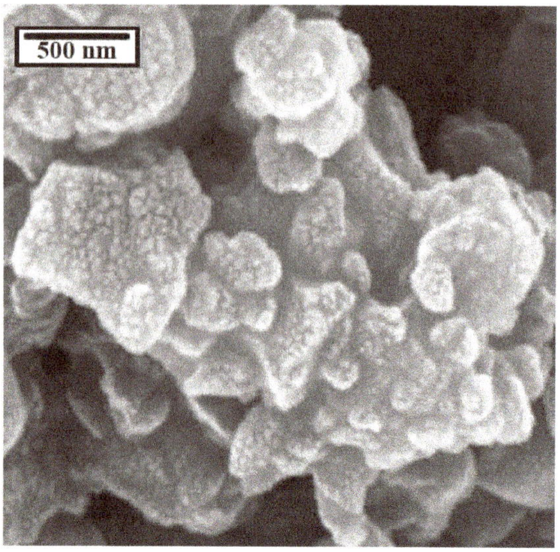

Figure 3A: SEM photomicrograph of glass particles before silanization

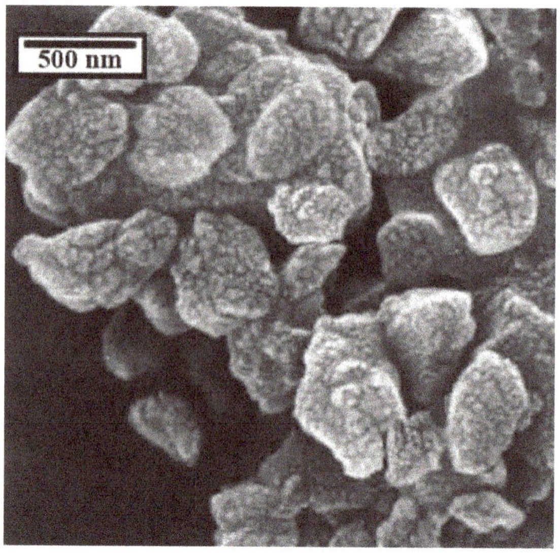

Figure 3B: SEM photomicrograph of silanized glass particles

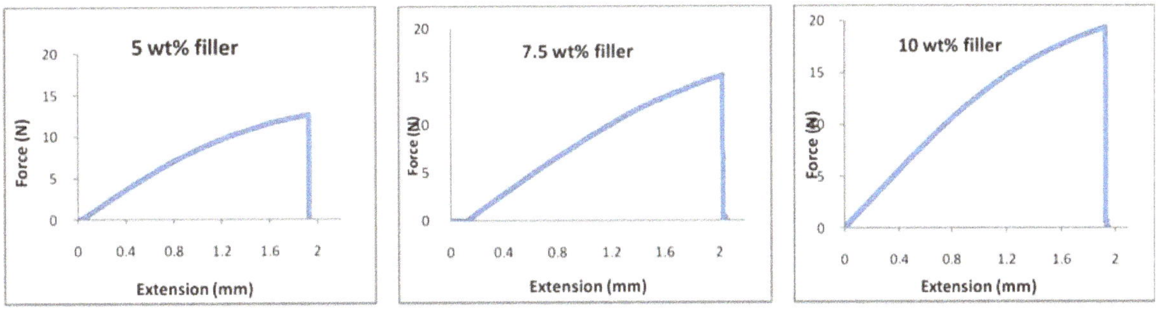

Figure 4: Force-displacement curves of the composites of each group achieved by flexural tests with 5, 7.5, 10 wt% filler

Discussion

Comparison of Figures 1 and 2 shows that there is a peak at 1714cm^{-1} wave number which is due to the existence of carbonyl (C = O) group and chemical bonds between glass and γ-MPTMS [18]. It can be concluded that modification of glass was successfully carried out through silanization process.

Micrographs 3A and 3B display that agglomerated particles were removed dramatically after modification. The particle size was analyzed in our previous study, showing that the mean particle size of the silanized glass particles was about 140 nm [16].

By increasing the fraction of glass filler from 5 to 10 wt%, the values of flexural strength increase from (64 ± 1.7) MPa to (75 ± 2.5) MPa and flexural moduli increase from (1.2 ± 0.01) GPa to (1.4 ± 0.02) GPa [16]. In other words, flexural strength and flexural modulus of the composites containing 10wt% filler improved by 17.2% and 16.7%, respectively.

The data in Table 1 indicate that work-of-fracture of composite samples increases from (4.07) kJ/m^2 to (5.33) kJ/m^2 with 5 wt% increase in the filler content. It means that work-of-fracture was improved by 30.9%. The results indicated that the impregnation of the silanized nano-glass particles into UDMA/TEGDMA resin could improve the mechanical properties considerably and enhance the resistance of this resin to brittle fracture.

Comparison of Figure 5 (a) with 5 (b) and 5 (c) reveals that the fractured surfaces of composites containing 5 wt% filler have a large smoother area, large hyperbolic marking, ribbon and fracture steps in the direction of crack propagation (from the bottom left side to top right side). These patterns are proportional to lower resistance to the crack propagation, and a minimum energy is required to fracture the specimen [19]. As calculated above, the composites in this group have the minimal work-of-fracture compared to the other ones; this indicates that this group has the lowest resistance to fracture.

On the other hand, by increasing the weight fraction of glass particles, the fractured surface area became rougher indicating more ductile fracture, which could be attributed to the crack deflection and crack pinning effects of the glass nano-particles [20]. The composites' fractured surfaces in Figures 5 (b) and (c) in contrast to Figure 5 (a) have rougher features such as out of the plane flaking and the thumbnail type marks, crack pinning, and shear yielding which requires additional energy to fail the materials.

As more energy was imparted from the deformation strain of the specimens for the creation of these features, corresponding increases in the flexural strength and work-of-fracture were obtained [19]. The higher values of flexural strength and work-of-fracture of the composites with 7.5 wt% and 10 wt% filler, concluded from force-extension curves are consistent with the morphology of the fractured surfaces of Figures 5 (b) and (c) .

In order to draw a conclusion about the amount of dissipated energy during the fracture, it is important to know how the cracks pass through the materials, and how the particles influence the crack propagation. Particles function as obstacles when cracks interacted them, so the crack front can deviate and branch or

Table1: The Maximum force, extension and work-of-fracture of the samples at break according to Figure 4

Glass filler content (wt%)	5	7.5	10
Maximum extension (mm)	1.92	2.02	1.92
Maximum force (N)	12.60	15.13	19.33
work-of-fracture (kJ/m^2)	4.07 ± 0.04	4.69 ± 0.28	5.33 ± 0.31

even pin in them, which leads to a higher energy absorption in the composite. In addition, the interface has a critical effect in deformation behavior so that under the strong bonding conditions high amounts of energy will be consumed at the interface of the particle and matrix [19].

The nano-composite reinforced with higher fraction modified glass nano-particles improved the

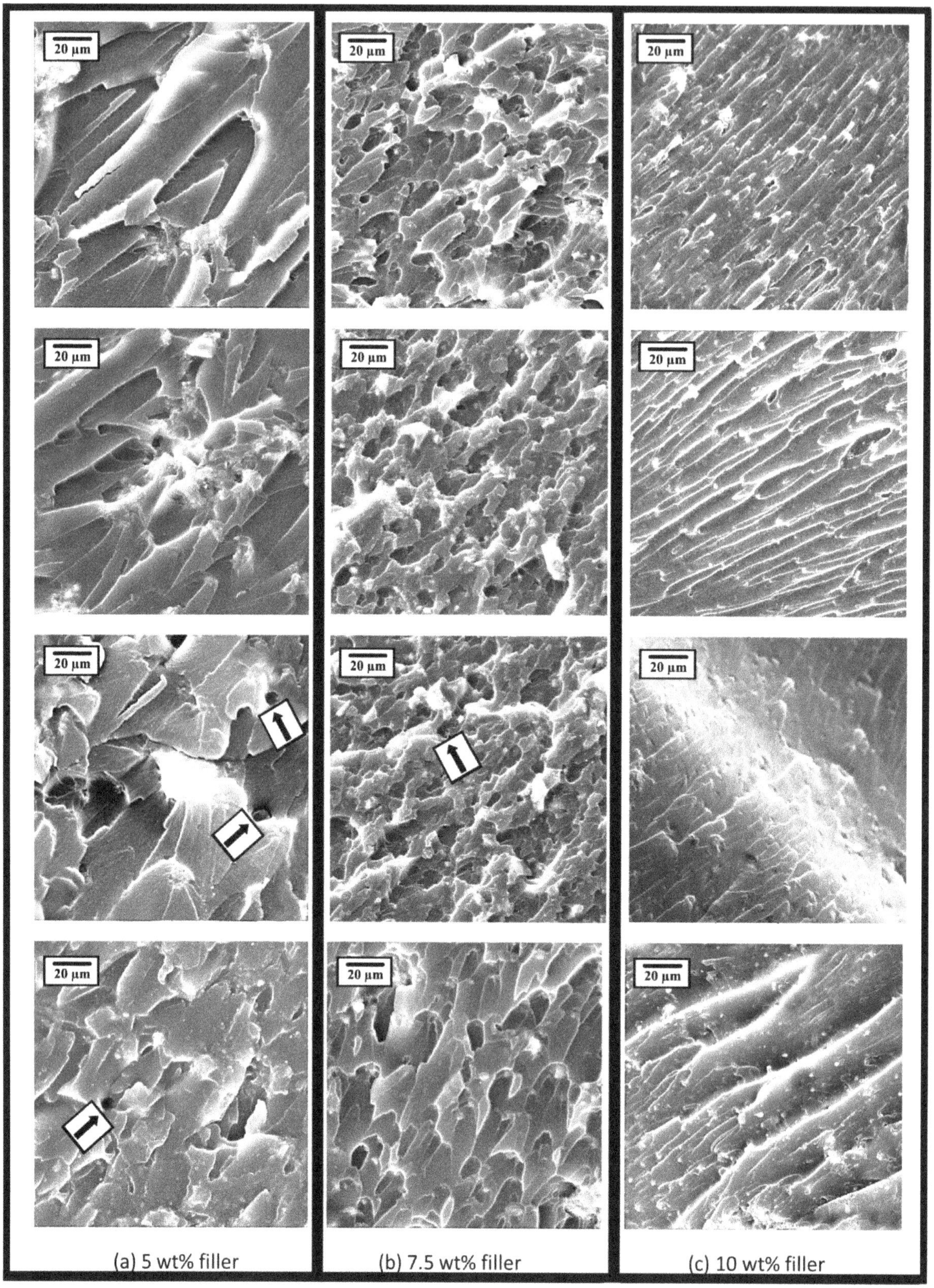

Figure 5: Representative fractured surfaces of three-point flexural specimens: (a): composites with 5 wt% glass filler; (b) composites with 7.5 wt% glass; (c) composites with 10 wt% glass filler. The arrows show voids formation due to failure of the glass particles in the composites with lower filler fractions.

interface and requires more energy to fracture. This leads to a higher flexural strength and a rougher fractured surface. In order to elaborate, it can be observed that some voids are formed on the fractured surface of the composites with lower filler fractions, especially in the composites with 5 wt% filler. These voids are indicated by arrows in Figures 5 (a) and (b). Formation of these voids results from failure of the glass particles. In fact, the filled resin is dramatically weakened because of the agglomeration which functions as structural defects [17].

According to SEM photos and the lower values of work-of-fracture and flexural strength in composites with less filler fraction, it may be concluded that lower content of glass filler in composites has much more tendency to agglomerate which results in weak interface and void formation. In other words, when the glass filler content in the resin matrix is low, the particles' tendency to interact with each other is more than the amount required to interact with the resin matrix. Hence, due to the lack of an efficient interface, the particles are pulled out and the voids are formed by lower forces.

Conclusions

In this study, glass nano-particles were produced via milling process. It was found that the silane modification has a significant effect on dispersion and stabilization of these particles and removes agglomeration due to the formation of the carbonyl group on the particles' surface.

It was discovered that a little increase in glass nano-particles' mass fraction dramatically improves the mechanical properties of the composite. This raise owes to the effective energy dissipation mechanisms such as crack pinning and deflection, as observed in SEM micrographs. Moreover, void formation in the low filler content composite is another mechanism to decrease the energy required for fracture of these composites and eventually weaken them.

Conflict of Interest: None declared.

References

1. Chao X, Zhong-Yi W, Hui-Ming H, *et al.* Study on the Structure and Mechanical Properties of Dental Barium Glass Particles Surface Modification with Silane Coupling Reagent. Polym-Plast Technol and Eng. 2008;47:858-864.
2. Liu Y, Tan Y, Lei T, *et al.* Effect of porous glass–ceramic fillers on mechanical properties of light-cured dental resin composites. Dent Mater. 2009;25:709-715.
3. Bowen RL. Particle distribution in reinforced polymer. J Am Dent Assoc. 1964;69:481-495.
4. Beyth N, Farah S, Domb AJ, *et al.* Antibacterial dental resin composites. React Func Polym. 2014; 75:81-88.
5. Chan K, Nicolella D, Furman B, *et al.* Fracture toughness of zirconia nanoparticle-filled dental composites. J Mater Sci. 2009;44:6117-6124.
6. Rozenberg B, Tenne R. Polymer-assisted fabrication of nanoparticles and nanocomposites. Prog Polym Sci. 2008;33:40-112.
7. Wang Li-Li, Jiang J-S. Preparation of α-Fe 2 O 3 nanoparticles by high-energy ball milling. Physica B Condens Matter. 2007;390:23-27.
8. Arbain R, Othman M, Palaniandy S. Preparation of iron oxide nanoparticles by mechanical milling. Miner Eng. 2011;24:1-9.
9. Garcia F, Le Bolay N, Trompette J-L, *et al.* On fragmentation and agglomeration phenomena in an ultrafine wet grinding process: the role of polyelectrolyte additives. Int J Miner Process. 2004;74:43-54.
10. Sabzi M, Mirabedini SM, Zohuriaan-Mehr J, *et al.* Surface modification of TiO_2 nano-particles with silane coupling agent and investigation of its effect on the properties of polyurethane composite coating. Prog Org Coat. 2009;65:222-228.
11. Kelly JR. Approaching clinical relevance in failure testing of restorations. J Prosthet Dent. 1999;81: 652-661.
12. Quinn GD, Morrell R. Design data for engineering ceramics: a review of the flexure test. J Am Ceram Soc. 1991;74:2037–2066.
13. Lewis D. Observations on the strength of a commercial glass-ceramic. Am Ceram Soc Bull. 1982;61:1208-1214.
14. Parrington RJ. Fractography of metals and plastics. Pract Fail Anal. 2002;2:16-19.
15. Rice RW. Ceramic fracture features, observations, mechanisms, and uses. Fractography of ceramic and metal failures. Am Soc Test Mater. 1984;827:5-103.
16. Monfared M, Mirdamadi S, Khavandi A. Synthesis of new dental nanocomposite with glass nanoparticles. Nanomedicine J. 2014;1:107-111.
17. Tian M, Gao Y, Liu Y, *et al.* Fabrication and

evaluation of Bis-GMA/TEGDMA dental resins/composites containing nano fibrillar silicate. Dent Mater. 2008;24:235-243.

18. Yuvaraj H, Shim JJ, Lim KT. Organic-inorganic polypyrrole-surface modified SiO2 hybrid nanocomposites: a facile and green synthetic approach. Polym Adv Technol. 2010;21:424-429.

19. Du M, Zheng Y. Modification of silica nanoparticles and their application in UDMA dental polymeric composites. Polym Composite. 2007;28:198-207.

20. Deng S, Ye L, Friedrich K. Fracture behaviours of epoxy nanocomposites with nano-silica at low and elevated temperatures. J Mater Sci. 2007;42:2766-2774.

21

The Effect of Four Commonly Used Root Conditioner Agents in Different Time Periods Applied on Periodontally Diseased and Healthy Teeth

Torkzaban P[a], Seyedzadeh Sabounchi S[b]

[a]Department of Periodontology, Member of Hamadan Dental Research Center, School of Dentistry, Hamadan University of Medical Sciences, Hamadan , Iran
[b]Department of Periodontology, School of Dentistry, Hamadan University of Medical Sciences, Hamadan , Iran

ARTICLE INFO

Key words:
Citric Acid
Doxycycline
Periodontal Debridement
Smear Layer
Tetracycline

Corresponding Author:
Sepideh Seyedzadeh Sabounchi
Department of Periodontology, School of Dentistry, Hamadan University of Medical Sciences, Hamadan , Iran
E-mail: sepideh1s@gmail.com

Abstract

***Statement of Problem*:** Root surface contamination or infection can potentially change the consequences of regenerative periodontal therapies and therefore the modification and disinfection of the contaminated root surfaces are necessary.
***Objectives*:** This study aimed to compare the surface characteristics of the extracted human teeth after exposure to four root conditioners in different time periods.
***Materials and Methods*:** The study samples were prepared from 40 freshly extracted teeth including 20 affected teeth with periodontal diseases and 20 healthy teeth. After performing root planning, 240 dentinal block samples were prepared and each affected and healthy sample was randomly allocated to receive one of the following root conditioners; Ethylenediaminetetraaceti acid (EDTA), citric acid, doxycycline, and tetracycline or rinsed with normal saline as the control agent. The prepared specimens were evaluated using scanning electron microscope and the inter-group differences and changes in study indices; dentin (%), tubular spaces (%), and diameter of dentinal tubules (μm^2) were compared using one-way ANOVA test.
***Results*:** In the control group receiving normal saline, the changes in the indicators of dentin, tubular spaces, and diameter of dentinal tubules remained insignificant in all time periods. EDTA, citric acid, and tetracycline had chelating effects on the study indices; however, doxycycline led to gradual decrease of the tubular space and diameter as well as increase in dentin percentage.
***Conclusions*:** In different time intervals and when considering healthy or affected tooth surfaces, the effect of conditioning agents could be different. Amongst the four agents used, EDTA and tetracycline consistently increased the diameter of tubules and percentage of patent tubules in both healthy and diseased teeth.

Introduction

One of the goals of periodontal therapy is predictable regeneration of the periodontium in areas previously affected by periodontal disease [1]. Root surfaces are potentially at risk for hypermineralization as well as contamination by different strains of bacteria and their endotoxins [2]. Root surface contamination or infection can potentially change the consequences of regenerative periodontal therapies and therefore for achieving optimal appropriate outcome the modification and disinfection of the contaminated root surfaces are necessary [3]. The most minimally invasive procedures for removing the bacterial deposits, accretions and endotoxins from the exposed root surface are scaling and root planning that removes the calculus below the gum line and cleans the root surface which allows the healing process to begin [4]. However, the potential limitations of scaling and root planning have been also described. First, by using this treatment, complete decontamination of the root surfaces affected by periodontitis seems to be impossible. In fact, scaling and root planning provides only a temporary solution to the periodontal disease. Moreover, it has been shown that these methods are less effective in deeper pockets in which removing the calculus is more difficult [1].

This is also true for the posterior teeth which are difficult to reach for mechanical root surface debridement. In order to overcome this difficulty, root conditioning could be considered as an adjunct to mechanical debridement [5]. Different materials and agents have been introduced for removing the smear layer and bacterial endotoxins from the root surface; many application times have been tested ranging from 0.5 to 10 min, and most of the studies have found the best results during 3 to 4 min of application [6].

A systematic review related to the subject was published by Mariotti [7] who concluded that the use of citric acid, tetracycline or EDTA to modify the root surface provides no benefit of clinical significance to regeneration in patients with chronic periodontitis. On the other hand, the author also states that since most of the included study designs are not fully developed, a definite conclusion should be taken into account [7]. There is still a remarkable controversy concerning the need to use chemical agents; this justifies the search for parameters that can support the selection for this procedure in periodontal treatments. In addition, knowing the effect of these agents in different time periods could be helpful for selecting the best application time.

Therefore, the present study aimed to compare the surface characteristics of both healthy and periodontally diseased extracted human teeth at different time periods after treatment with different root conditioning agents.

Materials and Methods

The study samples were 40 freshly extracted molars including 20 affected teeth with periodontal diseases and 20 healthy teeth that were extracted because of other reasons. None of the affected teeth had a history of periodontal treatment such as scaling or root planning within the last 6 months. Also, those with root surface caries and/or restoration, root surface abnormalities, or cervical abrasion and/or erosion were excluded.

Following the extraction, the teeth were thoroughly washed and then root planning was performed on the root surfaces using a curette to obtain smooth, shiny, and hard surface. For facilitating dehydration and coating, the teeth were divided longitudinally by a water cooled high speed fissure bur (Teeskavan, Tehran, Iran) and the pulp and canal spaces were removed. Then, the teeth were washed by soft brush and distilled water and then dehydrated. The crowns were separated and a total of 240 dentinal block sample sizes of 2x3x1 mm were obtained by sectioning the root on the planed area with a flexible double-faced diamond disc.

The samples were randomly allocated to one of the following treatment groups. The chelating agents were provided by the Department of Pharmacology in Hamedan University of Medical Sciences:

A. Control group – rinsed with normal saline

B. Group 1 – received EthyleneDiamineTetraAcetic Acid (EDTA) 24% (pH = 7.3)

C. Group 2 – received saturated citric acid (pH = 1.0)

D. Group 3 – received doxycycline 10% (pH = 2.2)

E. Group 4 – received tetracycline 10% (pH = 1.8)

In each group, 48 samples were included. The groups were divided into subgroups according to the tooth type. Two types of teeth (affected and healthy) were used (n = 24). Each of these two subgroups was further divided into the four application time intervals of 1, 2, 3 or 4 min (n = 6).

Application of the agents on the root was done by rubbing method using cotton pellets for 10 to 15 seconds and set on for 1,2,3 and 4 minutes after which the tooth specimens were flushed with distilled water to stop the reactions. Then, the specimens were dehydrated in an ascending concentration of alcohol solutions (40 min in alcohol 50%, 40 min in alcohol 75%, and finally 40 min in alcohol 100%); and air dried. Dried specimens were mounted on Scanning Electron Microscope (SEM) stubs and sputter coated with gold in a gold sputtering unit Balt-Tec SCD-050 (Balt-Tec, Cheshire, UK). With the gold coating procedure, a very thin layer of gold (about 200 Angstrom) covers the specimens by which the contrast increases in the SEM view.

Finally, the mounted specimens were evaluated using the SEM JSM8A (JEOL, Tokyo, Japan) by grouping them in 10 groups each consisting of 24 specimens and evaluating one group at each time. The SEM micrographs were transferred to a computer and analyzed by Image J software. The field shown at magnification of 1,000× was taken as a reference for the total area in which the percentage of the areas occupied by the enlarged dentinal tubules and by the dentin, and also the mean diameter of the patent dentinal tubules according to the scale bar 10 μm, were calculated (Figure 1). For better assessment of the changes in study parameters, the following ratio was defined indicating the efficacy of the applied agents (zero indicating no effectiveness of the agent):

$$\text{k index} = \frac{\sum \Delta y}{\sum \Delta x}$$

y: The difference of each study parameter (tubular space percentage, percentage of area occupied by dentin or tubular diameter measured on the 1,000× magnification SEM view) at different application time intervals

x: Time intervals (1-2 min, 2-3 min, and 3-4 min)

Inter-group differences and changes in study indices after interventions were compared using one-way ANOVA test.

Results

In the control group receiving normal saline, the changes in the indicators of the dentin (%) ($p = 0.730$), tubular spaces (%) ($p = 0.751$), and diameter of the dentinal tubules (μm^2) ($p = 0.867$) were insignificant in all time periods. Those who received EDTA experienced a significant linear and partial persistent increase in the tubular spaces ($p = 0.001$) and the mean diameter of the tubules ($p = 0.041$), as well as a decrease in the percentage of the dentins ($p = 0.001$) at 3-4 min time periods in both affected and healthy teeth. The use of citric acid led to a non-linear and inconsistent but increasing trend in root conditioning in the affected group ($p = 0.001$).

Doxycycline groups experienced non-linear and non- persistent decreasing trend in root conditioning which led to a gradual decrease in tubular space and diameter as well as an increase in the percentage of area occupied by dentin ($p = 0.001$). In tetracycline groups, although the observed trend in root conditioning was non-linear, it was persistent and increasing ($p = 0.001$) (Table 1,2). As shown in Table 3 and according to the measurement of K index, the use of EDTA, citric acid, and tetracycline had positive chelating effects on the study indices (increasing the tubular space or tubular diameter); however,

(a) (b)

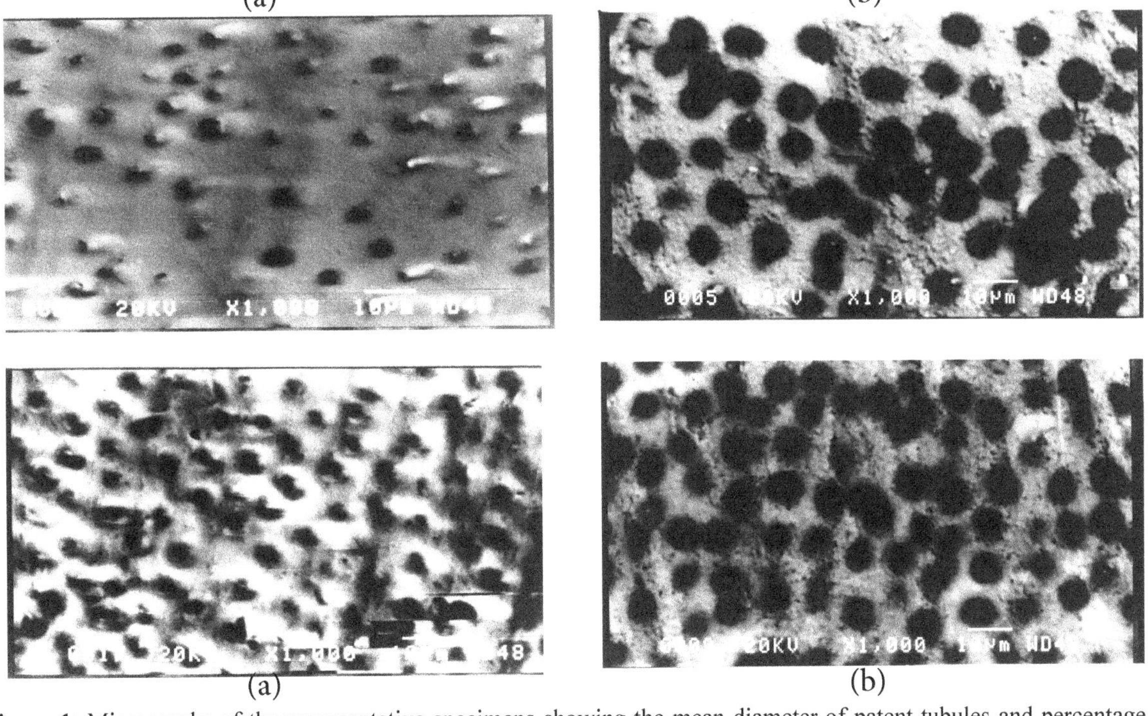

(a) (b)

Figure 1: Micrographs of the representative specimens showing the mean diameter of patent tubules and percentage of areas occupied by dentinal tubules and dentin before (a) and after (b) applying conditioning agent viewed by SEM (1,000X).ntin before (a) and after (b) applying conditioning agent viewed by SEM (1,000X).

Table 1: Changes in tubular space, dentin and tubular diameter indices in healthy groups at different time periods following the use of each conditioner

Group	Time (min)	Tubular space (%)		Dentin (%)		Tubular diameter (μm²)	
		Before	After	Before	After	Before	After
EDTA	4	42.7±0.6	52.0±0.3	57.3±0.6	47.9±0.6	4.4±0.5	6.2±0.5
	3	43.0±0.8	46.5±0.5	57.0±0.8	73.4±0.8	4.1±0.5	3.9±0.5
	2	43.2±0.7	43.0±5	56.8±0.7	76.9±0.7	3.8±0.5	4.0±0.6
	1	44.0±1	39.4±0.7	56.0±1.2	80.5±1.2	3.6±0.5	3.7±0.4
Citric acid	4	42.0±0.5	25.1±0.5	58.0±0.5	74.8±0.5	4.3±0.5	7.5±0.7
	3	42.4±0.8	30.2±0.5	57.6±0.8	69.7±0.5	4.1±0.6	6.2±0.5
	2	42.6±0.7	18.0±0.7	57.4±0.7	81.9±0.7	3.6±0.7	6.1±0.6
	1	43.0±0.6	21.3±0.5	57.0±0.6	78.6±0.5	3.7±0.5	4.4±0.7
Doxycy-cline	4	42.9±0.6	34.1±0.6	57.1±0.6	65.8±0.6	5.5±0.5	4.3±0.6
	3	43.0±0.7	35.4±0.5	56.9±0.7	64.5±0.5	5.1±0.4	4.2±0.7
	2	43.0±0.6	37.2±0.5	57.0±0.6	62.7±0.5	6.8±0.4	3.8±0.5
	1	43.0±0.6	35.8±0.8	57.0±0.6	64.1±0.8	7.8±0.6	3.5±0.5
Tetracy-cline	4	41.0±0.8	42.1±0.5	59.0±0.8	57.8±0.8	4.3±0.5	7.6±0.5
	3	43.2±0.7	34.8±0.6	56.8±0.7	65.1±0.7	4.2±0.5	4.9±0.7
	2	42.7±0.6	26.9±0.5	57.3±0.6	73.0±0.5	4.0±0.6	8.0±0.6
	1	41.2±0.4	43.3±0.6	58.8±0.4	56.6±0.6	4.1±0.4	7.2±0.5
Normal saline	4	42.2±0.5	43.3±0.5	57.7±0.5	56.6±0.5	4.4±0.6	4.4±0.4
	3	42.8±0.8	43.9±0.8	57.1±0.8	56.0±0.8	4.1±0.6	4.2±05
	2	43.0±0.8	44.0±0.6	57.0±0.8	56.0±0.6	3.7±0.4	3.9±0.6
	1	44.1±0.7	45.0±0.7	55.8±0.4	55.0±0.7	3.6±0.5	3.7±0.5

Table 2: Changes in tubular space, dentin and tubular diameter indices in affected groups at different time periods following the use of each conditioner

Group	Time (min)	Tubular space (%)		Dentin (%)		Tubular diameter (μm²)	
		Before	After	Before	After	Before	After
EDTA	4	42.7±0.6	49.9±1.2	57.3±0.6	50.0±1.2	4.4±0.5	7.6±0.4
	3	43.0±0.8	47.2±0.3	57.0±0.8	52.7±0.3	4.1±0.5	8.0±0.3
	2	43.2±•,7	42.1±0.7	56.8±0.7	57.9±0.7	3.8±0.5	8.0±0.4
	1	44.0±1.2	41.7±0.7	56.0±1.2	58.2±0.7	3.6±0.5	7.8±0.4
Citric acid	4	42.0±0.5	48.3±0.6	58.0±0.5	51.6±0.6	4.3±0.5	8.1±0.5
	3	42.4±0.8	39.9±0.8	57.6±0.8	60.0±0.8	4.1±0.6	6.2±0.6
	2	42.6±0.7	21.3±0.8	57.4±0.7	78.6±0.8	3.6±0.7	6.1±0.6
	1	43.0±0.6	18.0±0.6	57.0±0.6	81.1±0.6	3.7±0.5	4.5±0.7
Doxycy-cline	4	42.9±0.6	34.1±0.3	57.1±0.6	65.8±0.3	5.6±0.5	4.3±0.6
	3	43.0±0.7	29.5±0.6	56.9±0.7	70.4±0.6	5.1±0.4	4.2±0.5
	2	43.0±0.6	36.4±0.7	57.0±0.6	63.5±0.7	5.7±0.4	3.8±0.3
	1	43.0±0.6	55.6±0.6	57.0±0.6	44.3±0.6	3.5±0.6	7.9±0.3
Tetracy-cline	4	41.0±0.8	53.3±0.4	59.0±0.8	46.7±0.4	4.3±0.5	7.8±0.8
	3	43.2±0.7	27.8±0.7	56.8±.7	72.1±0.7	4.2±0.5	5.5±0.6
	2	42.7±0.6	23.8±0.7	57.3±0.6	76.1±0.7	4.0±0.6	8.2±0.4
	1	41.2±0.4	31.9±0.7	58.8±0.4	68.0±0.7	4.1±0.4	7.3±0.6
Normal saline	4	42.2±0.5	43.3±0.5	57.7±0.5	56.6±0.5	4.4±0.6	4.4±0.4
	3	42.8±0.8	43.9±0.8	57.1±0.8	56.0±0.8	4.1±0.6	4.2±0.5
	2	43.0±0.8	44.0±0.6	57.0±0.8	56.0±0.6	3.7±0.4	3.9±0.6
	1	44.1±0.7	45.0±0.7	55.8±0.4	55.0±0.7	3.6±0.5	3.7±0.5

doxycycline had adverse effects as a root conditioner in the affected teeth. The changes in the study indices across the four treatment regimens in different time periods are presented in Table 4. In each time interval the differences in study indices between treatment regimens were significant ($p = 0.001$).

Table 3: Changes of study indices according to the measurement of K

$\frac{\sum \Delta y}{\sum \Delta x}$	Tubular space (%)	Dentin (%)	Tubular diameter (μm^2)
EDTA			
Affected teeth	3.16	-3.17	0.33
Healthy teeth	4.63	-4.63	0.69
Citric acid			
Affected teeth	10.46	-10.60	0.94
Healthy teeth	-1.54	1.60	0.85
Doxycycline			
Affected teeth	-7.14	7.39	-1.06
Healthy teeth	0.55	-0.55	1.03
Tetracycline			
Affected teeth	7.23	-7.17	0.10
Healthy teeth	0.33	-0.33	0.09
Normal saline			
Affected teeth	0.11	0.65	-0.02
Healthy teeth	0.00	0.01	0.01

Discussion

To select the best therapeutic conditioning material for contaminated root surfaces, we compared the effectiveness of different materials applied in different time periods. Regarding the linear and consistent trend of the changes in the parameters, the use of EDTA, followed by tetracycline was preferable. In addition, EDTA and tetracycline samples had a greater percentage of patent tubules when compared with other treated samples.

The proper effectiveness of EDTA has been previously shown. In the study done by Gamal *et al.* [8] applying EDTA gel for 4 minutes after scaling and root planning removed the root surface smear layer and had the best result in adherence and growth of the PDL cells. In addition to the contact time, it has been shown that the curative effects of EDTA quickly become apparent so that it can remove the smear layer in less than 1 minute [9]. Moreover, EDTA can reduce the micro-hardness of the dentin by 17.33% to 29.48%, and this effect is considerably greater than other active and control solutions [10,11]. Thus, on the basis of our result and in comparison with the previous findings, the application of EDTA, even alone, had the maximum results in root conditioning. In fact, the natural pH along with the capability to remove the root surface smear layer makes the use of EDTA highly beneficial in clinical practice.

According to our results, the use of tetracycline can be the second choice for root conditioning. Different studies have evaluated and compared the

Table 4: Effects of treatment regimens on the study indices in different time periods in affected teeth

Material		EDTA	Citric acid	Doxycycline	Tetracycline	Normal saline	p value
min 1	TS	-2.2±1.1	-24.1±0.3	12.6±0.2	-9.2±0.3	0.8±0.1	*0.001
	D	2.2±1.1	24.1±0.3	-12.6±0.2	9.2±0.3	-0.8±0.1	*0.001
	TD	4.2±0.4	0.9±0.3	4.4±0.5	3.2±0.2	0.7±0.1	*0.001
min 2	TS	-1.1±0.9	-21.3±0.5	-6.5±0.3	-18.9±0.0	1.0±0.5	*0.001
	D	1.1±0.9	21.3±0.5	6.5±0.3	18.9±0.0	-1.0±0.5	*0.001
	TD	4.1±0.8	2.5±0.3	-1.9±0.4	4.2±0.7	0.1±0.6	*0.001
min 3	TS	4.2±0.7	-2.4±0.3	-13.4±0.2	-15.4±0.1	1.1±0.2	*0.001
	D	-4.2±0.7	2.4±0.3	13.4±0.2	15.4±0.1	-1.1±0.2	*0.001
	TD	3.9±0.8	2.0±0.7	-0.1±0.5	1.3±0.3	0.0±0.2	*0.001
min 4	TS	7.2±1.7	6.4±0.2	-8.8±0.2	12.3±0.7	1.1±0.3	*0.001
	D	-7.2±1.7	-6.4±0.2	8.8±0.2	-12.2±0.7	-1.1±0.3	*0.001
	TD	3.2±0.6	3.7±0.1	-1.2±1.0	3.5±0.3	0.0±0.6	*0.001

TS: Tubular Space, D: Dentin, TD: Tubular Diameter

*$p < 0.01$

efficacy of tetracycline with other materials such as citric acid [12-15]. According to the findings of Grover *et al.*, the number of patent tubules present in the citric acid and EDTA test groups was significantly higher than those in the tetracycline hydrochloride test group. However, in their study the average diameter of the patent tubules was greater in the tetracycline hydrochloride group compared with the citric acid and EDTA groups [4].

Shetty *et al.* also showed that the proportion of patent dentinal tubules was significantly higher in the tetracycline HCl group (74%) compared to minocycline (48.3%), doxycycline (42%) and citric acid (52%). The number of patent tubules was also higher in the tetracycline group compared to minocycline and doxycycline and the difference was statistically significant [16]. In fact, it can be concluded that with regard to root conditioning, tetracycline can be a good choice regarding its effects on the dentin smear layer removal and tubule exposure. Because of its efficacy against suspected causative microflora, anti-enzymatic properties, as well as antibiotic impacts, the use of this agent is preferred to other antibiotics [17].

Our results showed that applying tetracycline increased the tubular diameter in less than one minute and the tubular space after 3 minutes. However, a previous study suggested that the application time should be limited to 2-3 minutes [18] since long etching time of 3 minutes and above could impair periodontal healing [19]. Tetracycline is able to enhance fibrin clot adhesion by exposing collagen matrix [20] and it enhances fibroblast chemotaxis and binding leading to a more stable initial clot formation [21].

According to our results despite having the maximum increase in the tubular space and tubular diameter in the first minute, doxycycline had adverse effects as a root conditioner and decreased the tubular space and tubular diameter after 1 minutes of applying. Similarly Chahal *et al.* [22] reported that removal of smear layer by tetracycline and citric acid is better than doxycycline and the percentage of patent tubules and their diameter were lower in the doxycycline group. This finding could be attributed to the lower pH of tetracycline HCl (pH 1.8) and citric acid (pH 1) as compared to doxycycline (pH 2.2).

Citric acid has the ability to remove the smear layer, exposes the dentinal tubules and makes them wider with funnel shaped orifices. It may also act as a potent antibacterial agent [23]. In a study comparing the effect of citric acid applied for 1,2 and 3 minutes removing the smear layer, showed that the efficacy of this root conditioner was best after 3 minutes [24]. In comparison, our results also showed that citric acid increased the tubular diameter and tubular space significantly after 3 minutes in the affected teeth ($p < 0.01$). However some disadvantages have been addressed with applying citric acid such as the formation of extremely acidic environment in the surrounding tissues, which may result in unfavourable wound healing responses [25].

Conclusions

Because of more persistent effectiveness on early root conditioning (chelating effect in less than one minute of applying), EDTA and tetracycline are preferable root conditioner agents which could be used in regenerative periodontal therapies. The use of citric acid agent for surface conditioning showed different outcomes in the healthy and periodontally affected teeth with increasing tubular space significantly in the affected teeth after applying for 3 minutes. Doxycycline has adverse effects as a root conditioner after 1 minutes of application.

Conflict of Interest: None declared.

References

1. Lowenguth RA, Blieden TM. Periodontal regeneration: Root surface Demineralization. Periodontol 2000. 1993;1:54-68.
2. Blomlof JP, Blomlof LB, Lindskog SF. Smear removal and collagen exposure after non-surgical root planing followed by etching with an EDTA gel preparation. J Periodontol. 1996;67:841-845.
3. Hanes PJ, O'Brien NJ, Garnick JJ. A morphological comparison of radicular dentin following root planing and treatment with citric acid or tetracycline HCl. J Clin Periodontol. 1991;18:660-668.
4. Grover HS, Yadav A, Nanda P. A Comparative Evaluation of the Efficacy of Citric Acid, Ethylene Diamine Tetra Acetic Acid (EDTA) and Tetracycline Hydrochloride as Root Biomodification Agents: An In Vitro SEM Study. J Periodontol Implant Dent. 2011;3:73–78.
5. Balos K, Bal B, Eren K. The effects of various agents on root surfaces (a scanning electron

microscopy study). Newsl Int Acad Periodontol. 1991;1:13-16.

6. Amaral NG, Rezende ML, Hirata F, *et al.* Comparison among four commonly used demineralizing agents for root conditioning. A scanning electron microscopy. J Appl Oral Sci. 2011;19:469-475.
7. Mariotti A. Efficacy of chemical root surface modifiers in the treatment of periodontal disease. A systematic review. Ann Periodontol. 2003;8:205-226.
8. Gamal AY, Mailhot JM. The effects of EDTA gel conditioning exposure time on periodontitis-affected human root surfaces: surface topography and PDL cell adhesion. J Int Acad Periodontol. 2003;5:11-22.
9. Calt S, Serper A. Time-dependent effects of EDTA on dentin structures. J Endod. 2002; 28:17-19.
10. Scelza MF, Pierro V, Scelza P, *et al.* Effect of three different time periods of irrigation with EDTA-T, EDTA and citric acid on smear layer removal. Oral Surg Oral Med Oral Pathol Oral Radiol Endod. 2004;98:499-503.
11. Zehnder M, Schicht O, Sener B, *et al.* Reducing surface tension in endodontic chelator solutions has no effect on their ability to remove calcium from instrumented root canals. J Endod. 2005;31:590-592.
12. Madison JG, Hokett SD. The effect of different tetracyclines on the dentin root surface of instrumented, periodontally involved human teeth: A Comparative Scanning Electron Microscope study. J Periodontol. 1997;68:739-745.
13. Lafferty TA, Gher ME, Gray JL. Comparative SEM study on the effect of acid etching with tetracycline HCL or citric acid on Instrumented periodontally involved human root surfaces. J Periodontol. 1993;64:689–693.
14. Labhan R, Fahrenbach WH, Clark SM, *et al.* Root dentin morphology after different modes of citric acid and tetracycline hydrochloride conditioning. J Periodontol. 1992;63:303–309.
15. Parashis AO, Mitsis FJ. Clinical evaluation of the effect of tetracycline root preparation on guided tissue regeneration in the treatment of class II furcation defects. J Periodontol. 1993;64:133-136.
16. Shetty B, Dinesh A, Seshan H. Comparative effects of tetracyclines and citric acid on dentin root surface of periodontally involved human teeth: A scanning electron microscope study. J Indian Soc Periodontol. 2008;12:8–15.
17. Kao RT, Takei HH, Cochran DL, *et al.* Periodontal Regeneration and Reconstructive Surgery and Host Modulation In: Carranza FA, Newman MG, Glickman I. Clinical periodontology, 12th Edition. Philadelphia: Saunders; 2015.611,48 .
18. Penmatsa T, Varma S, Mythili , *et al.* Effect of various concentrations of tetracycline hydrochloride demineralization on root dentin surface: A scanning electron microscopic study. J Pharm Bioallied Sci. 2013;5:48-53.
19. Blomlof J, Jansson L, Blomlof L, *et al.* Long time etching at low pH jeopardizes periodontal healing. J Clin Periodontol. 1995;22:459-463.
20. Preeja C, Janam P, Nayar BR. Fibrin clot adhesion to root surface treated with tetracycline hydrochloride and ethylenediaminetetraacetic acid: A scanning electron microscopic study. Dent Res J. 2013;10:382-388.
21. Terranova VP, Franzetti LC, Hic S, *et al.* A biochemical approach to periodontal regeneration: Tetracycline treatment of dentin promotes fibroblast adhesion and growth. J Periodontal Res. 1986;21:330-337.
22. Chahal GS, Chhina K, Chhabra V, *et al.* Effect of citric acid, tetracycline, and doxycycline on instrumented periodontally involved root surfaces: A SEM study. J Indian Soc Periodontol. 2014;18:32-37.
23. Wen CR, Caffesse RG, Morrison EC, *et al.* In vitro effects of citric acid application techniques on dentin surfaces. J Periodontol. 1992;63:883-889.
24. Cavassim R, Leite FR, Zandim DL, *et al.* Influence of concentration, time and method of application of citric acid and sodium citrate in root conditioning. J Appl Oral Sci. 2012;20:376-383.
25. Bhushan K, Chauhan G, Prakash S. Root Biomodification in Periodontics - The Changing Concepts. J Dent Oral Care Med. 2016;2:105-113.

22

Effect of Shade and Light Curing Mode on the Degree of Conversion of Silorane-Based and Methacrylate-Based Resin Composites

Mousavinasab SM[a], Atai M[b], Salehi N[c], Salehi A[d*]

[a]Dental Materials Research Center and Department of Operative Dentistry, School of Dentistry, Isfahan University of Medical Sciences, Isfahan, Iran
[b]Department of Polymer Science, Iran Polymer and Petrochemical Institute, Tehran, Iran
[c]Department of Oral Medicine, School of Dentistry, Rafsanjan University of Medical Sciences, Rafsanjan, Iran
[d]Department of Operative Dentistry, School of Dentistry, Rafsanjan University of Medical Sciences, Rafsanjan, Iran

ARTICLE INFO

Key words:
Degree of Conversion
Methacrylate-Based Resin Composites
Silorane-Based Resin Composites
Soft-Start Curing

Corresponding Author:
Arman Salehi
Department of Operative Dentistry, School of Dentistry, Rafsanjan University of Medical Sciences, Rafsanjan, Iran
Email:armansalehi1984@gmail

Abstract

***Statement of Problem*:** The degree of conversion depends on the material composition, light source properties, distance from light source, light intensity, curing time, and other factors such as shade and translucency.

***Objectives*:** In the present study, we evaluated the effects of different light-curing modes and shades of methacrylate and silorane-based resin composites on the degree of conversion of resin composites (DC).

***Materials and Methods*:** The methacrylate-based (Filtek Z250, 3M, ESPE) and low-shrinkage silorane-based (Filtek P90, 3M, ESPE) resin composites were used in three groups as follows: group 1-Filtek Z250 (shade A3), group 2-Filtek Z250 (shade B2), and group 3-Filtek P90 (shade A3). We used a light-emitting diode (LED) curing unit for photopolymerization. 10 samples were prepared in each group to evaluate the degree of conversion; 5 samples were cured using soft-start curing mode, and the other 5 were cured using standard curing mode. The DC of the resin composites was measured using Fourier Transform Infrared Spectroscopy (FTIR). The data were analyzed using Kruskal Wallis and one-way ANOVA statistical tests.

Results: The degree of conversion of silorane-based resin composite was 70 - 75.8% and that of methacrylate-based resin composites was 60.2 - 68.2% ($p = 0.009$). The degree of conversion of the composite with brighter colour (B2) was statistically more than the darker composite (A3). Higher degree of conversion was achieved applying the standard curing mode.

Conclusions: The results of the study showed that the colour and type of the resin composite and also the curing mode influence the degree of conversion of resin composites.

Introduction

Direct resin composite restorations have been widely used in restorative dentistry procedures. However, it is desirable for a dental resin composite to convert all of its monomer units into a polymer, during the process of polymerization [1]. A well-known drawback of dental resin composites is incomplete monomer conversion, and the resulting monomer release could at least partially account for the failures observed clinically, including persistent post-operative sensitivity and/or the need for endodontic treatment, as well as secondary caries [2].

Moreover, unsuitable biological responses, like cytotoxicity or pulp progenitor/stem cellular differentiation disturbance even at non-toxic concentrations, were suggested to be caused by the release of non-reacted monomers [2,3]. Therefore, incomplete polymer conversion and the increased potential for monomer release can affect the pulp tissues [2]. Hence, the degree of conversion (DC) of dental resin composites is a key physical property of the polymer since functional material characteristics, such as mechanical properties, volumetric shrinkage, wear resistance, and monomer elution are significantly correlated [2].

Generally, a high DC is associated with higher shrinkage strain. However, polymerization shrinkage directly influences the compliance and results in the passage of bacteria, fluids, molecules, or ions between the cavity wall and resin composite restoration which is called "Micro-leakage" [4,5]. Tooth sensitivity, secondary caries, and pulp problems are some complications of micro-leakage [6,7]. For this reason, researchers constantly aim to reduce the shrinkage of resin composite materials.

In the part of polymer network polymerization stage "Gel Point" exists, and before this point, the resin composite acts as a viscous fluid and can partially release tensions ("Pre-Gel" stage). After the "Gel Point", however, the resin composite converts into a hard material lacking sufficient flow for releasing the tensions ("Post-Gel" stage) [8,9].

The assumption is that if further tension release is allowed by increasing the "Pre-Gel" duration, there will be a possibility to decrease the shrinkage stress caused by the polymerization; accordingly, the soft-start curing mode was introduced [10-12]. In this mode, first, the polymerization begins with low intensities of light-cure device energy, and after a certain period of time (5 second), this intensity increases and the rest of the polymerization continues with high energy [13].

On the other hand, silorane-based resin composites exhibit lower shrinkage strain due to the ring opening polymerization mechanism [14-16]. As derivatives of siloxane and oxirane monomers, silorane resins are composed of a hydrophobic siloxane backbone of oxirane rings. A reduced shrinkage of about 1 vol% is provided by the polymerization of these monomers with a cationic ring opening. [17]. The polymerization shrinkage in silorane systems is reduced as a result of a double ring-opening polymerization caused by an oxaspirocyclic core. It should be noted that this type of polymerization is required for volume expansion, which occurs through cationic intermediates [18,19].

The DC is also dependent on the material composition, light source properties, distance from light source, light intensity, curing time, and other factors such as shade and translucency [20,21]. Therefore, the present study was performed with the purpose of investigating the effect of the use of different resin composite colours and curing modes on the DC of resin composites. The null hypothesis was that there would be no difference in the DC between methacrylate- and silorane-based resin composites at different light curing modes and using different composite shades.

Materials and Methods

The materials in the present study consisted of methacrylate-based (Filtek Z250, 3M ESPE,St. Paul, MN,USA) and silorane-based (Filtek P90, 3M ESPE, St. Paul, MN,USA) resin composites, that were used in three groups as follows: group 1-Filtek Z250 (shade A3), group 2-Filtek Z250 (shade B2), and group 3-Filtek P90 (shade A3). 10 samples were prepared in each group to evaluate the DC; 5 samples were cured using soft-start curing mode, and the other 5 were cured using standard curing mode (Table 1).

A Bluephase LED light-curing unit (Ivoclar Vivadent, Schann, Liechtenstein) capable of applying three curing modes of low, soft start and standard was used for photopolymerization. In the

Table 1: Materials and their composition used in the study

Type	Material	Content	Manufacturer
Filtek Z250	Methacrylate-based composite	Matrix: Bis-GMA, Bis-EMA, UDMA, TEGDMA Filler: zirconia, silica (0.01 - 3.5 μm), 78 wt%, 60 vol%	
Filtek P90	Silorane-based composite	Matrix: 3,4 Epoxycyclohexyl ethyl cyclopoly-methylsiloxane, bis-3,4 epoxycyclohexyl-ethyl-phenyl-methylsilane Filler: silanized quartz, Yttrium fluoride (0.04 - 1.7 μm), 76 wt%, 55 vol%	3M ESPE, St. Paul, MN, USA

Bis-GMA, Bisphenol A glycidyl dimethacrylate; Bis-EMA, Ethoxylated Bisphenol A dimethacrylate; UDMA, Urethane dimethacrylate; TEGDMA, Triethylene glycol dimethacrylate.

present study, the soft-start and standard curing modes were utilized. The unit functions at two wavelengths of 470 and 500 nm. Soft-start curing method output energy was 200 mW cm^{-2} during the first 5s, which increased to 750 mW cm^{-2}. In the standard curing method, the output energy was 750 mW cm^{-2}. The light-curing time was 40s during all the study procedures. The output energy of the unit during the study was checked by a radiometer (LED Radiometer, Kerr, USA)

The DCs of the resin composite materials were measured using Fourier Transform Infrared Spectroscopy (FTIR) (EQUINOX 55, Bruker, Ettlingen, Germany). A very thin layer of the resin composite was placed between two polyethylene layers and the absorbance peaks of the uncured samples were obtained.

Subsequently, the samples were light-cured according to the specified procedure (Table 2). The FTIR spectrum of each light cured sample was then recorded. The DC (%) of methacrylate-based resin composites (Filtek Z250, 3M ESPE) was determined from the ratio of the absorbance intensities of aliphatic C = C (peak at 1,638 cm^{-1}) against the internal reference aromatic C = C (peak at 1,608 cm^{-1}) prior and subsequent to light-curing [22] . The DC was calculated as follows:

$$DC\% = \left(1 - \frac{(1637\ cm^{-1}/\ 1\,608\ cm^{-1})\text{peak area after curing}}{(1637\ cm^{-1}/\ 1\,608\ cm^{-1})\text{peak area before curing}}\right) \times 100$$

For silorane-based resin composites (Filtek P90,3M ESPE), the DC was calculated using the ratio of absorbance intensities of the reacting epoxy rings C-O-C (peak at 882 cm^{-1}) against the Si-CH3 internal reference (peak at 695 cm^{-1}) prior and subsequent to light-curing (Figure 1) [23]. The DC was calculated as follows:

$$DC\% = \left(1 - \frac{(882\ cm^{-1}/\ 695\ cm^{-1})\text{peak area after curing}}{(882\ cm^{-1}/\ 695\ cm^{-1})\text{peak area before curing}}\right) \times 100$$

The number of samples was determined according to similar studies [1,16,17]. Data were analyzed with SPSS 21 (SPSS Inc., Chicago, IL,

Table 2: The number of samples and the study groups

Group	Resin Composite Type	Shade	Curing Method	Number of Samples
				30
1	Filtek Z250 (Methacrylate-based)	A3	Standard curing	5
			Soft start curing	5
2	Filtek Z250 (Methacrylate-based)	B2	Standard curing	5
			Soft start curing	5
3	Filtek P90 (Silorane-based)	A3	Standard curing	5
			Soft start curing	5

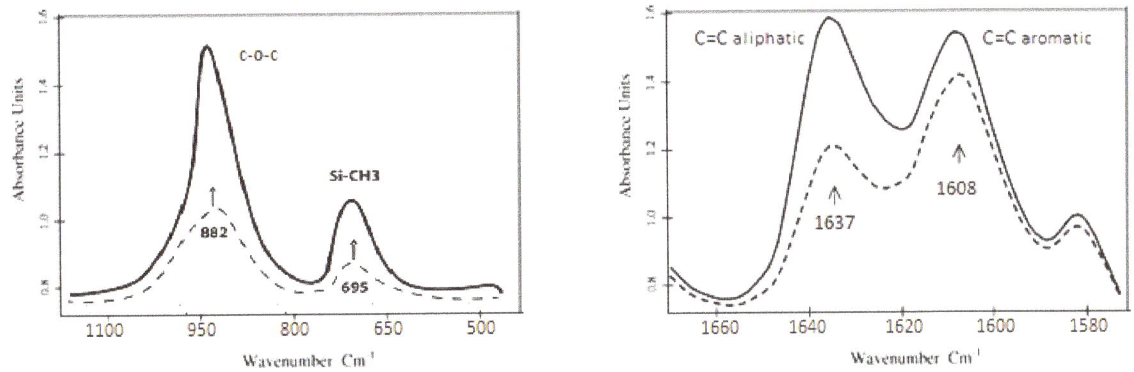

Figure 1: Infrared spectra of silorane-based (left) compared with methacrylate-based (right) resin composites.

USA). Statistical significance was set at $p < 0.05$. Kruskal Wallis H and Mann- Whitney U tests were used to compare the DC in different groups.

Results

The DCs of the study resin composites are given in Table 3 based on their group and curing mode. In the silorane-based resin composite (group 3) Filtek P90 (shade A3), the DC was higher than the methacrylate-based resin composite (group 1) Filtek Z250 with similar colour (shade A3) ($p = 0.009$). Standard curing mode in all the groups caused a higher DC increase compared to soft-start curing method ($p = 0.009$). Also, in group 2 Filtek Z250 (shade B2) with brighter colour compared to group 1 Filtek Z250 (shade A3), the DC was statistically higher ($p = 0.009$).

Discussion

In this study, the DC of the studied composites was investigated 40s after curing by standard and soft-start curing modes with the use of LED light-curing unit. The results showed that the silorane-based resin composite, the brighter colour and also in the standard curing mode, the DC is higher. In Xiong *et al.*'s study [23], which used a methodology similar to that of the current study to measure the DC of low-shrinkage silorane-based resin composites (maximum absorption 882 cm^{-1}), the DC of the silorane-based resin composites has been reported 62.3% to 69.1%. While in other studies in which the 1638 cm^{-1} maximum absorption has been considered to measure the DC [22,24], lower values (37.2% - 43.5%) was reported for the DC of silorane-based resin composite (Filtek P90, 3M, ESPE) which can be due to the use of a different methodology.

Base of Gao *et al.*'s study, it has been reported that Filtek P90 (3M, ESPE) takes the longest time to reach the gel points [25]. One hypothesis for this behavior is that siloranes are slowly polymerized, resulting in longer gel times so that siloranes have a polymerization reaction with a slow onset. Through slow polymerization, more time is allowed for increasing polymerization and higher DC [25]. On the contrary, the DC of methacrylate-based resin composites is in alignment with past studies [24,26]. In the study of Porto *et al.* [24], the DC with 44–71%

Table 3: The DC of the study resin composites

Group / Curing	1	2	3	*p*-value*
	Mean ± SD	Mean ± SD	Mean ± SD	
Standard	60.4 ± 2.0	68.2 ± 1.9	75.8 ± 1.7	.002
Soft start	60.2 ± 1.3	61.4 ± 1.6	70.0 ± 2.5	.006

Group 1: Methacrylate-based resin composite (Filtek Z250, 3M ESPE), shade A3

Group 2: Methacrylate-based resin composite (Filtek Z250, 3M ESPE), shade B2

Group 3: Silorane-based resin composite (Filtek P90,3M ESPE), shade A3

*: Kruskal-Wallis H test

for the Filtek Z250 (3M, ESPE) was obtained using (LED) standard curing mode.

The lower value of DC with the soft-start curing mode could be caused by the lower intensity of light at the beginning of this curing mode which results in the decrease in the polymerization rate. Al-Qudah *et al.* [27] also explained that the increase in resin composite viscosity in the early seconds of soft-start curing can cause rapid distribution of free radicals, and at the end, the polymerization degree would remain limited even after the increase of light intensity.

In Mousavinasab *et al.*'s study [21], the DC values of the methacrylate-based resin composites cured by the QTH and LED LCUs with different irradiation intensities were from 53 ± 0.11% to 60 ± 0.02%. Therefore, different light intensities can be a factor influencing the DC. However, Soares, *et al.* [10] reported that the soft-start curing mode produced the lowest DC at the bottom surface with a significant statistical difference from the normal protocol because the lower irradiance produced at the first 10s of polymerization reduced the total irradiance available to polymerization.

In our study, we classified resin composite shades from bright to dark based on the degree of brightness similar to what was proposed by Al-Qudah *et al.* [27]. However, due to limitations of availability of different shades in the market, and lack of similar shades between methacrylate and silorane based resin composites, we only used two shades across the spectrum of methacrylate based resin composites. Shade B2 was used as a lighter shade and shade A3 as a darker shade. The DC of Filtek Z250 (shade B2) was slightly higher than Filtek Z250 (shade A3).

The difference might be attributed to the type and amount of dark pigments which absorb more light; hence less free radical are available for polymerization resulting in lower DC [27]. In addition, it has been shown that darker shades need more irradiation, compared to lighter shades, to reach the same curing depth [28].

Aguiar *et al.*'s [29] study showed that shade is a factor that can alter the polymerization efficacy. In this study, lighter shade showed the highest DC. Due to the opacity of dark shades, light transmission is diminished when passing through them. The photopolymerization initiation rate depends on the incident light intensity, so the reduced intensity of light led to a decrease in DC.

Conclusions

1. The DC of silorane-based resin composite 40s after the LED curing is higher than methacrylate-based resin composite.
2. The DC of the resin composite in the standard curing method is higher than the soft-start curing method.
3. The DC of brighter colour resin composite (B2) is slightly higher than the darker resin composite (A3).

Acknowledgments

The authors gratefully acknowledge that this report is based on a part of thesis that was submitted to the School of Dentistry, Isfahan University of Medical Sciences, in partial fulfilment of the requirements for the MSc degree in Restorative Dentistry (#393392). This study was financially supported and approved by Isfahan University of Medical Sciences, Isfahan, Iran.

Conflict of Interest: None declared.

References

1. Yoon TH, Lee YK, Lim BS, *et al.* Degree of polymerization of resin composites by different light sources. J Oral Rehabil. 2002;29:1165-1173.
2. Randolph LD, Palin WM, Bebelman, *et al.* Ultra-fast light-curing resin composite with increased conversion and reduced monomer elution. Dent Mater. 2014;30:594-604.
3. Bakopoulou A, Leyhausen G, Voik J, *et al.* Effects of HEMA and TEDGMA on the in vitro odontogenic differentiation potential of human pulp stem/progenitor cells derived from deciduous teeth. Dent Mater. 2011;27:608-617.
4. Amirouche-Korichi A, Mouzali M, Watts DC. Effects of monomer ratios and highly radiopaque fillers on degree of conversion and shrinkage-strain of dental resin composites. Dent Mater. 2009;25:1411-1418.
5. Stansbury JW, Trujillo-Lemon M, Lu H, *et al.*

Conversion-dependent shrinkage stress and strain in dental resins and composites. Dent Mater. 2005;21:56-67.
6. Burke FJ, Cheung SW, Mjor IA, *et al.* Restoration longevity and analysis of reasons for the placement and replacement of restorations provided by vocational dental practitioners and their trainers in the United Kingdom. Quintessence Int. 1999;30:234-242.
7. Mjor IA. The reasons for replacement and the age of failed restorations in general dental practice. Acta Odontol Scand. 1997;55:58-63.
8. El-Korashy DI. Post-gel shrinkage strain and degree of conversion of preheated resin composite cured using different regimens. Oper Dent. 2010;35:172-179.
9. Sakaguchi RL, Berge HX. Reduced light energy density decreases post-gel contraction while maintaining degree of conversion in composites. J Dent. 1998;26:695-700.
10. Soares LE, Liporoni PC, Martin AA. The effect of soft-start polymerization by second generation LEDs on the degree of conversion of resin composite. Oper Dent. 2007;32:160-165.
11. Silikas N, Eliades G, Watts DC. Light intensity effects on resin-composite degree of conversion and shrinkage strain. Dent Mater. 2000;16:292-296.
12. Tarle Z, Meniga A, Knezevic A, *et al.* Composite conversion and temperature rise using a conventional, plasma arc, and an experimental blue LED curing unit. J Oral Rehabil. 2002;29:662-667.
13. Oliveira KM, Lancellotti AC, Ccahuana-Vasquez RA, *et al.* Shrinkage stress and degree of conversion of a dental composite submitted to different photoactivation protocols. Acta Odontol Latinoam. 2012;25:115-122.
14. Khosravi K, Mousavinasab SM, Samani MS. Comparison of microleakage in Class II cavities restored with silorane-based and methacrylate-based composite resins using different restorative techniques over time. Dent Res J. (Isfahan). 2015;12:150-156.
15. Giorgi MC, Hernandes NM, Sugii MM, *et al.* Influence of an intermediary base on the microleakage of simulated class II composite resin restorations. Oper Dent. 2014;39:301-307.
16. Boroujeni PM, Mousavinasab SM, Hasanli E. Effect of configuration factor on gap formation in hybrid composite resin, low-shrinkage composite resin and resin-modified glass ionomer. J Investig Clin Dent. 2015;6:156-160.
17. Eick JD, Kotha SP, Chappelow CC, *et al.* Properties of silorane-based dental resins and composites containing a stress-reducing monomer. Dent Mater. 2007;23:1011-1017.
18. Boaro LC, Goncalves F, Guimaraes TC, *et al.* Polymerization stress, shrinkage and elastic modulus of current low-shrinkage restorative composites. Dent Mater. 2010;26:1144-1150.
19. Karaman E, Ozgunaltay G. Polymerization shrinkage of different types of composite resins and microleakage with and without liner in class II cavities. Oper Dent. 2014;39:325-331.
20. Knezevic A, Tarle Z, Meniga A, *et al.* Degree of conversion and temperature rise during polymerization of composite resin samples with blue diodes. J Oral Rehabil. 2001;28:586-591.
21. Mousavinasab SM, Khoroushi M, Moharreri M, *et al.* Temperature changes under demineralized dentin during polymerization of three resin-based restorative materials using QTH and LED units. Restor Dent Endod. 2014;39:155-163.
22. Randolph LD, Palin WM, Watts DC, *et al.* The effect of ultra-fast photopolymerisation of experimental composites on shrinkage stress, network formation and pulpal temperature rise. Dent Mater. 2014;30:1280-1289.
23. Xiong J, Sun X, Li Y, *et al.* Polymerization shrinkage, stress, and degree of conversion in silorane-and dimethacrylate-based dental composites. J Appl Polym Sci. 2011;122:1882-1888.
24. Porto IC, de Aguiar FH, Brandt WC, *et al.* Mechanical and physical properties of silorane and methacrylate-based composites. J Dent. 2013;41:732-739.
25. Gao BT, Lin H, Zheng G, *et al.* Comparison between a silorane-based composite and methacrylate-based composites: shrinkage characteristics, thermal properties, gel point and vitrification point. Dent Mater J. 2012;31:76-85.
26. Porto IC, Soares LE, Martin AA, *et al.* Influence of the photoinitiator system and light photoactivation units on the degree of conversion of dental composites. Braz Oral

Res. 2010;24:475-481.

27. Al-Qudah AA, Mitchell CA, Biagioni PA, *et al.* Effect of composite shade, increment thickness and curing light on temperature rise during photocuring. J Dent. 2007;35:238-245.
28. Swartz ML, Phillips RW, Rhodes B. Visible light-activated resins-depth of cure. J Am Dent Assoc. 1983;106:634-637.
29. Aguiar FH, Lazzari CR, Lima DA, *et al.* Effect of light curing tip distance and resin shade on microhardness of a hybrid resin composite. Braz Oral Res. 2005;19:302-306.

23

Colour Stability of Various Types of Acrylic Teeth Exposed to Coffee, Tea and Cola

Mousavi S[a], Narimani S[b], Hekmatfar S[c], Jafari K[a*]

[a]Department of Prosthodontics, School of Dentistry, Ardabil University of Medical Science, Ardabil, Iran
[b]Department of Endodontics, School of Dentistry, Ardabil University of Medical Science, Ardabil, Iran
[c]Department of Pedodontics, School of Dentistry, Ardabil University of Medical Science, Ardabil, Iran

ARTICLE INFO

Key words:
Colour Stability
Acrylic Teeth
Spectrophotometer
Colouring Solutions

Corresponding Author:
Karim Jafari
Department of Prosthodontics, School of Dentistry, Ardabil University of Medical Science, Ardabil, Iran
Email: ddsjfr@gmail.com

Abstract

Statement of Problem: Acrylic teeth of dentures are prone to discoloration due to frequent exposure to different colouring solutions in the oral environment. Thus, in order to maintain their aesthetic appearance, they must possess high colour stability while exposed to colorant solutions.

Objectives: To compare the colour stability of three different brands of acrylic teeth following immersion in coffee, tea and cola.

Materials and Methods: This in vitro experimental study was conducted on 90 acrylic teeth in three groups (n = 30) of Ivoclar (Italy), PolyDent (Slovenia) and Apple (Iran). The teeth were immersed in coffee, cola and tea for one, three and six weeks (the teeth were not in contact with each other). Colour parameters were assessed before and after immersion using a spectrophotometer, and overall change in colour parameters was calculated. The overall colour change (ΔE) of the three groups at different time points was analyzed using one-way ANOVA. Pairwise comparisons were performed using Tukey's test.

Results: Coffee caused the greatest colour change in Apple acrylic teeth after six weeks (mean ΔE of 4.6 for coffee and 3.4 for tea and cola). Tea caused an almost equal colour change in the three groups. The greatest colour change in the Ivoclar teeth occurred in cola after six weeks (mean ΔE of 3.3, 3.4 and 2.8 for cola, tea and coffee, respectively). The greatest ΔE occurred at six weeks and was the highest in Apple, followed by PolyDent and then Ivoclar teeth in coffee (mean ΔE of 4.6, 3.4 and 3.3, respectively $p < 0.001$).

Conclusions: Despite the significant colour change in the three groups, ΔE in Ivoclar group was within the clinically acceptable range of ≤ 3.3. A slight colour change was expected regarding the Apple and PolyDent acrylic teeth clinically.

Introduction

Colour is among the most important factors for aesthetic appearance of prosthetic restorations. Aside from optimal chemo-mechanical properties of acrylic resins, their availability in different colour shades has increased their application in dentures. Denture materials must have optimal colour stability since they are constantly exposed to different foods and beverages in the oral environment [1,2]. Acrylic resins can pick up stains over time. Through the process of adsorption, liquid molecules adhere to resin materials depending on the environmental conditions and, consequently, possible discolorations may occur [3].

One major shortcoming of acrylic teeth is their gradual colour change over time. Colour change of acrylic resins may be due to internal or external factors. Internal or intrinsic factors are mainly related to chemical changes in the composition and formulation of materials while external factors mainly depend on the surface properties of the material and the environment in which the material is placed. It has been well documented that some beverages such as tea, coffee and fruit juice leave stains on dental materials. The magnitude of colour change also depends on the oral hygiene status and frequency of using cleaning agents by patients [4,5]. Extrinsic colouring agents include stains of foods, drinks or tobacco, which penetrate deep into the dental plaque and calculus and react with them [6].

Materials used for the fabrication of artificial teeth include porcelain, acrylic resin, reinforced acrylic resin and composite resins [7]. Reinforced acrylic and composite resin teeth were fabricated to overcome the problems due to the low wear resistance of acrylic resin teeth; however, some concerns exist regarding their colour stability when exposed to colouring materials [5,7].

This study aimed to compare the colour stability of three acrylic teeth (Ivoclar, PolyDent and Apple) exposed to coffee, tea and cola using a spectrophotometer.

The null hypothesis was that there is no difference between various brands of acrylic teeth in terms of color stability.

Materials and Methods

This in vitro experimental study assessed the colour change of three types of acrylic teeth of shade A1, namely Ivoclar (Ivoclar Vivadent AG FL-9494, Schaan, Liechtenstein), Apple (Ideal Macou, Tehran, Iran), and PolyDent (Denal Products Industry Vilcja Draga 42 Pri Novi Gorici). We preferred to use acrylic artificial teeth because they have more advantages such as pleasant esthetic, chemically bonding to acrylic base and easily grounding and polishing .Thirty samples in each group were evaluated (a total of 90).

The tea solution was prepared by immersing 2 prefabricated doses (2 x 2 g) of tea (Yellow Label Tea; Lipton, Rize, Turkey) in 200mL of boiling water at 100°C for one minute. After removing the tea waste, the final volume of the solution reached 200mL. To make coffee solution, 6 g of ground coffee powder(Nescafe Classic, Nestle,Switzerland) was poured in coffee filter and 200mL of water at 100°C was added. The obtained solution was passed through another filter and the final volume reached 200mL. In cola group, specimens were stored in 37°C cola (Coca-Cola;Coca-Cola Co, Istanbul, Turkey).

Baseline colour measurements of samples were performed before immersing them in colouring solutions, using a spectrophotometer. To simulate laboratory heating, ninety teeth were mounted in a flask containing gypsum and subjected to acrylic resin heat polymerization process. Ten teeth were immersed in each solution in such a way that they were not in contact with each other. The teeth were immersed in the solutions for one, three and six weeks. To prevent sedimentation, the solutions were replaced every three days.

Change in colour parameters was calculated using a spectrophotometer and reported. Colour parameters were measured at baseline and at one, three and six weeks after immersion. Spectrophotometer was calibrated prior to the onset of the study. Changes in CIE L*a*b* colour parameters were calculated and reported. Total colour change was also calculated using the formula below:

$$\Delta E = \sqrt{[(\Delta a)^2 + (\Delta L)^2 + (\Delta b)^2]}$$

The data were analyzed using SPSS, version 21.0. The mean and standard deviation of colour change in the acrylic teeth after immersion in coffee, tea and cola were calculated and reported at one, three and six weeks. Comparison of colour change of the acrylic teeth was done using one-way two ANOVA. Pairwise comparisons of acrylic teeth and solutions were made using Tukey's HSD test. ($\alpha = 0.05$)

Results

The mean and standard deviation of colour change of Apple, Ivoclar and PolyDent acrylic teeth following immersion in tea, coffee and cola solutions are presented in Table 1, respectively.

The results showed that all three types of acrylic teeth experienced some degrees of colour change after immersion in the colouring solutions. The colour change was smaller in the first week but increased by prolongation of immersion time. The greatest colour change occurred at six weeks and was the highest in Apple followed by PolyDent and Ivoclar acrylic teeth in coffee (mean ΔE of 4.6, 3.4 and 3.3 respectively).

Discussion

Several studies have assessed the effect of different solutions on the colour of dental materials. Jafari *et al.* evaluated the effect of different mouthwashes on the colour of porcelain [8]. Studies on stainability of the acrylic teeth following immersion in different colouring solutions have all shown variable degrees of colour change [9-11]. However, variations in the staining of acrylic teeth following immersion in colouring solutions have been documented. Colour change due to exposure to colouring agents often occurs due to extrinsic accumulation of stains on the surface or in the subsurface of restorations. Overall, stain adsorption due to exposure to colouring solutions

Table 1: The mean and standard deviation of colour change of the acrylic teeth in tea, cola and coffee solutions at one, three and six weeks

Solutions	Time	Type of tooth	Mean ± SD	*p*-value
Tea	One week	Apple	3.1 ± 0.9	0.400
		Ivoclar	3.4 ± 0.02	
		PolyDent	3.4 ± 0.07	
	Three weeks	Apple	3.4 ± 0.05	0.001
		Ivoclar	3.4 ± 0.01	
		PolyDent	3.4 ± 0.01	
	Six weeks	Apple	3.4 ± 0.07	0.140
		Ivoclar	3.4 ± 0.01	
		PolyDent	3.5 ± 0.01	
Cola	One week	Apple	2.65 ± 0.01	0.007
		Ivoclar	2.4 ± 0.3	
		PolyDent	2.6 ± 0.1	
	Three weeks	Apple	2.7 ± 0.3	0.001
		Ivoclar	3.4 ± 0.4	
		PolyDent	2.7 ± 0.3	
	Six weeks	Apple	3.4 ± 0.01	0.001
		Ivoclar	3.6 ± 0.08	
		PolyDent	3.4 ± 0.02	
Coffee	One week	Apple	2.5 ± 0.2	0.001
		Ivoclar	2.3 ± 0.01	
		PolyDent	2.7 ± 0.01	
	Three weeks	Apple	4.8 ± 0.01	0.001
		Ivoclar	2.7 ± 0.03	
		PolyDent	3.4 ± 0.01	
	Six weeks	Apple	4.6 ± 0.04	0.001
		Ivoclar	2.8 ± 0.02	
		PolyDent	3.5 ± 0.01	

SD: Standard Deviation

has been more commonly reported in the acrylic teeth of dentures, and dental composites and porcelain rank next. Based on the results, colour change following immersion of the acrylic teeth in colouring agents was significant [12,13].

Variable thresholds have been set for the perception of colour change by a normal observer. Raecke *et al.* reported that colour change was detectable in values of $\Delta E \geq 4$ [14]. Seghi *et al.* and the National Bureau of Standards reported $\Delta E = 1.5$ to be visually detectable [15]. However, a consensus has been reached by most studies on $\Delta E \leq 3.3$ to be clinically acceptable [16,17]. This threshold is often used to assess the efficacy and suitability of dental materials for restorative treatments.

Considering the above mentioned values, it appears that colour change following immersion of the Ivoclar acrylic teeth in colouring solutions, slightly more than acceptable value which is 3.2. However, some concerns exist regarding the colour change of Apple and PolyDent. The difference in colour change values and the standard threshold was close in all the three groups. However, ΔE of samples in colouring solutions would be lower considering the in vitro design of the study and frequent refreshing of solutions.

Mutlu-Sagesen *et al.* assessed the colour change of porcelain, reinforced acrylic and conventional acrylic teeth following immersion in coffee, tea and cola and reported results similar to ours [10]. Koksal and Dikbas reported a significant colour change in the porcelain and acrylic teeth after immersion in coffee, cola and tea for one and two weeks and one month [5]. However, the colour change in the acrylic teeth was higher in the current study.

In this study, we measured colour changes after the acrylic denture processing was done according to the manufacturer's instructions. We used Iranian brands to compare with foreign ones to be able to answer the patients' questions about Iranian artificial teeth qualities.

In the present study, colour change of the acrylic teeth at one and three weeks was greater but between three and six weeks it was lower in value. This finding is probably related to the absorption properties of acrylic resins, which experience severe colour change immediately after immersion in colouring solutions, but after a while they become saturated in terms of the presence of pigments and experience no further colour change [18].

Keskin *et al.* evaluated the colour stability of polymer-based dentures and showed a reduction in colour parameters after an initial increase in the values [19]. This finding may also be attributed to the removal of sediments of solution accumulated on the surface of restorations because tea and coffee accumulate on the surface of the samples to reach a certain thickness and after that they are dissolved back into the solution.

In the current study, coffee caused the greatest colour change in the Apple acrylic teeth after six weeks of immersion (mean ΔE of 4.6 for coffee and 3.4 for tea and cola) while tea caused almost an equal colour change in all acrylic teeth. The greatest colour change in the Ivoclar acrylic teeth occurred after six weeks of immersion in cola solution (mean ΔE of 3.6 for cola, 3.4 for tea and 2.8 for coffee).

Tea, coffee and cola colouring solutions were selected due to their frequent use by the Iranian population. These drinks have also been used for evaluation of colour change of the acrylic, composite and porcelain teeth in previous studies [8,20-22].

It has been reported that colour change due to exposure to tea is very superficial and can be easily removed by tooth brushing [23]. With regard to coffee, colour change occurs due to the superficial and deep absorption of stains and, thus, cleaning is more difficult. However, only a small number of polar coffee stains penetrate deep into the restorative material [9]. Since tea is a highly popular drink, especially in the Middle Eastern countries, dentists must inform the patients regarding the colour change of the acrylic teeth due to exposure to tea. It has been recommended that patients should brush their teeth immediately after drinking tea.

In the current study, cola caused a relatively small change in the colour of the acrylic teeth and only the Ivoclar acrylic teeth experienced a significant colour change following immersion in cola. Insignificant colour change due to immersion in cola has been attributed to its relatively low pH [23] (about 2 according to the manufacturer). Cola takes its colour from the caramel colour additive, which is prepared by heating sugar or glucose in the presence of a mineral or alkilic acid. Its colour is in the range of light yellow to dark brown [24].

Tannin is a common constituent of colouring solutions such as tea and coffee, which is highly chromogenic [25]. Other factors affecting colour change following immersion in coffee include addition of sugar and its processing procedures such as filtering

[26]. Colour change due to immersion in coffee also occurs due to the superficial and deep absorption of colouring agents mediated by the compatibility of the polymer phase with the yellow coffee stains. Moreover, there is a possibility that polymers in the structure of acrylic resins absorb water molecules in this beverage. It has been documented that both tea and coffee are capable of causing a significant change in the aesthetic appearance of acrylic resins [4], which was also noted in the current study.

Mutlu-Sagesen *et al.* reported that coffee caused the greatest colour change in porcelain, resin reinforced acrylic and acrylic denture base materials used in removable dentures [10]. This finding has also been discussed by some other studies such as the study by Oguz *et al.* [5,27].

Tea leaves have considerable amounts of flavonoids, which are responsible for taste as well as staining caused by tea. Caffeine and caffeic acid in the formulation of coffee are related to the colour change of polymer materials [19]. Another study reported that tea, compared to coffee, caused more considerable colour change in resin-based materials [11].

Imirzalioglu *et al.* demonstrated an almost equal colour change in denture base acrylic resins caused by coffee and tea [9]. Due to the colouring effects of coffee, cola and tea on the acrylic teeth, limiting their consumption can have advantages in terms of colour stability of denture materials for patients [9].

One, three and six-week time points were chosen in this study since four weeks and longer periods of time have been evaluated in previous studies to determine the effect of immersion in colouring agents on different restorations [5,10,13,18,21]. Guller *et al.* reported that the mean time of drinking a cup of coffee was 15 minutes and people often drank 3.2 cups of tea or coffee per day. Thus, one-week storage in coffee or tea corresponds to seven months of their daily consumption. Three weeks of storage corresponds to 21 months and six weeks of storage corresponds to 42 months of consumption [28].

A limitation of this study was that the impact of saliva and similar temperature condition in the oral environment was not considered.

Conclusions

Considering the $\Delta E \leq 3.3$ as the clinically acceptable colour change, it appears that despite the considerable colour change in all the three groups these changes in the Ivoclar acrylic teeth were in the clinically acceptable range. A slight colour change was expected regarding the Apple and PolyDent acrylic teeth clinically.

Conflict of Interest: None declared.

References

1. Craig RG. Restorative dental materials. 12th Edition. St. Louis: The CV Mosby Co. 2012;91-92,125-162,537-539.
2. Vergani CE, Ginmpaolo ET, Cucci AL. Composite occlusal surface for acrylic resin denture teeth. J Prosthet Dent. 1997;77:328-331.
3. Hersek N, Canay S, Uzun G, *et al.* Color stability of denture base acrylic resins in three food colorants. J Prosthet Dent. 1999;81:375-379.
4. Keyfa F, Etikan I. Evaluation of gloss changes of two denture acrylic resin materials in four different beverages. Dent Mater. 2004;20:244-251.
5. Koksal T, Dikbas I. Color stability of different denture teeth materials against various staining agents. Dent Mater J. 2008;27:139-144.
6. Alvin G. Description of color, color-replication process and esthetics. In: Contemporary Fixed Prosthodontics. 4th Edition. St. Louis: Mosby. 2006. p. 709-739.
7. Randa RD. Materials prescribed in the management for edentulous patients: Prosthodontic treatment for edentulous patients. 12th Edition. 2004.
8. Jafari K, Hekmatfar S, Badakhsh S. The effect of mouthwashes on surface hardness of dental ceramics. J Dent Biomater. 2014;1:23-26.
9. Imirzalioglu P, Karacaer O, Yilmaz B, *et al.* Color stability of denture acrylic resins and a soft lining materials against tea, coffee, and nicotine. J Prosthodont. 2010;19:118-124.
10. Mutlu-Sagesen L, Ergün G, Ozkan Y, *et al.* Color stability of different denture teeth materials: an in vitro study. J Oral Sci. 2001;43:193-205.
11. Um CM, Ruyter IE. Staining of resin-based veneering materials with coffee and tea. Quintessence Int. 1991;22:377–386.
12. Caranza FA, Newman MG. Clinical periodontology. 12th Edition. WB Saunders, Philadelphia 2010:87-155.
13. Omata Y, Uno S, Nakaoki Y, *et al.* Staining of

hybrid composites with coffee, oolong tea, or red wine. Dent Mater J. 2006;25:125-131.

14. Raecke H. Farbveranderungen von sahnarztlichen kunststoffen durch bestrahlung mit xenonlampen. Dissertation, FU: Berlin, 1979.
15. Seghi RR, Hwelett ER, Kim J. Visual and instrumental colorimetric assessment of small color differences on translucent dental porcelain. J Dent Res. 1989;68:1760-1764.
16. Vichi A, Ferrari M, Dadidson CL. Color and opacity variations in three different resin-based composite products after water aging. Dent Mater. 2004;20:530-534.
17. Kim HS, Um CM. Color differences between resin composites and shade guides. Quintessence Int. 1996;27:559-567.
18. Singh SV, Aggarwal P. Effect of Tea, Coffee and Turmeric Solutions on the Colour of Denture Base Acrylic Resin: An In Vitro Study. J Indian Prosthodont Soc. 2012;12:149-153.
19. Keskin S. The treatment of prosthetic dental materials with hypchlorite. MSc thesis, 2002 Middle East Technical University, Ankara, Turkey.
20. Goiato MC, Nóbrega AS, dos Santos DM, *et al.* Effect of different solutions on color stability of acrylic resin-based dentures. Braz Oral Res. 2014;28:1-7.
21. Sepulveda-Navarro WF, Arana-Correa BE, Ferreira Borges CP, *et al.* Color stability of resins and nylon as denture base material in beverages. J Prosthodont. 2011;20:632-638.
22. Turker SB, Kocak A, Aktepe E. Effect of five staining solutions on the color stability of two acrylics and three composite resins based provisional restorations. Eur J Prosthodont Restor Dent. 2006;14:121-125.
23. Gupta R, Parkash H, Shah N, *et al.* A spectrophotometric evaluation of color changes of various tooth colored veneering materials after exposure to commonly consumed beverages. J Indian Prosthodont Soc. 2005;5:72-78.
24. O'Neil MJ. The Merck index. 13th Edition. Whitehouse Station, NJ Merck, 2001:297.
25. Nordbo H, Attramadal A, Eriksen HM. Iron discoloration of acrylic resin exposed to chlorhexidine or tannic acid: a model study. J Prosthet Dent. 1983;49:126-129.
26. Guler AU, Yilmaz F, Kulunk T, *et al.* Effects of different drinks on stainability of resin composite provisional restorative materials. J Prosthet Dent. 2005;94:118-124.
27. Oguz S, Mutluat MM, Dogan OM, Bek B. Color change evaluation of denture soft lining materials in coffee and tea. Dent Mater J 2007;26(2): 209-216.
28. Guller AU, Guller E, Yucel AC, *et al.* Effects of polishing procedures on color stability of composite resins. J Appl Oral Sci. 2009;17:108-112.

24

Comparison of Wear Resistance of Hawley and Vacuum Formed Retainers: An In-Vitro Study

Moshkelgosha V[a], Shomali M[b], Momeni M[c]

[a]Orthodontic Research Center and Department of Orthodontics, School of Dentistry, Shiraz University of Medical Sciences, Shiraz, Iran.
[b]Orthodontic Research Center, School of Dentistry, Shiraz University of Medical Sciences, Shiraz, Iran
[c] Students Research Committee, School of Dentistry, International Branch, Shiraz University of Medical Sciences, Shiraz, Iran.

ARTICLE INFO

Key words:
Hawley Retainer
Vacuum-formed Retainer
Wear Resistance

Corresponding Author:
Masoomeh Momeni
Students Research Committee, School of Dentistry, International Branch, Shiraz University of Medical Sciences, and Shiraz, Iran.
Email: sepidehmomeni91@yahoo.com

Abstract

***Statement of Problem*:** As a physical property, wear resistance of the materials used in the fabrication of orthodontic retainers play a significant role in the stability and long term use of the appliances.

***Objectives*:** To evaluate the wear resistance of two commonly used materials for orthodontic retainers: Acropars OP, i.e. a polymethyl methacrylate based material, and 3A-GS060, i.e. a polyethylene based material.

***Materials and Methods*:** For each material, 30 orthodontic retainers were made according to the manufacturers' instructions and a 30×30×2 mm block was cut out from the mid- palatal area of each retainer. Each specimen underwent 1000 cycles of wear stimulation in a pin on disc machine. The depth of wear of each specimen was measured using a Nano Wizard II atomic force microscope in 3 random points of each specimen's wear trough. The average of these three measurements was calculated and considered as mean value wear depth of each specimen (μm).

Results: The mean wear depth was 6.10μm and 2.15μm for 3A-GS060 and Acropars OP groups respectively. Independent t-test showed a significant difference between the two groups ($p < 0.001$). The results show Polymethyl methacrylate base (Acropars) is more wear resistance than the polyethylene based material (3A-GS060).

Conclusions: As the higher wear resistance of the fabrication material can improve the retainers' survival time and its cost-effectiveness, VFRs should be avoided in situations that the appliance needs high wear resistance such as bite blocks opposing occlusal forces.

Introduction

Orthodontic removable appliances such as bite plates, active plates and retainers are the most commonly made of Polymethyl methacrylate polymer materials. However, two other based materials were recently introduced to orthodontics as thermoplastic appliances: the Essix retainer and the Invisacryl [1]. They have different reported physical characteristics in terms of life span and resistance to wear, fatigue, and fracture [2].

Vacuum formed appliances (VFRs), first introduced by Ponitz in 1971 [3], are more widely used compared to the more traditional Hawley appliances in the fabrication of orthodontic retainers. Vacuum formed appliances have advantages such as higher aesthetics, lower costs, ease of fabrication, and minimal thickness [4,5]. To fabricate a VFR, a vacuum forming machine pulls a thermoplastic plastic sheet onto working / study cast (made by gypsum plaster) and makes a vacuum to adapt the heat-softened plastic sheet to the cast by negative pressure [6].

From the structural aspect, two materials commonly used for VFR are polyethylene polymers and polypropylene polymers. These polymers are different in flexibility, durability, translucency and ability to bond acrylic resin. Polyethylene polymers have the advantages of transparency (aesthetic), beauty and are the choice, when we want to bond acrylic to posterior bite plane [7]. The polypropylene polymers do not have the beauty of the polyethylene polymers but are considered to be more durable and flexible. These benefits of the polyethylene polymer based appliances over the polypropylene polymer appliances have recently been a subject of controversy since some recent studies performed showed that some physical properties of these appliances may be problematic [1,8,9].

Only few published studies have compared the physical properties of VFR materials. In one study, Gardner *et al.* [1] put polyethylene and polypropylene polymer vacuum appliances under cyclic pressure and reported a higher resistance for the polyethylene polymer appliances. Lindauer *et al.* [8] compared the physical properties and survival of the Essix and Hawley appliances in clinical practice and found that in the Essix appliances, cracks appear after the placement during the follow-up period. Campbell *et al.* [9] showed that in a high number of patients (38%) with vacuum formed retainers, the main cause for the replacement was that the appliances had been worn out. Mai *et al.* [10] conducted a systematic review to compare the VFRs and Hawley appliances; they reported that with respect to changes in inter canine and inter molar widths after orthodontic retention; there was no difference between the appliances used. They also reported that in terms of occlusal contacts, cost effectiveness, patient satisfaction, and survival time, there was insufficient evidence to support the use of VFRs over Hawley retainers.

Among all physical properties, wear resistance is an important physical characteristic. Wear is considered as the removal of material from a solid surface when undergoing mechanical interaction; however, clinical wear is a more complex process [11,12]. The physical characteristics of the material used in the vacuum made appliances play an important role in defining the stability and long term use of them [13,14], also orthodontic retainers which have posterior bite plan usually get mechanical wear because of occlusal contact with teeth. This emphasizes the importance of appropriate comparison between these appliances. Therefore, in this in vitro study there was an attempt to evaluate and make a comparison between the wear resistance in acrylic and VFRs.

Materials and Methods

A total of sixty 30×30×2 mm blocks of Acropars OP (n = 30), and 3A-GS060 (n = 30) specimens were cut out of the mid-palatal area of premade orthodontic retainers. The retainers were made in the laboratory of Shiraz University of Medical sciences, School of dentistry. Acropars OP (Marlik Co., Iran) is a polymethilmethacrylic polymer used to prepare Hawley appliances, following the manufacturer's instructions. 3A-GS060 (3A Medes, Korea) is a polyethylene polymer used in the preparation of vacuum formed appliances (VFR), using a vacuum forming machine (Biostar, Scheu Inc., Germany). The manufacturer's instructions were followed in vacuum forming of each block (Figure 1-A).

To compare the two types of retainers, we evaluated 30 Acropars OP and 30 3A-GS060 blocks in two groups. For assessing the wear resistance, a Pin-on-disk device (Model TE 79; Phoenix tribology Ltd, Kingsclere, England) was used similar to the method used by Raja *et al.* [7] (Figure 1-B). The samples were secured on a custom made base plate that was moving on a horizontal plane via an electrical motor. Above all, 10 steel rods were holding the antagonist material- a steatite ball

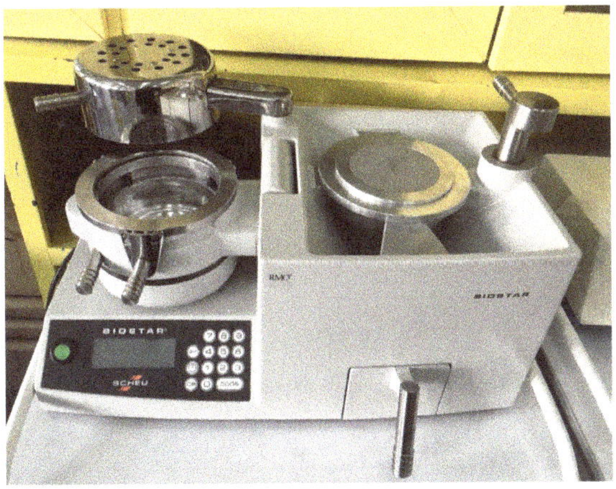

Figure 1-A: A vacuum forming machine for which the heating element is acting on the vacuum-formed retainers.

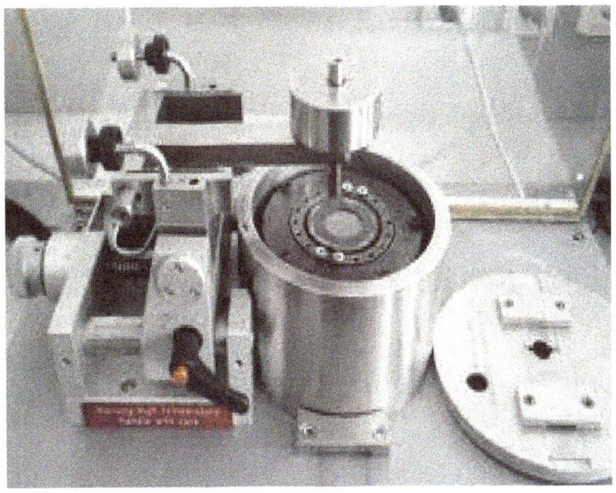

Figure 1-B: The pin-on-disk machine used to test the wear resistance

with 8 mm diameter. At the superior end of the rods, there were weights that applied a load of 460 g as the steatite antagonist drops down 3mm and contact our block samples. The duration of contact was 0.2 seconds and each sample was abraded for 1000 cycles. In our study, a cycle was defined as the horizontal cycle of the base plate that was moving from a start point and then reaching its start position again in a circular path with 16 mm diameter. After each abrasion process, a circular abrasion trough was clearly created on each sample, the wear machine was cleaned and lubricated, and new abraders were used for the next specimen. Then each specimen was washed with distilled water spray to remove and clear all debris from its surfaces.

The wear depth of the trough was measured using a Nano Wizard II atomic force microscope (Figure 2) (JPK Instruments AG, Berlin, Germany). The atomic force microscope (AFM) was used to generate an accurate topographic map of the surface features of each specimen. A three-area wear-depth analysis was used to measure the depth of the trough in 3 points of each specimen. The operator selects three points on 2D topographic images of the trough made by AFM on computer screen (Figure 3-A). 3D topographic images of each marked point were then generated automatically by the accompanying AFM software and the depth of wear in each of three points of the specimen was measured by a computer algorithm (Figure 3-B). The mean of three measurements made on each specimen was used in the statistical analysis as that sample wear depth.

Data were analyzed using the Statistical Software Package for the Social Sciences SPSS, version 18.0, (SPSS Inc., Chicago, IL, USA). Data achieved from the AFM for the two groups were compared using the Student's *t*-test. A p value of less than 0.05 was considered statistically significant.

Results

Table 1 shows the results of descriptive statistics on the wear depth in Acropars OP and 30 3A-GS060 groups. The measured wear depths of the study groups shows that 3A-GS060 group had a greater median wear depth and the range of measurements were also greater compared to the other group. The median wear depth for 3A-GS060 group was 6.00μm, which was higher than the Acropars OP group (2.00 μm).

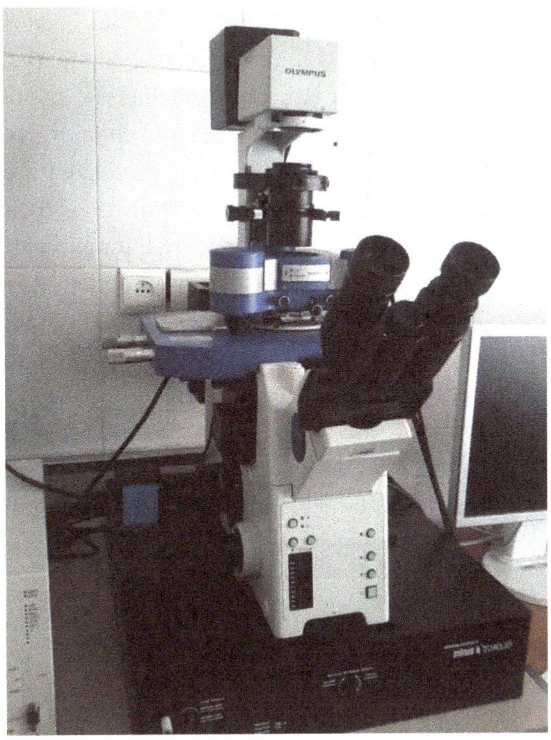

Figure 2. Nano Wizard II atomic force microscope

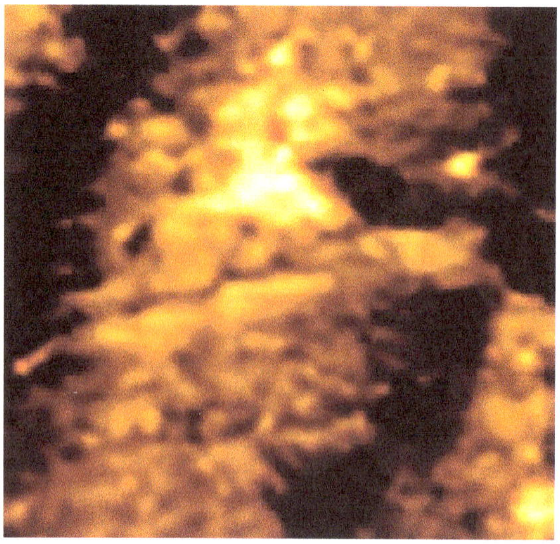

Figure 3-A: 2D topographic image of 3A-GS060 specimen

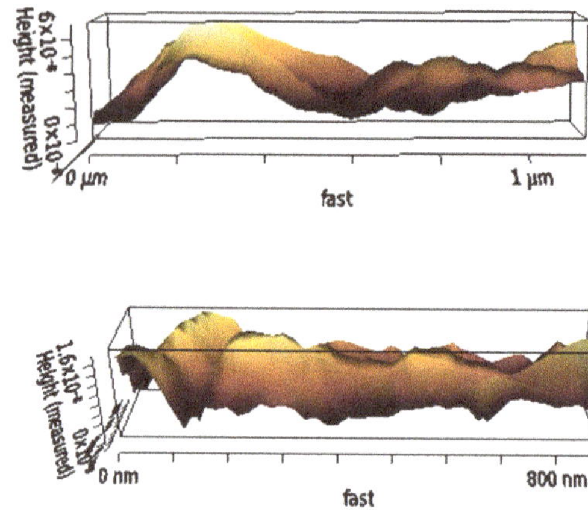

Figure 3-B: 3D topographic images of points selected in specimen trough (upper: 3A-GS060,lower:Acropars OP)

The mean wear depth was also higher in 3A-GS060 group (6.10 µm) compared to Acropars OP group (2.15µm). The Student's *t*-test showed a significant difference between mean wear depths of two groups of the study ($p < 0.001$). These results showed that 3A-GS060 group is less wear resistant than Acropars OP group.

Discussion

Retention is one of the main challenges the clinicians are faced in orthodontics, and choosing the proper methods and materials can be crucial in this regard [13,15,16]. There are various factors affecting the patients' cooperation and satisfaction in using orthodontic removable retainers. Some of these factors are aesthetics, cost, and comfort [4]. One of the factors that affects the prolonged use and cost-effectiveness of these retainers is their durability, and wear resistance of the appliance is one of the factors affecting its durability. The main focus of this study was to compare the wear resistance of two materials commonly used to make orthodontic retainers.

There are some studies comparing the patients' satisfaction, cost-effectiveness, and survival time of more traditional Hawley retainers and VFR materials, but according to a systematic review done by Mai *et al.* [10] the choice between them is still a matter of controversy; also, in terms of occlusal contacts, there is insufficient evidence to support the use of VFRs rather than Hawley retainers. Further studies are recommended to come to better conclusion in this regard. In our study, polymethyl methacrylate material was more wear resistant than polyethylene material, so it may be more wear resistant in clinical conditions, and higher wear resistance may improve the retainers' survival time and also cost-effectiveness. It was reported by Campbel *et al.* [9] that in a large number (38%) of patients, VFRs need to be replaced because they are worn too much. The high amount of wear in VFRs reported in their study reduces the retainers' service time and causes additional costs to patients. Lindauer *et al.* [8] also reported that VFRs break more than Hawley retainers. In contrast to them, Hichens *et al.* [4] compared the cost-effectiveness of Hawley retainers and VFRs, indicating that VFRs are more cost-effective in all aspects, such as patient satisfaction, comfort and fewer breakages. Sun *et al.* [17] and Capote [18] have both compared the clinical survival of these two retainers and reported that there was no significant difference between the percentage of breakage in the two types of retainers. One explanation for the differences between our results

Table 1: Descriptive statistics on the wear depth in Acropars OP and 3A-GS060 groups in µm

Group	Median	Mean (SD)	IQR	95% C.I Lower	95% C.I Upper	*p* value
Acropars	2.00	2.15 (0.46)	0.70	1.815	2.484	<0.001
3A-GS060	6.00	6.10 (1.44)	2.50	5.063	7.136	

n = 30 per group. IQR indicates interquartile range; SD, standard deviation; CI, confidence interval for mean.

and others can be the complex nature of clinical wear; this is the net result of a number of fundamental processes, such as abrasion, adhesive effects of the contacting surfaces, fatigue, and corrosive effects, which act in various combinations depending on the physical properties of the contacting surfaces and materials [19]. Therefore, the lack of some clinical factors can affect the results of any laboratory study, similar to ours.

In this study, we used a 460 g weight on the antagonist balls and an experimental run of 1000 cycles, which was just similar to that of the Raja *et al.* [7], but the mean values for polyethylene materials in their study was about 11.4 μm, which is about two times the mean measurements of the present study (6 μm). The reason for this difference can be the difference between the wear machines cycles used in the two studies. In our current study, in each cycle the antagonist was wearing the circumference of a circle once, but in their study it was wearing a 16mm line twice as much, because in one cycle their base plate was moving 16mm to the right on a straight line and then 16mm to left on the same line to its start position [7].

Conclusions

- Acropars polymethyl methacrylate material was more wear resistant than 3A-GS060 polyethylene material, so in clinical conditions, Hawley appliances made by Acropars OP may have more durability than VFRs made by 3A-GS060.
- An appropriately designed, randomized, controlled clinical trial may be helpful to determine whether these findings are replicated in vivo.

Acknowledgements

The present article was extracted from the thesis written by Masoomeh Momeni and was financially supported by Shiraz university of Medical Sciences, International Branch (Grant#8795156).

References

1. Gardner GD, Dunn WJ, Taloumis L. Wear comparison of thermoplastic materials used for orthodontic retainers. Am J Orthod Dentofacial Orthop. 2003;124:294-297.
2. Anbuselvan G, Senthil Kumar K, Tamilzharasi S, *et al.* Essix Appliance Revisited. Natl J Integr Res Med. 2012;3:125-138.
3. Ponitz RJ. Invisible retainers. Am J Orthod Dentofacial Orthop. 1971;59:266-272.
4. Hichens L, Rowland H, Williams A, *et al.* Cost-effectiveness and patient satisfaction: Hawley and vacuum-formed retainers. Eur J Orthod. 2007;29:372-378.
5. Rowland H, Hichens L, Williams A, *et al.* The effectiveness of Hawley and vacuum-formed retainers: a single-center randomized controlled trial. Am J Orthod Dentofacial Orthop. 2007;132:730-737.
6. Schwartz DA, Sheridan JJ. Thermoformed plastic dental retainer and method of construction. Patent US5692894. 1997.
7. Raja TA, Littlewood SJ, Munyombwe T, *et al.* Wear resistance of four types of vacuum-formed retainer materials: a laboratory study. Angle Orthod. 2014;84:656-664.
8. Lindauer SJ, Shoff RC. Comparison of Essix and Hawley retainers. J Clin Orthod. 1998;32:95-97.
9. Campbell AM, McMullan RE, Winning L, *et al.* Retention regimes following fixed appliance therapy-a change of practice re-audited. Br Orthod Soc Clin Effectiveness Bull. 2009;23:20-22.
10. Mai W, He J, Meng H, *et al.* Comparison of vacuum-formed and Hawley retainers: a systematic review. Am J Orthod Dentofacial Orthop. 2014;145:720-727.
11. Arnell RD, Davies PB, Halling J, *et al.* Tribology: Principles and design applications. New York; Springer-Verlag; 1991. p.266.
12. Peters M, Delong R, Pintado M, *et al.* Comparison of two measurement techniques for clinical wear. J Dent. 1999;27:479-485.
13. Ryokawa H, Miyazaki Y, Fujishima A, *et al.* The mechanical properties of dental thermoplastic materials in a simulated intraoral environment. Orthod Waves. 2006;65:64-72.
14. Kohda N, Iijima M, Muguruma T, *et al.* Effects of mechanical properties of thermoplastic materials on the initial force of thermoplastic appliances. Angle Orthod. 2013;83:476-483.
15. Melrose C, Millett DT. Toward a perspective on orthodontic retention? Am J Orthod Dentofacial Orthop. 1998;113:507-514.
16. Johnston C, Littlewood S. Retention in orthodontics. Br Dent J. 2015;218:119-122.
17. Sun J, Yu Y, Liu M, , *et al.* Survival Time Com-

parison between Hawley and Clear Overlay Retainers A Randomized Trial. J Dent Res. 2011;90:1197-1201.

18. Capote RT. Survival time comparison between Hawley and clear overlay retainers may not influence retainer choice. J Evid Based Dent Pract. 2012;12:222-224.

19. Casey J, Dunn WJ, Wright E. In vitro wear of various orthotic device materials. J Prosthet Dent. 2003;90:498-502.

Fracture Toughness of Nanohybrid and Hybrid Composites Stored Wet and Dry up to 60 Days

Sookhakiyan M[a], Tavana S[a], Azarnia Y[a], Bagheri R[b*]

[a]Shiraz Dental School, Shiraz University of Medical Sciences, Shiraz, Iran
[b]Dental Materials Department and Biomaterials Research Centre, Shiraz Dental School, Shiraz University of Medical Sciences, Shiraz, Iran

ARTICLE INFO

Key words:
Nanohybrid
Hybrid Composite
Fracture Toughness
Wet/Dry Storage

Corresponding Author:
Rafat Bagheri
Dental Materials Department and Biomaterials Research Centre, Shiraz Dental School, Shiraz University of Medical Sciences, Shiraz, Iran
Email: bagherir@unimelb.edu.au

Abstract

Statement of Problem: Patients' demand for tooth-colored restoratives in the posterior region is increasing. Clinicians use universal nanohybrid resin composites for both anterior and posterior regions. There are few published reports comparing fracture toughness of nonohybrids and that of hybrid composite stored wet and dry.

Objectives: To investigate the fracture toughness of three nanohybrids compared to that of a hybrid resin composite stored dry or wet up to 60 days, using four-point bending test.

Materials and Methods: Four resin composites were used: three nanohybrids; Filtek Supreme (3M), Ice (SDI), TPH3 (Dentsply) and one hybrid Filtek P60 (3M). For each material, 40 rectangular notched beam specimens were prepared with dimensions of 30 mm × 5mm × 2mm. The specimens were randomly divided into 4 groups (n = 10) and stored at 37°C either in distilled water or dry for 1 and 60 days. The specimens were placed on the four-point test jig and subjected to force (N) using universal testing machine loaded at a crosshead speed of 0.5mm/min and maximum load at specimen failure was recorded and K_{Ic} was calculated.

Results: Three-way ANOVA showed a significant interaction between all the factors (all $p < .0001$). Except for TPH3, all tested materials showed significantly higher K_{Ic} when stored dry than stored wet ($p < 0.05$). After 1 day of dry storage, Ice showed the highest K_{Ic} (2.04 ± 0.32) followed by Filtek P60 and the lowest was for Filtek Supreme (1.39 ± 0.13). The effect of time on fracture toughness was material dependent.

Conclusions: Wet storage adversely affected the fracture toughness of almost all materials. Keeping the restoration dry in the mouth may increase their fracture toughness. Therefore, using a coating agent on the surface of restoration may protect them from early water uptake and increase their strength during a time period.

Introduction

Fracture toughness of aesthetic restorative materials has grown significantly since they are used for posterior restoration in the load bearing area. On the other hand, the patients' increasing demand for having tooth-colored restoratives in the posterior region motivated the manufacturers to introduce and market a stronger resin composite. These composites consist of higher filler volume and smaller particle sizes of nanoscale, such as nanohybrids have shown to withstand greater mastication forces than the older composites [1].

A variety of resin composites are available in the market, being categorized into hybrid, microfilled, microhybrid, and nanohybrid with different physical and mechanical properties. Nowadays, nanohybrid composites are extensively used due to their mechanical improvement that makes them suitable for use in anterior and posterior restorations [2-4]. Nanohybrid is a hybrid resin composite with nanofiller in a prepolymerised filler form [5,6]. Nanotechnology, at a scale of 0.1–100 nanometers, is the invention of functional materials and structures by numerous physical and chemical methods [7].

The oral cavity restorations are subjected to complex forces such as bending, shear, fatigue and fracture. Fracture toughness (K_{Ic}) is an important mechanical property of dental materials that signifies the ability of a material against crack propagation [4]. In order to measure fracture toughness of resin composites, single edge V-notched beam (SEVNB), ISO 6872 is one of the reliable recommended methods [2]. A recent study [3] evaluated three different fracture toughness methods of seven resin composites and found that the four-point method was a more perceptive method determining the fracture toughness (K_{Ic}) value for resin composites with different percent filler contents. The results of this study [3] showed that hybrid resin composite with the highest filler vol% and the largest filler sizes had significantly higher fracture toughness compared to the nanohybrid, microhybrid and microfill composites.

In addition, water sorption by resin composites has been shown to have a degradation effect on the fracture toughness of the materials [8]. Dental restorative materials are exposed to saliva and beverages in the oral environment that could adversely affect their strength due to aging [9,10]. It has been shown that storing resin composites in dry condition increased their load bearing capacity in comparison to storing them in the wet condition [11]. Others also showed a significant decrease in fracture toughness or resin composites following water uptake [12,13]. Curtis *et al.* [13] in their study investigated the influence of water uptake and mechanical properties of a nano-filled compared with a conventional resin composite, reporting a decrease in fracture toughness following 3-12 months of water immersion. They revealed that strength degradation occurred at different rates between material types. The size and morphology of nanoparticles were important factors in water uptake and mechanical properties of the tested materials [13].

There are a few studies comparing the fracture toughness of glass fiber-reinforced resin composites stored dry and wet with conventional resin composites [14-17], but there are no published reports on the comparison of fracture toughness of nanohybrid and hybrid composites stored dry and wet. Therefore, this study aimed to compare the effect of water uptake on the fracture toughness of three nanohybrid resin composites to that of a hybrid composite up to 60 days of immersion. The null hypothesis is that storing resin composites in dry or wet condition does not affect their fracture toughness after one or 60 days.

Materials and Methods

In this study, four different resin composites (Table 1) were selected to be used in the four-point fracture toughness test. A four-point bending mould consists of a stainless steel detachable set up and prefabricated notch placed in the center of the beam (1 mm long and 0.1 mm wide) to enable the fabrication of tests specimens. A total of 40 rectangular notched beam specimens were constructed with dimensions of 30 mm × 5mm × 2mm for each material. The resin composite was placed into the mould using a flat double-ended stainless steel instrument and compressed, then covered by a clear plastic strip and a stainless steel metal plate was used to level out the material and extrude the excess. The stainless steel plate was then removed and the specimen was light cured along its length in 20 sec intervals using a SDI Radii plus LED light curing unit, (SDI, Bays water, Victoria, Australia) with a wavelength of 440-480 nm/output of 1500 mW/cm^2. The mould was then dismantled and the specimen was turned over to cure the bottom surface again using the same curing regimen. The excess (flash) was clipped from the edges and the sides were polished using fine 1200 grit silicon carbide paper (Tufbak waterproof sanding

Table 1: Detail information of the materials used

Material	Filler type /content	Matrix content	Batch No	Manufacturer	Classification
Filtek Supreme XT	78.5 w% Zirconia/ silica clusters (0.6-1.4 µm)	Bis-GMA, UDM, TEGDMA, Bis-EMA	N599645	3M /ESPE, St Paul, MN, USA	Nanohybrid
Filtek P60	61 v % Zirconia/silica (0.01-3.5) µm	Bis-GMA, UDMA, Bis-EMA	N511095	3M /ESPE, St Paul, MN, USA	Hybrid
Ice	77 w% inorganic filler SAS, AS (40nm-1.5 µm)	UDMA/ Bis-EMA/ TEGDMA	131194T	SDI, Vic, Australia	Nanohybrid
TPH3	76 w% Barium glass (0.8), Nano silicon dioxide particles (10-20nm)	Bis-GMA, Bis-EMAand TEGDMA	1109241	Dentsply	Nanohybrid

UDMA: urethane dimethacrylate, Bis-GMA: bisphenol A glycidyl dimethacrylate, TEGDMA: triethyleneglycol dimethacrylate, Bis-EMA: ethoxylated bisphenol-A dimethacrylate, SAS= Strontium alumino silicate, AS= amorphous silica

sheets; Scour Pads, Melbourne, Victo- ria, Australia).

The specimens were then divided into four groups of 10 and stored either dry or wet (in distilled water) for one or 60 days in a vented container at 37°C. The specimens were tested after each time interval in universal testing machine (Zwick/Roll Z020, Zwick GmbH & Co, Germany) using a four-point bend test jig, loaded at a crosshead speed of 0.5mm/min, and the maximum load at specimen failure was recorded.

Before testing, a new razor blade was used under hand pressure to create a sharp crack in the notch. Crack length was measured using a stereomicroscope (BS-3060C, Beijing, China) at 60x. The width and height of each specimen was measured using a digital calliper with accuracy of 0.1mm (mini Electronic Caliper, Qingdao Preco Imp. & Exp. Co., Ltd., Zhejiang, China). The K_{Ic} ($MPa.m^{0.5}$) was calculated using the following equation:

Where: L_{max} = fracture load,

$$K_{Ic} = \frac{L_{max}}{w\sqrt{h}} \cdot \frac{I_0 - I_1}{h} \cdot \frac{3 . r_M \sqrt{d/h}}{2.(1-d/h)^{3/2}}$$

$$r_M = 1.9887\text{-}1.326\frac{d}{h} \cdot \frac{[3.49-0.68\, d/h + 1.35(d/h)^2]\, d/h(1-d/h)}{(1+d/h)^2}$$

l_0: outer span; l_1: inner span,

w = specimen width, $\alpha = a/w$,

d = notch depth, h = specimen height

Statistical analysis

Data were analyzed using SPSS version 21.0 (SPSS Inc., Chicago, IL, USA). Three-way ANOVA was used to find if any interaction is found between materials, times and conditions. One-way ANOVA and Tukey's post-hoc test were conducted for sub-group analysis comparing each factor individually. $p < 0.05$ was considered as statistically significant.

Results

Three-way ANOVA showed a significant interaction among all three factors of material, time, and wet/dry condition (all $p < 0.001$). Results of one-way ANOVA and pairwise comparisons are shown in Table 2 and graphically in Figure 1 All materials had higher fracture toughness when kept dried after either 1 or 60 days of storage with an exception of TPH3 that

Table 2: Mean ($MPa.m^{0.5}$) and standard deviation of K_{Ic} after one and 60 days of wet and dry storage for all resin composites (n=10)

Material	One Day Wet	One Day Dry	60 Days Wet	60 Days Dry
Filtek Supreme	$^{Ba}1.28 \pm 0.11$	$^{Bb}1.39 \pm 0.13$	$^{Bab}1.34 \pm 0.33$	$^{Bc}1.54 \pm 0.48$
Filtek P60	$^{Aa}1.52 \pm 0.13$	$^{Ab}1.81 \pm 0.17$	$^{Ab}1.78 \pm 0.40$	$^{Ac}1.93 \pm 0.25$
Ice	$^{Aa}1.62 \pm 0.15$	$^{Ab}2.04 \pm 0.32$	$^{Cc}1.09 \pm 0.29$	$^{Ba}1.63 \pm 0.34$
TPH3	$^{Aa}1.7 \pm 0.13$	$^{Bb}1.43 \pm 0.17$	$^{Bb}1.39 \pm 0.69$	$^{Cc}1.06 \pm 0.33$

Different upper case letters show significant differences between materials in a column

Different upper case letters show significant differences between conditions in a row

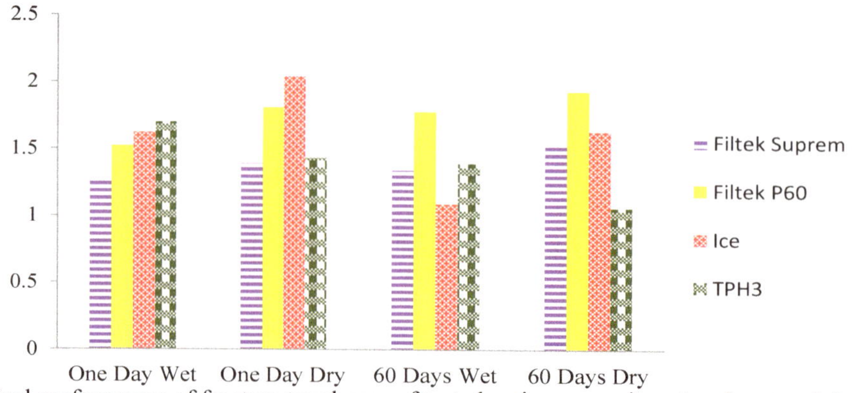

Figure 1: Graphical performance of fracture toughness of tested resin composites stored wet and dry at one or 6o days

showed a higher resistance when stored in distilled water. The effect of time on fracture toughness was material dependent. Filtek Supreme and Filtek P60 showed a significant increase after 60 days of storage in both wet and dry condition while Ice and TPH3 showed a significant decrease in the same condition ($p < 0.05$). Among the materials, in dry condition, Ice showed significantly higher fracture toughness (2.04 ± 0.32) than Filtek P60 (1.81 ± 0.17) followed by TPH3 (1.43 ± 0.17) and Filtek Supreme having the lowest K_{Ic} value (1.39 ± 0.13). A similar trend was observed at wet condition. However, after 6o days of storage in water, Ice had the most decrease in fracture toughness value compared to all other materials (1.09 ± 0.29).

Discussion

Comparison of the fracture toughness of three nanohybrids with that of hybrid composite revealed comparable fracture toughness in different times and conditions. Filtek P60 showed significantly greater K_{Ic} values than Filtek Supreme but slightly lower than Ice and TPH3. However, after 60 days of water storage, Filtek P60 showed significantly higher fracture toughness than all other nanohybrids. That is, the K_{Ic} values of two nanohybrids (Ice and TPH3) decreased significantly after 60 days of immersion in water while Filtek P60 and Filtek Supreme showed a significant increase in toughness This result indicated that the midterm water storage adversely affected the fracture toughness of the nanohybrids compared to the hybrid composite. This effect may be related to less water uptake of hybrid than the others. Curtis *et al.* [13] in their study of water uptake and strength characteristics of a nanofilled composite found an increased water uptake and degradation of the filler/matrix interface for nanofilled. They speculated that it could be due to the larger surface area to volume ratio of the fillers in nanofilled compared with those of the microhybrid composite. They also concluded that the presence of nanoparticles and clusters in the nanofilled led to diverse mechanical and physical properties of this material [13].

In general, almost all resin composites performed with higher K_{Ic} values when stored dry in both time intervals of one or 60 days. This result is in agreement with those of other recent studies [11,14-17]. Farmani *et al.* [11], under hertzian indentation test, showed that nanohybrid composites had comparable or even higher load bearing capacity than that of hybrid composite. Specimens stored in distilled water showed significantly lower load bearing capacity in comparison with dry condition. Bijelic-Donova *et al.* [16] compared fracture toughness and some other mechanical properties of short fiber-reinforced composite (everX Posterior, eXP) with that of microfilled, nanofilled and bulk-fill composites. The specimens were stored dry for 7 days or in water for 30 days. They showed that water storage weakened the fracture toughness of all materials and this reduction of K_{Ic} was material dependent. Higher fracture toughness of the resin composites reveals the fact that immersion in water probably facilitates and accelerates the crack propagation by water diffusion in the interface between the resin matrix and the filler, leads to softening the polymer matrix by swelling the network and reducing the frictional forces between the polymer chains [18,19].

On the other hand, Hoshika *et al.* [18] evaluated the degree of conversion and mechanical properties of Bis-GMA / TEGDMA / HEMA (60:30:10) containing 0–15 mass% QAMs (quaternary ammonium-methacrylates) after 3 days of dry or water storage. They reported higher fracture toughness for wet specimens ($p < 0.05$). The author [18] speculated that the significant increase in fracture toughness seen after water immersion for three days might have been due to slight decreases in the elastic modulus of the resins after water plasticization. This may have increased the ability of the matrix in absorbing water to resist crack propagation. Indrani *et al.* [19] assessed the effect of aging in water on the K_{Ic}, elastic modulus and fracture energy. The results indicated an increase in the fracture toughness and fracture energy as well as a decrease in the elastic modulus. The reported that water sorption also occurred mainly during the first 2 weeks. They interpreted variations in the mechanical properties to be due to plasticization of the resin matrix by water, which seems to lower the yield stress and increase in the size of the plastic zone ahead of the crack, thus leading to an increase in K_{Ic} and fracture energy [19].

Among all the tested resin composites, TPH3 behaved differently in terms of the effect of the condition, i.e. specimens stored in water had higher K_{Ic} values (1.7 and 1.39) than that of those stored dry (1.39 and 1.06). Polymeric matrix composition of TPH3 may justify the dissimilar results for this material compared to others. Although the exact percentages of oligomers in each material is not released by the manufacturer, it seems that TPH3 consisted of less amount of TEGDMA in which more water is absorbed compared to Bis-EMA and Bis-GMA; therefore, less degradation of the oligomer occurs in water [20,21,22]. It has been found that physical and mechanical properties of resin composites are affected by different monomer structures of the materials. Gonçalves *et al.* [23] in their study determined the influence of variety of concentration of Bis-GMA/ TEGDMA/Bis-EMA on the flexural strength of resin composites. The result revealed that Bis-EMA mixtures presented a statistically lower flextural strength followed by TEGDMA + Bis-EMA mixtures, and then by TEGDMA mixtures [23].

In general, the results of this study showed that water storage for up to 60 days reduced the fracture toughness of almost all the tested resin composites in comparison to dry specimens. One of the limitations of this study was the dry and wet storage of the specimens in a short time. Further long-term studies of more than a year are needed to find out if aging and wet storage in the fracture toughness of resin composites affects the fracture toughness of resin composites more objectively.

Conclusions

Within the limitations of this study, the following conclusions are drawn. Hybrid composite (Filtek P60) showed higher fracture toughness than one of the nanohybrids (Filtek Supreme) and less than the other two nanohybrids after one day of storage in distilled water but higher toughness than all the three nanohybrids after 60 days of aging. In general, dry specimens had greater K_{Ic} values than wet specimens after one or 6o days with an exception of TPH3. The results revealed that keeping the restoration dry in the mouth may increase their fracture toughness. Therefore, using a resin-coating agent on the surface of the restoration may protect them against early water uptake and increase their strength during a time period.

Conflict of Interest: None declared.

References

1. Klapdohr S, Moszner N. New inorganic components for dental filling composites. Monatshefte für Chemie. 2005;136:21-45.
2. International organization for standardization. ISO/ FDIS 6872, 2007. Dentistry-Ceramic materials. Switzerland. Available at: https://www.iso.org/standard/41385.html
3. Fani M, Farmani S, Bagheri R. Fracture Toughness of Resin Composites under Different Modes and Media: Review of Articles. J Dent Biomater. 2015;2:73-82.
4. Knobloch LA, Kerby RE, Seghi R, *et al.* Fracture toughness of packable and conventional composite materials. J Prosthet Dent. 2002;88: 307-313.
5. Senawongse P, Pongprueksa P. Surface roughness of nanofill and nanohybrid resin composites after polishing and brushing. J Esthet Restor Dent. 2007;19:274-275.
6. Ertas E, Guler AU, Yucel AC, *et al.* Color stability of resin composites after immersion in different drinks. Dent Mater J. 2006;25:371-376.
7. Mitra SB, Wu D, Holmes BN. An application of nanotechnology in advanced dental materials. J Am Dent Assoc. 2003;134:1382-1390.
8. Torabi Ardakani M, Atashkar B, Bagheri R, *et al.* Impact of bleaching agents on water sorption and solubility of resin luting cements. J Invest and

Clinic Dent. 2016.

9. Ferooz M, Azadeh N, Barahman N, *et al*. The Role of home bleaching agent on the fracture toughness of resin composites using four-point bending test. J Dent Biomater. 2014;1:9-15.
10. Bagheri R, Azar MR, Tyas MJ, *et al.* The effect of aging on the fracture toughness of esthetic restorative materials. Am J Dent. 2010;23:142-146.
11. Farmani S, Orandi S, Sookhakiyan M, *et al.* Hertzian Load-bearing Capacity of Hybrid and Nano-hybrid Resin Composites Stored Dry and Wet. J Dent Biomater. 2016;3:162-168.
12. Kalachandra S, Turner DT. Water sorption of polymethacrylate networks: bis-GMA/TEGDM copolymers. J Biomed Mater Res. 1987;21:329-338.
13. Curtis A, Shortall A, Marquis P, *et al.* Water uptake and strength characteristics of a nanofilled resin-based composite. J Dent. 2008;36:186-193.
14. Garoushi S, Vallittu PK, Lassila LV. Fracture toughness, compressive strength and load-bearing capacity of short glass fibre-reinforced composite resin. Chin J Dent Res. 2011;14:15-19.
15. Wang T, Tsoi JK, Matinlinna JP. A novel zirconia fibre-reinforced resin composite for dental use. J Mech Behav Biomed Mater. 2016;53:151-160.
16. Bijelic-Donova J, Garoushi S, Lassila LV, *et al.* Mechanical and structural characterization of discontinuous fiber-reinforced dental resin composite. J Dent. 2016;52:70-78.
17. Debnath S, Ranade R, Wunder S, *et al.* Interface effects on mechanical properties of particle-reinforced composites. Dent Mater. 2004;20:677-686.
18. Hoshika T, Nishitani Y, Yoshiyama M, *et al.* Effects of quaternary ammonium-methacrylates on the mechanical properties of unfilled resins. Dent Mater. 2014;30:1213-1223.
19. Indrani DJ, Cook WD, Televantos F, *et al.* Fracture toughness of water-aged resin composite restorative materials. Dent Mater. 1995;11:201-207.
20. Ferracane J, Berge H, Condon J. In vitro aging of dental composites in water-effect of degree of conversion, filler volume, and filler/matrix coupling. J Biomed Mater Res. 1998;42:465-472.
21. Pearson GJ, Longman CM. Water sorption and solubility of resin-based materials following inadequate polymerization by a visible-light curing system. J Oral Rehabil. 1989;16:57–61.
22. Taha Na, Ghanim A, Tavangar MS. Comparison of Mechanical Properties of Resin Composites with Resin Modified Glass Ionomers. J Dent Biomater. 2015;2:47-53.
23. Gonçalves F, Kawano Y, Pfeifer C, *et al.* Influence of BisGMA, TEGDMA, and BisEMA contents on viscosity, conversion, and flexural strength of experimental resins and composites. Eur J Oral Sci. 2009;117:442-446.

Permissions

All chapters in this book were first published in JDB, by Shiraz University of Medical Sciences; hereby published with permission under the Creative Commons Attribution License or equivalent. Every chapter published in this book has been scrutinized by our experts. Their significance has been extensively debated. The topics covered herein carry significant findings which will fuel the growth of the discipline. They may even be implemented as practical applications or may be referred to as a beginning point for another development.

The contributors of this book come from diverse backgrounds, making this book a truly international effort. This book will bring forth new frontiers with its revolutionizing research information and detailed analysis of the nascent developments around the world.

We would like to thank all the contributing authors for lending their expertise to make the book truly unique. They have played a crucial role in the development of this book. Without their invaluable contributions this book wouldn't have been possible. They have made vital efforts to compile up to date information on the varied aspects of this subject to make this book a valuable addition to the collection of many professionals and students.

This book was conceptualized with the vision of imparting up-to-date information and advanced data in this field. To ensure the same, a matchless editorial board was set up. Every individual on the board went through rigorous rounds of assessment to prove their worth. After which they invested a large part of their time researching and compiling the most relevant data for our readers.

The editorial board has been involved in producing this book since its inception. They have spent rigorous hours researching and exploring the diverse topics which have resulted in the successful publishing of this book. They have passed on their knowledge of decades through this book. To expedite this challenging task, the publisher supported the team at every step. A small team of assistant editors was also appointed to further simplify the editing procedure and attain best results for the readers.

Apart from the editorial board, the designing team has also invested a significant amount of their time in understanding the subject and creating the most relevant covers. They scrutinized every image to scout for the most suitable representation of the subject and create an appropriate cover for the book.

The publishing team has been an ardent support to the editorial, designing and production team. Their endless efforts to recruit the best for this project, has resulted in the accomplishment of this book. They are a veteran in the field of academics and their pool of knowledge is as vast as their experience in printing. Their expertise and guidance has proved useful at every step. Their uncompromising quality standards have made this book an exceptional effort. Their encouragement from time to time has been an inspiration for everyone.

The publisher and the editorial board hope that this book will prove to be a valuable piece of knowledge for researchers, students, practitioners and scholars across the globe.

List of Contributors

Alizadeh Oskoee P
Professor, Department of operative dentistry, Dental School, Tabriz University of Medical Science, Tabriz, Iran

Ebrahimi Chaharom ME
Associate professor, Department of operative dentistry, Dental School, Tabriz University of Medical Science, Tabriz, Iran

Abed Kahnemui M
Associate professor, Department of operative dentistry, Dental School, Tabriz University of Medical Science, Tabriz, Iran

Mohammadi N
Professor, Department of operative dentistry, Dental School, Tabriz University of Medical Science, Tabriz, Iran

Pournaghi Azar F
Assistant professor, Department of operative dentistry, research center for evidence-based medicine, Dental School, Tabriz University of medical science, Tabriz, Iran

Vahedpour H
Assistant professor, Department of operative dentistry, Dental School, Urmia University of Medical Science, Urmia, Iran

Saadat M
Department of Periodontology, Dental School, Tabriz University of Medical Science, Tabriz, Iran

Mousavinasab SM
Dental Materials Research Center and Department of Operative Dentistry, School of Dentistry, Isfahan University of Medical Sciences, Isfahan, Iran

Atai M
Department of Polymer Science, Iran Polymer and Petrochemical Institute, Tehran, Iran

Salehi N
Department of Oral Medicine, School of Dentistry, Rafsanjan University of Medical Sciences, Rafsanjan, Iran

Salehi A
Department of Operative Dentistry, School of Dentistry, Rafsanjan University of Medical Sciences, Rafsanjan, Iran

Mousavi S and Jafari K
Department of Prosthodontics, School of Dentistry, Ardabil University of Medical Science, Ardabil, Iran

Narimani S
Department of Endodontics, School of Dentistry, Ardabil University of Medical Science, Ardabil, Iran

Hekmatfar S
Department of Pedodontics, School of Dentistry, Ardabil University of Medical Science, Ardabil, Iran

Safari S, Vossoghi Sheshkalani Ma, Hoseini Ghavam F and Hamedi M
Department of Prosthodontics, School of Dentistry, Kerman University of Medical Sciences, Kerman, Iran

Vossoghi Sheshkalani Mi
Department of Endodontics, School of Dentistry, Ilam University of Medical Sciences, Ilam, Iran

Malek Mohammadi T
Social Determinants of Health Research Center, Institute for Futures Studies in Health, Department of Dental Public Health, Kerman University of Medical Sciences, Kerman, Iran

Derakhshani R
Department of Geology, Shahid Bahonar University, Kerman, Iran

Tavallaie M
Oral and Dental Diseases Research Center and Kerman Social Determinants on Oral Health Research Center, Kerman University of Medical Sciences, Kerman, Iran

Raoof M
Department of Endodontic, School of Dentistry, Kerman University of Medical Sciences, Kerman, Iran

Hasheminejad N
Oral and Dental Diseases Research Center and Kerman Social Determinants on Oral Health Research Center, Kerman University of Medical Sciences, Kerman, Iran

Haghdoost AA
Modeling in Health Research Center, Institute for Futures Studies in Health, Kerman University of Medical Sciences, Kerman, Iran

Monfared M and Bahrololoom ME
Department of Materials Science and Engineering, School of Engineering, Shiraz University, Shiraz, Iran

Shaghaghian S
Department of Dental Public Heath, School of Dentistry, Non-communicable Diseases Research Center, Shiraz University of Medical Sciences, Shiraz, Iran

Zeraatkar M
Department of Dental Public Health, School of Dentistry, Shiraz University of Medical Sciences, Shiraz, Iran

Moazzami SM and Amiri Daluyi R
Dental Research Center and Department of Operative and Esthetic Dentistry, Mashhad Dental School, Mashhad University of Medical Sciences, Mashhad, Iran

Sadid Zadeh R
Department of Restorative Dentistry, School of Dental Medicine, Buffalo, NY

Kianoush K
Biomedical Engineering Student, Biomechanics Research Assistant, Adelaide, SA, Australia

Sarmad M
Faculty of Mathematical Sciences, Ferdowsi University of Mashhad, Mashhad, Iran

Barani Karbaski F
Dental Research Center and Department of Pediatric Dentistry, Mashhad Dental School, Mashhad University of Medical Sciences, Mashhad, Iran

Kazemi RB
Operative Dentistry D200, Department of Craniofacial Sciences, UCONN Health, School of Dental Medicine, Farmington CT, USA

Zarei I and Khajehpour S
Department Of Mechanical Engineering, Collage of Engineering, Shiraz Branch, Islamic Azad University, Shiraz, Iran

Sabouri A
Department of Prosthodontics, School of Dentistry, Shiraz University of Medical Sciences, Shiraz, Iran

Haghnegahdar AZ
Department of Oral and Maxillofacial Radiology, School of Dentistry, Shiraz University of Medical Sciences, Shiraz, Iran

Jafari K
Department of Prosthodontics, School of Dentistry, Ardabil University of Medical Sciences, Ardabil, Iran

Sobhnamayan F and Ghanbaran S
Department of Endodontics, School of Dentistry, Shiraz University of Medical Sciences, Shiraz, Iran

Adl A
Department of Endodontics and Biomaterials Research Center, School of Dentistry, Shiraz University of Medical Sciences, Shiraz, Iran

Farhadpour H
Department of Dental Materials, School of Dentistry, Shiraz University of Medical Sciences, Shiraz, Iran

Sharafeddin F
Department of Operative Dentistry and Biomaterials Research Center, School of Dentistry, Shiraz University of Medical Sciences, Shiraz, Iran

Akbarian S
Department of Operative Dentistry, School of Dentistry, Shiraz University of Medical Sciences, Shiraz, Iran

Azarian B
Tohid high school, Shiraz, Iran

Sobhnamayan F and Sadat Shojaee N
Department of Endodontics, School of Dentistry, Shiraz University of Medical Sciences, Shiraz, Iran

Bakhtiar M and Golkari A
Oral and Dental Disease Research Center, and Department of Dental Public Health, School of Dentistry, Shiraz University of Medical Sciences, Shiraz, Iran

Azadi N
Student Research Committee, School of Dentistry, Shiraz University of Medical Sciences, Shiraz, Iran

Deljoo Z and Sadeghi M
Shiraz Dental School, Shiraz University of Medical Sciences, Shiraz, Iran

Azar MR
Department of Endodontics and Prevention of Oral and Dental Disease Research Center, School of Dentistry, Shiraz University of Medical Sciences, Shiraz, Iran

Bagheri R
Department of Dental Materials and Biomaterials Research Centre, School of Dentistry, Shiraz University of Medical Sciences, Shiraz, Iran

Peyravi A
Student Research Committee, School of Dentistry, Shiraz University of Medical Sciences, Shiraz, Iran

Movahhedian N
Assistant Professor, Department of Oral and Maxillofacial Radiology, School of Dentistry, Shiraz University of Medial Science, Shiraz, Iran

Shahidi SH
Professor, Department of Oral and Maxillofacial Radiology, School of Dentistry, Shiraz University of Medial Science, Shiraz, Iran

Bahadori Jahromi M
Student Research Committee, School of Dentistry, Shiraz University of Medical Sciences, Shiraz, Iran

Sahebi S
Associate Professor, Department of Endodontics, School of Dentistry, Shiraz University of Medical Sciences, Shiraz, Iran

Pourhatami N and Ahzan SH
Department of Endodontics, School of Dentistry, Shiraz University of Medical Sciences, Shiraz, Iran

Salehi P
Professor, Orthodontics Research Center, Department of Orthodontics, School of Dentistry, Shiraz University of Medical Sciences, Shiraz, Iran

Malekpour B
Department of Orthodontics, School of Dentistry, Shiraz University of Medical Sciences, Shiraz, Iran

Roshan A
Department of Orthodontics, School of Dentistry, Shiraz University of Medical Sciences, Shiraz, Iran

Hamedani Sh
Dental Research Development Center, School of Dentistry, Shiraz University of Medical Sciences, Shiraz, Iran

Torkzaban P
Department of Periodontology, Member of Hamadan Dental Research Center, School of Dentistry, Hamadan University of Medical Sciences, Hamadan, Iran

Vossoughi M
Oral and Dental Disease Research Center, Department of Dental Public Health, School of Dentistry, Shiraz University of Medical Sciences, Shiraz, Iran

Teymoorienik Z
Student Research Committee, Shiraz University of Medical Sciences, Shiraz, Iran

Seyedzadeh Sabounchi S
Department of Periodontology, School of Dentistry, Hamadan University of Medical Sciences, Hamadan, Iran

Moshkelgosha V
Orthodontic Research Center and Department of Orthodontics, School of Dentistry, Shiraz University of Medical Sciences, Shiraz, Iran

Shomali M
Orthodontic Research Center, School of Dentistry, Shiraz University of Medical Sciences, Shiraz, Iran

Momeni M
Students Research Committee, School of Dentistry, International Branch, Shiraz University of Medical Sciences, Shiraz, Iran

Ghavami-Lahiji M
Research Center for Science and Technology in Medicine, Department of Dental Biomaterials, School of Dentistry, Tehran University of Medical Sciences, Tehran, Iran

Benedicenti S
Professor, Department of Surgical Sciences and Integrated Diagnostics, University of Genoa, Genoa, Italy

Karimian R
Department of Dental Biomaterials, School of Dentistry, Tehran University of Medical Sciences, Tehran, Iran

Shahabi S
Professor, Laser Research Center of Dentistry, Dentistry Research Institute, Department of Dental Biomaterials, School of Dentistry, Tehran University of Medical Sciences, Tehran, Iran

Koohpeima F
Assistant Professor, Department of Operative Dentistry, School of Dentistry, Shiraz University of Medical Sciences, Shiraz, Iran

Sobhnamayan F
Assistant Professor, Department of Endodontics, School of Dentistry, Shiraz University of Medical Sciences, Shiraz, Iran

Bagheri R
Department of Dental Materials and Biomaterials Research Centre, School of Dentistry, Shiraz University of Medical Sciences, Shiraz, Iran

Esfandiari M
School of Dentistry, Shiraz University of Medical Sciences, Shiraz, Iran

Siabani S
Department of Operative Dentistry, School of Dentistry, Shiraz University of Medical Sciences, Shiraz, Iran

Topcuoglu HS
DDS, PhD Department of Endodontics, Faculty of Dentistry, Erciyes University, Kayseri, Turkey

Sener I
DDS, Department of Endodontics, Faculty of Dentistry, Erciyes University, Kayseri, Turkey

Demirbuga S
DDS, PhD Department of Restorative Dentistry, Erciyes University, Kayseri, Turkey

Çakir NN
DDS, PhD Department of Restorative Dentistry, Kayseri, Turkey

Topcuoglu G
DDS, PhD Oral and Dental Health Hospital, Kayseri, Turkey

Khaghaninejad MS
Assistant Professor, Department of Oral and Maxillofacial Surgery, School of Dentistry, Shiraz University of Medical Sciences, Shiraz, Iran

Khosravifard A
Assistant Professor, Department of Solid Mechanics, School of Mechanical Engineering, Shiraz University, Shiraz, Iran

Peyravi E
Student Research Committee, School of Medicine, Shiraz University of Medical Sciences, Shiraz, Iran

Eftekharian HR
Associate professor, Department of Oral and maxillofacial surgery, School of Dentistry, Shiraz University of Medical Sciences, Shiraz, Iran

Peyravi MR
Assistant Professor, Department of Health in Emergencies and Disasters, School of Management and Medical Informatics, Shiraz University of Medical Sciences, Shiraz, Iran

Haghnegahdar AA and Khojastepour L
Department of Oral and Maxillofacial Radiology, School of Dentistry, Shiraz University of Medical Sciences, Shiraz, Iran

Sookhakiyan M, Tavana S and Azarnia Y
Shiraz Dental School, Shiraz University of Medical Sciences, Shiraz, Iran

Bagheri R
Dental Materials Department and Biomaterials Research Centre, Shiraz Dental School, Shiraz University of Medical Sciences, Shiraz, Iran

Index